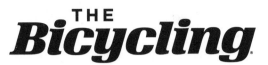

THE Bicycling

BIG BOOK

of CYCLING

for WOMEN

Everything You Need to Know for
Whatever, Whenever, and Wherever You Ride

SELENE YEAGER

RODALE

Copyright © 2015 by Rodale Inc.

All rights reserved. No part of this publication may be reproduced or transmitted in any form or by any means, electronic or mechanical, including photocopying, recording, or any other information storage and retrieval system, without the written permission of the publisher.

Rodale books may be purchased for business or promotional use or for special sales. For information, please write to: Special Markets Department, Rodale Inc., 733 Third Avenue, New York, NY 10017.

Bicycling magazine is a registered trademark of Rodale Inc.

Printed in the United States of America

Rodale Inc. makes every effort to use acid-free ♾, recycled paper ♾.

Library of Congress Cataloging-in-Publication Data is on file with the publisher.

ISBN: 978–1–62336–486–1   paperback

Distributed to the trade by Macmillan

2 4 6 8 10 9 7 5 3 1   paperback

RODALE.

We inspire and enable people to improve their lives and the world around them.

rodalebooks.com

Photo/Illustration Credits

Beth Bischoff, 180–182
Cannondale Bicycle Corporation, 19 (touring bike)
Colnago, 23 (cyclocross bike)
Jennifer Daniel, 124–125
Michael Darter, 103
Tim De Waele/www.tdwsport.com, 279
Pat Dishinger, 75
Trevor Dixon, 55 (socks),
Troy Doolittle, 80
Felt Racing, LLC, 21, (racing bike)
Gallery Stock/Mike Tittel, 113
Getty Images/Erik Isakson, 84
Getty Images/Foodcollection RF, 240
Getty Images/Gorfer, 91
Getty Images/Johner Images, 68
Getty Images/Heather Shimmi, 185
Giant Bicycle USA, 21 (mountain bike)
Jered Gruber, 88
Linda Guerrette Photography, 188
Hacob Khodaverdian, 60
Image Club Graphics, 26
Charlie Layton, 294, 295
Mel Lindstrom, 291 (levers)
Thomas MacDonald, 49 (helmet), 51 (shorts)
Mitch Mandel, 18 (endurance bike), 19 (triathlon bike), 25 (gravel bike), 49 (jersey), 53, 54, 55, 56, 58, 161–171, 212, 290, 292 (shock pump)
Heather McGrath, 62, 271
James Michelfelder and Therese Somme, 174 (photo), 175 (photo), 176 (photo), 177 (photo), 178 (photo), 179 (photo)
Norco Performance Bikes, 22 (downhill mountain bike)
Kent Pell, 57, 59, 63, 291, 292 (multitool)
Richard Pierce, 205
Embry Rucker, 97
Daniel Sharp, 61
Shutterstock/gresei, 151
Angie Smith, 95
Specialized Bicycle Components, 51 (shoe)
Trek Bicycle Corporation, 25 (flat bar road bike)
Adam Wallenta, 17, 20, 23, 40
Waterford Precision Cycles, 18
Kyle Webster, 174 (illus.), 175 (illus.), 176 (illus.), 177 (illus.), 178 (illus.), 179 (illus.)
Yasu & Junko, 22 (fat tire bike)

*For all the women
who ride to be free*

Contents

INTRODUCTION   vii

PART I:
SPINNING WHEELS AND WEAVING DREAMS

Chapter 1: Why Women Ride—And Why More Should   3

PART II:
GEARING UP

Chapter 2: Bikes, Bikes, and Women's Specific Bikes   15

Chapter 3: Fitting a Bike to the Female Form   38

Chapter 4: Essentials, Accessories, and Bling   47

Chapter 5: The Cycling Lifestyle: Take Time to Make Time   64

PART III:
SKILLS, DRILLS, AND RULES OF THE ROAD

Chapter 6: You and the Machine   73

Chapter 7: Climbing, Descending, and Cornering   83

Chapter 8: Pacelines, Packs, and Group Riding   93

Chapter 9: Life on the Road   100

PART IV:
OFF THE BEATEN PATH

Chapter 10: Take to the Trails   111

Chapter 11: Cyclocross Fever   122

Chapter 12: Dirt, Gravel, and Cinders Galore   127

Chapter 13: Try the Track   132

PART V:
GET FIT, GO FAST!

Chapter 14: Why and How to Train   140

Chapter 15: Strengthen Your Human Frame   158

Chapter 16: Flexible Benefits   172

Chapter 17: Off to the Races   183

Chapter 18: Conquer the Century   195

PART VI:
EAT TO RIDE, RIDE TO EAT

Chapter 19: Fuel for Life and the Ride of Your Life   203

Chapter 20: Drink Up!   216

Chapter 21: Pedal Off the Pounds   224

Chapter 22: Performance Enhancers   238

PART VII: FOR WOMEN ONLY

Chapter 23: Menstrual Cycle Facts, Myths, and Management   249

Chapter 24: Riding for Two: Pregnancy   254

Chapter 25: Menopause   258

Chapter 26: Lady Parts   262

PART VIII: GO BY BIKE!

Chapter 27: Commuting   268

Chapter 28: Charity Rides   273

Chapter 29: Bike Touring   277

Chapter 30: Cycling as a Family Affair   282

PART IX: MAINTAINING YOUR MACHINE

Chapter 31: Basic Maintenance and Repair   289

Chapter 32: Shop Talk   297

ACKNOWLEDGMENTS   302

INDEX   303

Introduction

WHAT IS WOMEN'S CYCLING ANYWAY?

DO WOMEN NEED THEIR OWN CYCLING BOOK? DO WOMEN NEED THEIR own women's specific bikes? Do women need their own group rides, clothing, and gear? After all, aren't we all just cyclists at this point, not *women* cyclists?

Yes . . . and no.

Yes, we all—men and women who love and ride bikes—are cyclists. We share the same loves. We all love the sun in our face, slicing through the air, the sound of our tires whirring on the ground. We love feeling like we're flying. We love the freedom. We love the camaraderie, the spirited competition, the satisfaction of a mountain pass conquered and a hard ride completed. We love how irrationally delicious peanut butter tastes 65 miles into a 100-mile day. We love beautiful bikes and sweet new shoes. You don't need any particular chromosome combinations to appreciate all that.

But let's face it, the cycling experience still has and will always have some significant gender differences, even as the sport evolves. Though more women than ever are pedaling bikes of all kinds, we're still a minority in the sport. Depending on where you live, it can still be hard to find other women to ride and train with. Most shops are still male dominated, and though the guys who work there may be very nice and accommodating, it can still be kind of awkward and maybe even impossible to get all your women's specific questions answered—or more importantly, to have women's specific needs you may not even know you have addressed by a man, even a sensitive, knowledgeable one.

So, though we all are "cyclists," all those not so insignificant differences in our anatomy and our very DNA do make us different from our male counterparts. Or as cyclist, triathlete, and nutrition and exercise physiology researcher Stacy Sims, PhD, likes to say:

"Women Are Not Small Men"

I love that saying. It's so simple and so obvious, yet so scientific and complex all in five little words. There are the blatant differences—we have breasts, we can get pregnant, we have vaginas—that can influence our gear and cycling needs. There are also the less obvious differences. Our ever-changing hormones, whether over the course of a month or our lifetime (or both, really), change the way we burn fuel, and even what fuel we burn, before, during, and after we ride. Our nutrition needs are different, as are our hydration requirements.

Though we are not just small men, by and large we *are* smaller than men. Our weight is distributed differently, too. All of that changes how we fit on a bike and how a bike might behave under our female frame. Speaking of frames, the female one has special needs to stay strong. Our muscles, bones, and ligaments are under the influence of our hormones and demand a uniquely female touch when we ride, race, and train.

Our relationships and our relationship to the sport are often different, as well. We have a different history with cycling. We live in a different present. Inevitably, we will have a different future in the sport than men will, despite all we have in common. With all of the unique wants, needs, challenges, and opportunities that women riders have and face, it only makes sense that women should indeed have their own cycling book—a big book, one that answers all the questions a woman who rides a bike wants to know, including many she never even thought to ask.

FROM CLIPPING IN TO TOEING THE LINE, AT EVERY LEVEL

I want to be clear that though this book is very beginner friendly, it is *not* just for beginners. Somewhere along the way, "woman cyclist" became almost synonymous with "beginner cyclist." Women find that insulting and alienating, and with good reason. The goal of this book is to cover everything a cyclist needs to know, regardless of experience level, and to tell it through a female prism.

For instance, you'll find a soup-to-nuts discussion of gear: helmets, shoes, clothing, bikes—the works. That includes the evolution from "unisex" to women's specific designs, so you understand where we started and where we're going. But it doesn't stop there. You'll also learn industry-insider information—much of it from women themselves—that will help you discern when women's specific is right for you, and when it may not be the best buy.

We'll talk women's specific bike fit, too. Com-

Cycling Herstory

Cycling has always been and continues to be a vehicle for freedom. This was particularly true in the late 1800s, during the "New Woman" movement. The "new woman" was a suffragette. She worked outside the home, pushed back against traditional gender roles, and saw herself as an equal of men.

New Women loved bicycles. They not only could get around more easily by riding two-wheelers, but also then had a reason to shed the ridiculous layers (and layers and layers) of corsets, hoops, petticoats, and collared shirts that made walking, let alone pedaling a bike, a nearly insurmountable chore.

As women took to bikes, they slipped into more sensible—and empowering—clothes like split skirts and even (gasp) trousers. The more women pedaled, the more powerful they felt—and became. They discovered untapped athleticism and strength, which transcended the bike and spilled into daily life.

There was a lot of pushback, of course. Women were warned that cycling could harm their internal organs and lead to painful menstruation problems. Conservatives cautioned against the prudence of a woman straddling a bicycle saddle, lest she get too "stimulated." The hue and cry continued for some time, but it was too late. Women had felt the wind in their hair and the freedom in their hearts. There was no turning back. Ultimately, the queen of the suffragette movement, Susan B. Anthony herself, famously said: "I'll tell you what I think of bicycling. I think it has done more to emancipate woman than any one thing in the world. I rejoice every time I see a woman ride by on a wheel. It gives her a feeling of self-reliance and independence the moment she takes her seat; and away she goes, the picture of untrammelled womanhood."

To that, we should all simply say, Amen.

mon discomforts among women are neck and back pain, as well as pain in the rear and nether regions. Sure, that's common among the fellas, too, but you may carry your weight in a way that calls for different fixes to put you in the proper position and eliminate the aches and pains.

Did you know that women respond differently than men to both resistance and high-intensity interval training? You do now. And you'll learn even more in the sections that cover getting fit and going fast. Whether you want to try cyclocross, ride off-road, race, or train for a century (or maybe even a double), everything you need to know about bike handling, training, and racing, particularly as it pertains to you as a woman, is in here.

Women are often more limber than men; they're definitely more prone to connective tissue injuries, and, on the plus side, may actually be more fatigue resistant. We also age differently in endurance sports than our male counterparts. For far too long we've been viewed as the "weaker" sex, simply because we have less sheer muscle mass and generally produce less power. However, we have many of our own unique strengths that are actually, well, stronger. You'll be sure to learn all about those, too.

Trying to shed some unwanted pounds? It's not your imagination. Guys actually do lose weight faster than women. It's a matter of basic physiology: testosterone gives them more muscle, more muscle helps them burn more calories, so once they put themselves in action and watch what they eat, the weight comes off more quickly. Science also shows that women's brains appear to be hardwired to make us more susceptible to cravings—and more inclined to be hungry when we see food—likely because we're the ones who carry the next generation and perpetuate the species. But that doesn't mean we're doomed to stare down a perpetually stuck scale. We just have to outsmart Mother Nature a bit. You'll learn how.

Of course, then there's commuting, bike fashion, lifestyle cycling, touring, vacations, charity rides, advocacy, riding with your partner and your kids, finding the right bike shop to suit your needs—the list goes on and on. That's why we call it a BIG BOOK.

And we haven't even gotten to the *real* women's issues yet. Nope, it's not in your head. Your hormones have a profound effect not just on your moods (you don't need me to tell you that), but also on your training, riding, and racing. Fortunately, you're not at the mercy of your menstrual cycle. You'll see what smart (yes, women) scientists have to say on that subject. Speaking of hormones, no one in the industry ever talks about perimenopause or menopause. But consid-

ering that surveys show that women between the ages of 45 and 54 actually ride more days than their male counterparts, we sure will. After all, it's pretty tough to perform at your best with hot flashes, lousy sleep, and muscle loss, right? We can't help you turn back time, but we can certainly help you stave off some of the harsher symptoms that come with its passing. And of course there's your vagina. When it's not happy, you're not happy. You'll find all the info to keep you comfortable and healthy down below.

Finally, from beginning to end, you'll find our story. From Susan B. Anthony waxing poetic about her views on emancipation as seen from her bike saddle to former Wall Street wonder turned American cycling sensation Evie Stevens inspiring women to follow their hearts and ride like the wind, we women have a unique history—or shall we say "herstory"—in the sport. You'll find that here, too.

R-E-S-P-E-C-T

Aretha sang about it. Decades later, Pink sang about it. Respect. It's really all women want, especially as we try to make our way through traditionally male-dominated domains, like cycling. That's one of the goals of this book. To give women their due respect as they saddle up and go out and ride.

After all, there's room under this big tent for all of us. Do you hate pink and glitter and all things girlie? That's okay. Do you own your own BeDazzler and put rhinestones on your cycling socks? You're welcome on the ride, too. No matter where you're coming from, where you want to go, or how fast or slow you want to get there, there's room for you in the pack.

Now is our moment. You can feel it in the air. It's a really exciting time for women in the sport of cycling. Superstar riders like Dutch Marianne Vos and American Katie Compton are making history with blistering performances in nearly every cycling discipline. Teams like Velocio-SRAM Pro Cycling, formerly known as Specialized-lululemon, are blazing a path to success that generations of young girls will be able to follow for decades to come. Women have joined forces to work together in the Women's Cycling Association to push for equality in the professional ranks—equal pay, equal opportunities to race and to be seen racing, and more women's grand Tours and cycling festivals. Our efforts are working.

Statistics from the National Sporting Goods Association reveal that while males still make up the majority of cyclists, the gap is closing fast. The NSGA's latest figures show that among recreational riders, 20.2 million are men and 19.1 million female—a sizable gap, but not a chasm. And female participation in cycling is growing, up by 4 percent last year. All you have to do is look around and you can see there are many more women on shop rides, charity rides, and out and about than there were just 5 or 10 years ago. More women are buying bikes, riding, and racing. They may still be in the minority, but they're there, and increasing in number. In fact, among those under age 28, *more* women than men own bikes. For the first time in US history, 60 percent of bicycle owners between the ages of 18 and 27 are women.

We have most definitely come a long way, baby, and the journey is nowhere near over. So grab your bike and a friend or two, and let's keep this ride going strong for years to come.

PART I

SPINNING WHEELS AND WEAVING DREAMS

Women come to cycling for many reasons and in many ways: because of a significant other, because of a friend, or of their own volition. But the joys, the sense of accomplishment, and the places they go outside and deep within themselves follow a common trajectory. It might sound clichéd to say that bikes change women's lives, maybe even empower them to make their dreams come true. But from what I've seen in my travels and read in the many stories that have crossed my desk these 20 years of writing about cycling and fitness, it's no exaggeration. There are so many reasons for women to pick up a bike and ride, ranging from boosting mental health to, yes, shedding those unwanted pounds. We'll talk about them all in this section. But I'll stop talking for the moment and let Elizabeth Seifert, 47, mother of two and information tech specialist and business owner from Woodstock, Georgia, kick it off in her own words.

After not riding a bike since I was 18, I started again just before turning 42. I was looking to get rid of the last few pounds of baby weight and was completely bored with speedwalking and working out in the gym. My husband had been riding for a few years, so I figured I'd follow his lead. I went on the cheap and picked up a 35-pound hybrid and started riding that on the road. The weight dropped off and I discovered a love of riding. The following year, I upgraded to a road bike and joined a small group of women who ride . . . and eventually started leading that group. Two years ago, I added mountain biking to my repertoire and am in love with the woods and dirt! Getting covered in mud is one of my favorite things to do.

I am 47 now and am so thankful that biking has added so much to my life. I now easily have 100 cycling friends and acquaintances, and that number just keeps on growing. This, for a person who tends to be on the shy and quiet side in larger social settings, is simply amazing to me. It's as if cycling opened up my world and brought a massive sun to shine in my life. Never once has riding ever felt like exercise. Jeez, "exercise"? That sounds too much like work. Who wants to work? No, riding is a freedom.

It's a freedom from what ails you. If I feel down, sad, or even angry, riding is the cure. When I'm done, my spirits are lifted, and I feel at peace, a very much "all's well with the world" type of feeling. At times, I'm even giddy and riding a high with a grateful attitude. Riding is also freedom from boredom. If I want an adventure, I get outside and explore new roads or paths. It's been a great way to see new places and even gives me a new way to see old ones. You notice things that you miss when you're in a car.

Riding is also a social freedom, too. Too many times in life, we get stuck in social ruts and endure situations that can make us want to find a cave and hide away from humankind. That's the best time to go riding with a buddy. Fellow cyclists are some of the nicest folks I've met on this earth, and I enjoy more laughs while out on rides with friends than I do at any other time during the week. Lastly, as a busy mom and business owner among other things, it's hard to find the time to just be me. This last one is an especially important freedom I feel while on the bike. I spend so much of the rest of my life doing things for others that it can be hard to break out of the mold and remember there's a me in here. When I pull out my bike and start pedaling, I remember who I am and I get to enjoy being her. That's a treasure, right there. It does not matter who you are, where you are, what kind of bike you have, or how old you are (I have met and ridden with folks in their 60s and 70s and know of folks in their 80s who still ride!), you can find enjoyment and like-minded friends on two wheels.

Thanks, Elizabeth. I couldn't have said it any better myself.

CHAPTER 1

Why Women Ride—And Why More Should

IF YOU'RE JUST GETTING INTO CYCLING, WELCOME. IF YOU'VE been here a while, very happy to have you. No matter where you fall on the cycling spectrum, you're part of a growing movement and everyone from bicycle manufacturers to event organizers to most certainly other women are happy to have you along for the ride.

Women, somewhat like frogs but cuter, are considered an "indicator species" for the health of cycling communities—the more women you see pedaling about, the healthier the community is and the more likely it is that cycling will continue to grow and thrive. And, well, everyone in the sport and affected by the sport wants it to flourish. How much we're flourishing right now depends on where you look. But in general, "indications" are looking up.

According to a raft of survey stats from the League of American Bicyclists, more women than ever are out there enjoying cycling in every shape and form. In 2012, women made up 37 percent of MS 150 (a classic 2-day charity ride) riders, 40 percent of American Diabetes Association Tour de Cure riders, and 39 percent of New York City's Five Boro Bike Tour participants. In the same year, 38 percent of participants in multiday bike tours hosted by Adventure Cycling, the largest bike-touring group in the United States, were women. Though women are still a clear minority in most bike-racing disciplines, the numbers are rising in both road and mountain bike racing. In the case of cyclocross, some places have reported a staggering 65 percent increase in women's fields over the past 5 years. And women continue to pour into triathlon, making up 36 percent of USA Triathlon membership.

We're also simply pedaling more from here to there. The total number of women bike commuters in 2012 grew by almost 11 percent from 2011. Impressively, women commuting by bike has skyrocketed nearly 59 percent in the past 6 years—outpacing the growth among their male counterparts. And let me repeat—because it bears repeating—60 percent of bike owners between the ages of 17 and 28 are women.

Purely anecdotally, you can see the groundswell in women's cycling. Back in the early '90s, when I became fully bitten by the cycling bug and crossed the bridge from sometime rider to "cyclist," there weren't many women on the scene. In fact, I won my very first local road race in 1994 because I was the only woman who showed up. Back then you could barely find cycling clothes that fit the female frame, let alone ones made for and by females. Those days are very thankfully in the past.

A Mutually Satisfying Relationship

Good things are happening to the sport because women are in it. I'd also argue that more women should participate as often as they can in cycling, because, well, good things—really good things—happen to women when they toss a leg over a bike and ride.

The medical literature is filled with reams of scientific evidence on the benefits of cycling for everyone, particularly women. But more importantly, many women themselves can tell you how their lives were completely transformed simply by getting on a bike. We talked to dozens of women just like yourself about how they got into the sport and what they got and continue to get out of it. Their replies, woven into the discussion of the benefits appearing below, will make you want to grab your bike and go for a ride—and take every woman you know with you.

FREEDOM

For many of us, a bicycle was our first ticket to freedom—a vehicle allowing us to explore on our own and cover far more ground in a much more fun way than we ever could on foot. Turns out that really never changes. Nearly every woman I talked to praised the feeling of freedom that cycling gives them, despite their being passport-carrying, car-driving, relatively free adults now.

Here's how Sharon Castle sums up her lifelong relationship with cycling.

My two brothers and I shared an old Schwinn cruiser before getting our brand-new Schwinn Sting-Rays for Christmas when I was in the fifth grade. I lived in rural West Virginia, and the world just got bigger. From that point on, I cannot tell you an adventure story without a bicycle being involved. Mom had no idea where we were, or how far we had ridden. We would scavenge lost golf balls from the neighboring woods and hustle them to golfers at the city park. Then we'd race over to the concession stand, where our quarter could buy a bag of chips and a Coke. Freedom . . . absolute, uninhibited freedom! To this day I use my bike to go out on long rides and find adventure. My bicycle is definitive of my personality.

Elizabeth Seifert, who picked up the sport later, echoes those sentiments.

I muse regularly about the fantastic luck I have had by taking up this sport. I cannot think of another sport—or form of exercise, for that matter—that gives you all the freedom, fun, and adventure that cycling does.

I think it's because cycling feels like flying. The wind in your hair as you're sailing down the road. The rush of speed as you sweep down a long, windy descent. It's like spreading your wings and soaring—and let's face it, nothing says freedom like a soaring bird . . . or a bicycle.

EMPOWERMENT

A bike has carried me out of pretty much every bad relationship I've ever had—romantic ones with not very nice men, dead-end jobs, and even some bad spells with myself—and taken me to a better place. From the first time our suffragette sisters pulled up their petticoats and pedaled off to fight for equality, bicycles have been helping women unearth their inner badass.

My friend Jill recently confided to me that personal empowerment is exactly what made her fall in love with the sport nearly 20 years ago.

At the ripe old age of 27, I was carrying 155 pounds on my 5-foot-2 frame, supporting a two-pack-a-day Marlboro 100's habit, and living with my alcoholic, verbally abusive boyfriend of 4 years. My other roommate (who I actually later married) was a fitness guy and had just started mountain biking. So my boyfriend bought us matching Trek hybrids. I drove over to Valley Forge on a warm spring day and threw my fat leg over the top tube and started pedaling.

After about 2 hours of riding around the paved trails, I was back at my car, where a serious mountain biking woman was packing up her car. She said I should hit the dirt trails. I did, and I loved it. Two months later, I entered my first mountain bike race. I stood there in the 98°F heat and humidity and got goose bumps, I was so excited! I finished mid-pack [in the beginner category] and had the time of my life. After the race, the same woman came up to me and said, "It's in your blood now, isn't it?" It was—more than she knew! I never looked back. Biking empowered me to leave that horrible relationship and get a career with a Fortune 500 company, and has led me to the best friends any soul could ask for.

Even if life is rosy and you've got nothing to pedal away from, cycling can still boost your confidence and empower you to do things you never thought possible, says Robin Dunn.

I started riding because of a boy. I had a miserable first ride with him and vowed to never ride with him again. I then met an incredible group of ladies who took me under their wing and guided me to be the rider I am today. I am thankful for the cycling community and all the support. I've earned my mountain bike and cyclocross racing categories! I still don't ride with the boy (now my husband) because I'm devoted to my own goals and accomplishing them. It's been incredibly empowering.

SHED STRESS

You can't run away from your problems, but you can sure as heck ride away from the stress they cause, says Teresa DiSessa-Johnson.

I got started because I needed an outlet for the stress in my life. My dad had a massive stroke in 2004 and then my sister passed away in a tragic car accident Christmas Eve morning of 2005. I was always an athlete growing up and then a kickboxer after college. But I needed something where I could feel free and at peace with the world. I saw a group of cyclists riding one day in these awesome kits. They looked fast and fit and free. I told myself, That is something I can do. I did. The rest was history.

That history includes forming Riptide Cycling in 2005, a women's cycling team devoted to encouraging women riders in road, track, cyclocross, and mountain biking and helping everyone from newbies to elite racers compete at their highest level. "All my team kits have a sunflower on the back pocket in memory of my sister. I'm so grateful to have found this sport. It's been life-altering [and] -saving," she says.

No matter what the source of your stress, cycling can help. It's scientifically proven. Riding your bike lowers your stress level by burning off stress hormones like adrenaline and cortisol. It also makes you stress resilient. Though healthy, exercise itself is a stressor, especially when you're newly active. When you first start exerting yourself, your body releases cortisol to raise your heart rate, blood pressure, and blood sugar levels, says Monika Fleshner, PhD, professor of integrative physiology at the University of Colorado Boulder. As you get fitter, it takes a longer, harder ride to trigger that same exercise stress response. That training effect doesn't stop after you rack your bike. It carries over into the rest of your day.

"People who are active have decreased cortisol response to emotional crisis compared to sedentary people," says Fleshner. "So now you can go into a stressful environment and be okay. You can just endure a lot more before you kick off a stress response," she says.

BODY IMAGE

I'll speak personally here: I've always had a pretty rocky relationship with my body. I was always bigger than I wanted to be, more muscular than other girls, and just plain uncomfortable in my skin. In college, that discomfort (combined with other insecurities) led to a pretty nasty eating disorder. Once I finally rediscovered my love of bikes and became a cyclist, that all went away. I learned to love the legs that could sprint down country lanes and conquer mountains. I'm far from alone in that regard.

HAPPINESS

As little as 10 minutes of cycling can significantly improve your mood, according to research from Bowling Green State University. Longtime depression researcher James Blumenthal, PhD, professor of psychology and neuroscience at Duke University, agrees and prescribes exercise for better mental health. "Exercise works as well as psychotherapy and antidepressants in the treatment of depression, maybe better," he says. A recent study analyzing 26 years of research on depression and exercise finds that even just a little exercise—like 20 to 30 minutes a day—can prevent depression long term.

The exact mechanisms aren't entirely understood, but it's clear that exercise like cycling boosts production of feel-good chemicals like serotonin and dopamine. "As soon as our rats start running on their wheels, they get a 100 to 200 percent increase in serotonin levels," says brain chemistry researcher J. David Glass, PhD, of Kent State University.

As you pedal past the 20- to 30-minute mark, other mood-lifting chemicals like endorphins and cannabinoids (which, as the word implies, are in the same family of chemicals that give pot smokers their high) kick in. When researchers asked 24 men to either run or bicycle at a moderate intensity or sit for about 50 minutes, they found high blood levels of anandamide, a natural cannabinoid, in the exercisers, but not in the sedentary volunteers.

A group of researchers from the University of Texas Southwestern Medical Center recently came up with an exercise prescription for happiness. To ward off depression with aerobic exercise, they recommend three to five sessions a week. Each session should be 45 to 60 minutes long and keep your heart rate at between 50 and 85 percent of your max. That's a spin class or a spirited ride.

"Cycling is a Zen state for me. From bike commuting to mountain biking and some road riding, this lifetime love of ours is therapy, fitness, and love all wrapped together," says Elizabeth Hunter, who is the parent of a special needs child. "Rolling over sweet singletrack brings me peace and is the greatest thing ever."

INCREASED ENERGY

It's like you learned in 11th-grade physics: An object in motion wants to remain in motion. That's how it is with cycling. It charges you up so you're still buzzing with energy long after you've racked your bike and hit the showers. Again, not just me talking here.

In a research analysis of 70 studies on exercise fatigue that involved more than 6,800 people, University of Georgia scientists reported that more than 90 percent of the studies turned out the same result: Formerly sedentary people who started participating in an exercise program experienced less fatigue and more energy compared to their still-sedentary counterparts. What's more, the average energy boost was greater than the improvements they reported getting from stimulant medications like the ones used for ADHD and narcolepsy. And everyone benefited: healthy adults, chronically ill men and women, folks with heart disease, cancer, and diabetes.

One bout is all it takes for an instant lift. When researchers at the University of Georgia in Athens had volunteers engage in a single 30-minute cycling session, the men and women reported an immediate boost in energy. When the scientists examined the volunteers' brain activity, they discovered why. Pedaling trips circuits in the brain that are related to energy and leave you feeling, well, energized. Are you tired of being tired? Get on a bike and ride.

BETTER SLEEP

You probably know sleep is important for cell regeneration and weight control. But you may not know that, according to the National Sleep Foundation, women are more likely than men to have trouble both falling and staying asleep and, unsurprisingly, are more likely to be sleepy during the daytime. Worse, women are more likely than men to be saddled with the ill consequences of too little sleep.

Sleep-deprived women are at higher risk for heart disease, depression, blood clots, and stroke than their male peers. Some sleep experts believe that we women actually need more sleep than men because we work our brains harder. Women are known to be multitaskers. Our brains are actually hardwired to allow us to do so. But that demands an awful lot of your brainpower, which in turn demands an awful lot of recovery—i.e., sleep, the only time your brain, especially the cerebral cortex (the part of the brain responsible for complex thought, memory, and language), goes into recovery mode. Bad sleep, bad brains.

Bicycling to the rescue. Research from Stanford University found that regular riding can help you fall asleep faster, sleep more soundly, and get a whole lot more shut-eye overall. When researchers there asked 43 men and women with mild sleep troubles to do 30 to 40 minutes of aerobic exercise, which included bike riding, 4 days a week, they found that after 16 weeks, the volunteers were able to fall asleep about 15 minutes faster and slept about 45 minutes longer each night. That's a full hour of slumber for very little exercise. Though scientists are still teasing out the exact mechanism behind exercise's slumber-inducing effects, they believe it's a combination of stress reduction and regulation of circadian rhythms. Bicycling also gets you out into the fresh air and sunshine, both of which have been shown to improve biological rhythms as well.

MORE SMARTS

As Einstein (who, it's said, may have come up with the theory of relativity while riding his bike) could have told you, cycling also makes you smarter. In a recent study published in the *Journal of Clinical and Diagnostic Research*, scientists from India found that volunteers scored better on tests of memory, reasoning, and planning after just 30 minutes of spinning on a stationary bike. They also completed the tests much more quickly postexercise.

In a nutshell, exercise is like fertilizer for your brain. It starts with irrigation. Just as those hours spent turning your cranks create rich capillary beds in your legs, they do the same in your brain. "More blood vessels in your brain means more oxygen and nutrients to help it work," says Canadian neuroscientist Brian Christie, PhD.

As you pedal away, you're also forcing more nerve cells to fire, which increases the creation of proteins like brain-derived neurotrophic factor, as well as a compound aptly named noggin, which promotes stem cell division and neurogenesis (new brain cell formation). The result: You double or triple the production of neurons—literally building your brain, says Christie. You also increase your synthesis of neurotransmitters (the messengers between your brain cells), so all those brain cells, new and old, can communicate with each other for better, faster functioning.

Brain growth is especially important with each passing birthday, because with age our brains shrink and those connections shrivel away. Exercise, like cycling, restores and protects them, says researcher Arthur Kramer, PhD, of the University of Illinois at Urbana-Champaign. "Our research finds that after only 3 months, those who were exercising had the brain volume of people 3 years younger," says Kramer, referring to a study that examined the brains of 59 sedentary volunteers ages 60 through 79, who either started exercising or did no exercise for 6 months.

Aerobic exercise like cycling can also fend off degenerative brain diseases like Alzheimer's, stroke, and dementia, says Kramer, by safeguarding your telomeres, the protective ends on your chromosomes that act like shoelace tubing, safeguarding your chromosomes from the tangling and fraying that lead to disease. In a study of 2,400 twins, those who did the most exercise, 199 minutes a week (just about 30 minutes a day), had telomeres that looked a full decade younger than those of people who did just 16 minutes of activity a week.

A bigger, better-connected, healthier brain simply works better. "Adults who exercise display sharper memory skills, higher concentration levels, more fluid thinking and reasoning, and greater problem solving than those who are sedentary," says Kramer.

GENERAL HEALTH

Moderate aerobic exercise is good for you. Vigorous exercise that makes you huff and puff and sears your muscles with a warm burn is good for you. Easy aerobic exercise is good for you. The beauty of cycling is that it can be all of those things for every body. Even if your knees (or heart and lungs) won't let you sprint half a block on your feet, you can push hard for half a mile (or much more) on your bike.

Of course everybody knows that exercise is "good for you." But just a few stats to show how much: Every single ride positively affects your levels of triglycerides (a potentially dangerous group of fatty acids that circulate in your blood). Riding for just 30 minutes on most of the days in a week—enough to burn about 1,200 calories—can drop levels of these blood fats by 25 percent. The National Institutes of Health reports that aerobic exercise like cycling can lower your systolic blood pressure (the top number) by an average of 11 points and your diastolic (the bottom number) by an average of 9 points. Cardio activity like cycling also helps keep blood sugar in check. And, of course, cycling helps you lose weight. All of that helps protect your heart and reduce your risks of diabetes and cardiovascular ills such as stroke.

A bonus for women: Exercise also reduces the risk of breast cancer. A 12-year landmark study of 110,559 women reported that those who do vigorous exercise like brisk cycling for at least 5 hours a week have a 20 percent lower risk of invasive breast cancer and a 31 percent lower risk of early-stage breast cancer than their more sedentary peers. A related study of 15,000 women between the ages of 20 and 69 yielded similar findings, showing that women who did 6 hours of heart-pumping exercise a week reduced their risk of malignant breast cancer by 23 percent. The latter study also noted that the disease protection kicked in no matter how late in life the women started exercising—great news for latecomers to the sport.

At the end of the day, riding a bike may help you enjoy a longer life. A study of more than 5,000 Americans reported that people who enjoyed moderate exercise like cycling for most of their lives racked up about 4 more years at the end of the line.

FINDING SELF

We women have a tendency to lose ourselves—and not in a nice bubble-bath, escapist kind of way, but rather in an "I'm taking care of everyone else 24/7, who the hell am I again?" sort of situation. One of the things I heard over and over from women was that cycling helped them remember who they were, to find themselves and actually enjoy being themselves again.

Like Laura Sock-Nardelli, a 45-year-old mom of four—who homeschooled all of them—said, "I rode in my 20s, but it fell to the wayside when my children were very young. I picked it back up again 2 years ago and haven't looked back since! I'm training for my first triathlon this summer. My bike helped me find myself again!"

Sometimes cycling can even help you find a self you didn't know you had. Like Diane Bauer, who didn't toss a leg over a bike until well into her adult life. "I am a mother of seven children, all of whom I have homeschooled. I got my first bike at 48. I have lost more than 40 pounds and did my first sprint triathlon at 49. I just rode 57 miles today with a friend and just celebrated the 1-year anniversary with my bike. It's given me a whole new lease on life."

And it's never too late to take this journey to

inner/new/new-and-improved selfhood, as Susan Keys, 65, told me.

I started mountain biking at age 60. I love being outdoors and I like the physical and mental challenge of mountain biking. It keeps me young. I road cycle, too, but mountain biking is my favorite. I ride in Bend, Oregon, with a couple of more experienced friends. Both have encouraged me and taught me tons. I also have a few good riding friends who challenge me to continue to do better. I feel lucky. Now I just wish I had a cycling team just for amateur women over 60 and more opportunities to race with women in my age category.

I'd like to see Susan's dream come true, for sure.

Let's Keep Rolling

In the pages that follow, you'll find pretty much everything you need to know about our great big sport of cycling, no matter what your favorite form or flavor. As you read and learn and train and become more active, consider bringing a friend or two or five with you.

Stats from the League of American Bicyclists indicate that with just a little support and education, more women are willing to get out and swing a leg over a bike. For instance, the group reports that 58 percent of women compared to 81 percent of men say they feel "very confident" riding a bike. We can change that by riding together and encouraging each other, or maybe joining a local cycling club to learn from more experienced riders.

In a survey of six cities, just 29 percent of women versus 83 percent of men said they could fix a flat tire; only 3 percent of women versus 34 percent of men said they could fix pretty much any problem. Basic bike maintenance and repair aren't any more complicated than pulling your morning espresso. You'll find everything you need to know starting on page 289. Feel free to share it with others.

Just one-third of women said it was "no problem" to find clothing and gear that matched their personal style. *That's* a very easy one to change with all the options available today. In fact, we'll tackle that right out of the gate in Part 2.

Get involved and get your stories out there. The sport has grown an awful lot among women in just the past 5 or 6 years, following the same rising trajectory as social media. Some experts don't think that's a coincidence. You're less likely to feel like the only woman out there if you log on to Facebook or Instagram and see a feed full of smiling women riding bikes all over the country.

Imagery is powerful. Your messages are powerful. And everyone is listening, from rank-and-file riders on the street to Olympic pros to the very manufacturers who make our bikes and the politicians who help secure safe places to ride. Ride loud. Ride proud. Bring a friend and let's keep this party going strong. Turn the page and let's roll.

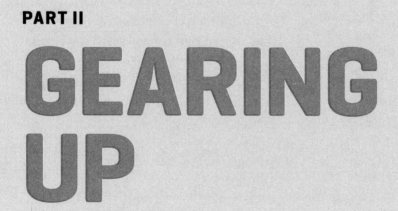

PART II

GEARING UP

Few topics are as polarizing in the cycling industry as "women's specific" gear. When *Bicycling* magazine surveyed women who read the magazine about their cycling to help shape future content, the responses were all over the map.

Some women bristled at the term "women's specific," regarding it as a marketing tool for selling inferior bikes (as I mentioned earlier, many women's specific bikes are indeed outfitted with mid- to low-range components; we'll get to that later). Others begged to differ, saying they were grateful for the surge in women's specific design because they felt it made them able to brake and steer and feel in control of a bike for the first time. The fact is that it is nearly impossible to define what's ideal women's cycling gear because women are every bit as diverse as the men on the roads and trails we share.

Sure, some of our wants are universal. Women want bikes that are a joy to ride and clothes that fit well and look nice. What does all that mean? That's where it seems to get sticky. In trying to answer the question, I called some of the brightest female brains in the industry, including none other than Anna Schwinn (yes, of *that* Schwinn family), bike designer and engineer, and even they couldn't agree on whether or not women's specific bikes are necessary, let alone what defines them.

Here's what they did agree on and what you, as a woman who rides a bicycle, should keep in mind as you gear up for your rides.

OUR PROPORTIONS MAY NOT BE ALL THAT DIFFERENT. Much of women's specific bike geometry revolves around the notion that women generally have shorter torsos and longer legs than men, so they need their handlebars to be closer and higher up to reach them. This is actually a shockingly controversial point. Many experts stand by it, stating that men typically have inseams that are 46.5 to 47.5 percent of their height, while women's are in the range of 47.5 to 49.0 percent of their height. But others refute it. In either event, it is a sweeping generalization rather than a defining difference between us. So in the end, many women skew that way, but not all do, and the same is true for men, for that matter. That doesn't mean you can't benefit from a switch to a women's specific bike, but the point is that first and foremost, you want a bike that fits your particular body. You'll learn all about that in the chapters that follow.

BUT WE ARE BUILT DIFFERENTLY. Probably more important than how we are proportioned is how we are built, which *is* notably different from men. By and large we are shorter—an average of 6 inches shorter than the average man, according to stats from the Centers for Disease Control and Prevention. And we tend to be lighter at any given height. As you'd expect, we're generally smaller in other areas, too, like our hands. That's important because you brake, shift, and generally control the bike with them. Women also tend to have narrower shoulders and less-muscular upper bodies, which doesn't factor into road riding too much but is significant in mountain biking, where you need to put weight on the front wheel to carve corners and pull up the front of the bike to work through technical terrain.

SADDLES ARE EVERYTHING. No matter whom you talk to, there's agreement on one thing: Women need to be sure they find a saddle that fits their anatomy, which *is* different from a man's (and not just in the obvious ways). Our pelvises are shaped and structured for childbirth, which ultimately means that we end up positioned differently on a saddle than men. "I found one of my great-grandfather's notebooks from the 1940s, and he had a whole chapter dedicated to saddles," says Schwinn. "His words: 'If we don't figure out saddles, we'll never get women on bikes.'" We've come a *long* way since then, and now there's an option for every body. This section will help you find yours.

WE HAVE CURVES. Before manufacturers got serious about developing women's specific cycling clothing, it was a challenge to find shorts that didn't come down to your knees or jerseys that weren't boxy or baggy. Nowadays you can find women's specific clothes, including shoes, helmets, gloves, and even arm warmers. You'll learn about everything you need—or maybe just everything you want—in this section as well.

Once you have all the gear you need to ride, you'll want people to ride with, and more time to ride. This section wraps up with a look at the cycling lifestyle and how, as a woman, you can get even more involved.

CHAPTER 2

Bikes, Bikes, and Women's Specific Bikes

WHAT BIKE (OR BIKES) YOU BUY AND RIDE DEPENDS ON WHERE and how you ride. Seems kind of obvious. But there is a stunning array of bikes available in every category, and it's surprisingly easy to screw it up. I know. I've done it more than once, as have many well-intentioned riders I know.

It goes like this. You walk into a bike shop, cash in hand, determined to get yourself a "good bike." Like my friend Steven C. who was completely bitten by the cycling bug. The man waltzed into his local boutique bike shop with six grand burning a hole in his pocket. He laid it down on the lightest, sweetest, fastest whip on the floor—a Specialized Venge. Big mistake. Not because the Venge isn't a featherlight, superfast, really hot bike. It is. But it's extremely aerodynamic, highly responsive, and specially designed to be raced at blistering speeds, so it actually handles better the faster you go and less confidently when you're just cruising along. In short, it wasn't the bike for Steve, who was an extremely enthusiastic but more casual rider. Steve needed comfort and stability rather than sheer racing speed. He went back within a week to make a change.

I was sympathetic to Steve's situation, as I'd done the same thing—twice. The first time was in my early 20s, when I'd just gotten back into riding. The only bikes I'd ever had were the ones my parents had given me, so when I walked in, I was dumbfounded by all the choices. When the salesperson came up to me, I just muttered, "I want a bike." To his credit, he did ask a few questions about what kind of riding I'd be doing. I said I didn't really know. So he pursued, "Roads? Maybe paths?" I thought they both sounded like fun, so I said, "Yes!" and ended up giving him all the money in my pocket (which was $700; not small change at the time) and walking out the door with a decent hybrid (which means a bike that's designed half like a road bike and half like a mountain bike). Problem is, I couldn't keep up riding with anyone on the road with it and it didn't handle anything more off-road than a cinder path. I ditched it 6 months later for a real road bike, and then later I added a real mountain bike to my bike stable.

Despite being 10 years wiser *and* working in the industry *and* even having race experience, I blew it again a few years back when upgrading my mountain bike (adjusting for inflation, the mistake was equally costly). Swayed by marketing hype, I bought a bike that was more plush than fast and was better suited to cruising than hammering rough terrain and spent months with buyer's remorse because I didn't follow the fundamental rule of buying a bike: *Know where and how you want to ride.*

"But I Already Have a Bike"

You may be thinking you can skip this section because you already have a bike. But I'd encourage you to at least skim through it, especially if your bike is more than a few years old and/or has been collecting dust and rust because you don't ride as much as you'd like. You may find that, like so many unwitting riders, you don't have the right bike to satisfy your riding goals, especially if the one you have came from a department store or was a hand-me-down.

While almost any bike is fine for bumming around town or tooling around your local park with your kids, if you want to ride any kind of distance or take to the open road, riding a heavy cruiser or old mountain bike may end up feeling more like a chore than joyful exercise. Bike technology has exploded during the past decade, and today's bikes are lighter, perform better, and are a whole lot more fun to ride than their predecessors.

Note: Even if your current bike is perfectly suited to your riding needs and style, it's always wise to take it to your local shop for regular tune-ups, especially if you stash it away for months at a time (like during the winter months). Time and disuse can take a toll on a bike's key components (like brakes and shifters), bolts can loosen, and parts you'd never even think of checking can rust or degrade. Your local bike mechanic will think of checking them all, and then some. You'll be safer and happier knowing that all the nuts and bolts are tight, the moving parts are lubed, and everything is in top working order. She can also suggest upgrades that will extend the enjoyable life span of your current bike.

Without further ado, here's a guide to nearly every type of ride.

ROAD BIKES

As the name implies, these bikes are designed to be ridden on pavement. They're generally constructed from lightweight materials like high-grade steel, aluminum, titanium, or carbon fiber (for more on that, see "Materials Matter," page 36) and are generally outfitted with

aerodynamic features like curved "drop" handlebars that allow you to tuck into a fast, aerodynamic position and skinny tires for the least amount of rolling resistance on the road.

This category is enormous, offering a wide variety of subcategories to choose from, from ultraresponsive top-shelf race bikes to sturdier, more stable touring bikes to full-on aerodynamic machines made for crushing Ironman bike courses, and everything in between. Below is a generic silhouette of a road bike.

Here's what you need to know to pick the right one for you.

Diagram of a road bike

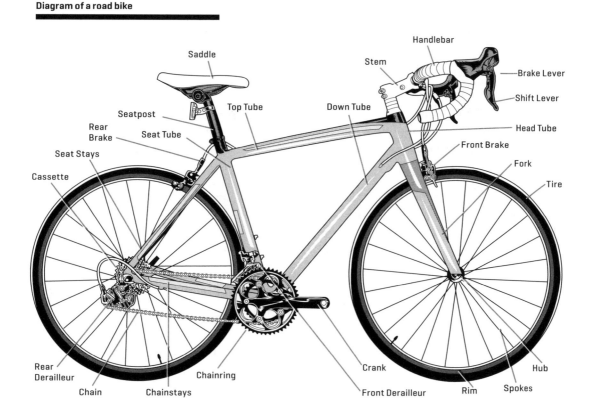

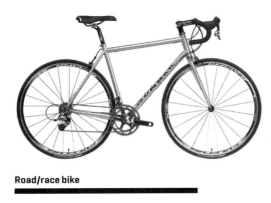

Road/race bike

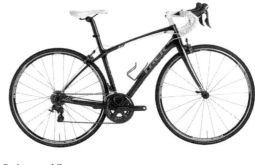

Endurance bike

RACE

This is an oversimplification of this category, because racers use all types of bikes, depending on the course conditions and demands. But in general race bikes have shorter head tubes, shorter seat stays, and other specific design characteristics that make the rider more aerodynamic and the bike more responsive to steering. They also tend to be "stiffer," which means that when you put the pedal down, most of your power goes directly into making the bike shoot forward. Race bikes also have high-end components, light wheels, and a higher price tag to pay for it all. These bikes are fun because they're fast. They're sexy because they're fast. But some riders find them "nervous"—too responsive for their needs—and they may be so stiff and aggressive that they're uncomfortable over long rides.

ENTHUSIAST/ENDURANCE

First, let's set the record straight. Just because these bikes are a bit more relaxed and put you in a more upright position, it does not mean they are not plenty fast and fun. They are. And because you're more comfortable, you might even go faster and have more fun in the long run than if you were on a less forgiving, more aggressive race bike. Sometimes also called "plush" or recreation bikes, these generally have a longer head tube and slightly shorter top tube, which is what makes your positioning more upright than the low and stretched-out orientation you have on a race bike. The bottom bracket is generally lower, which drops the center of gravity and increases your feeling of stability while riding. They also have some vibration absorption built into the frame, so the ride isn't as rigid as a more aggressive road race bike gives you. Yet, the bikes are still relatively light and their overall geometry is responsive, so when you want to open it up, the bike goes fast.

TIME TRIAL/TRIATHLON

Interest in these bikes has risen with the soaring popularity of triathlon, especially among women, who now make up about 40 percent of the race field at any given tri. The primary thing to keep in mind when you're contemplating buying one of these aero-missiles is that they are highly specialized race machines. They're designed with one thing in mind—making you more aerodynamic so you can more easily maintain a higher speed on the generally flat to rolling, nontechnical courses you find in these events. One of the defining characteristics of these bikes is the low front end that is dressed with aerobars, which cause you to place your elbows close to your sides while extending your hands in front of you to minimize wind resistance. This means you can't get to the brakes as easily. You are also less stable in that position. Triathletes have a terrible reputation as bike handlers, but I'd argue it's often the bikes, not the riders. Many charity rides, group rides, and all road races prohibit time trial bikes because they're simply not safe in mass-start, group-riding situations.

This is a very specific tool for a very specific job. It does it better than the rest. But if you're just dabbling in tri competition, stick to a road bike. Particularly well-endowed women who decide to go ahead with this type of bike sometimes complain that their knees knock against their breasts as they're hammering down the road, so ensuring that you have a good fit is definitely in order.

TOURING/COMMUTING

You don't need a special bike for commuting or even light touring, but if you see yourself packing up your steed for lots of self-supported saddle time, they're definitely worth a look. Touring bikes often have racks (or at least braze-on mounts for attaching them) or fenders (or braze-ons so you can easily attach them), and room for fatter tires. They also tend to have lower bottom brackets for a more upright position so they're stable and comfortable for the long haul.

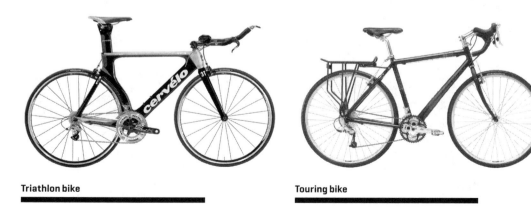

Triathlon bike

Touring bike

MOUNTAIN BIKES

Going off-road? Get a mountain bike. Mountain bikes are specifically crafted for riding on dirt paths and mountain trails, which include stream crossings, fallen trees, and often lots of rocks and roots along the way. If you're new to the sport, you'll recognize mountain bikes by their very beefy tires and upright design. They usually have at least one shock absorber (generally in the front) to absorb the impact from bumpy terrain. The handlebars are straight and wide, so you have better steering control. The bike's design puts you in a more upright position, so you can easily maneuver the bike around trees and other obstacles. Though they're built for off-road riding, you can (and many people do) use them to ride on roads. The upside of riding a mountain bike is that they're very stable, so even the sketchiest beginner will feel confident behind the bars. The downside is that they're heavier and slower on the pavement than a road-specific bike, so you won't experience the joy of rolling along really fast—until you take it on the trail.

Mountain biking is as easy or as gnarly as the terrain you ride, and there are bikes specially designed for every type of riding and rider, whether you stick to buttery-smooth singletrack—a narrow trail—or bomb down boulder-strewn mountainsides. One of the defining characteristics of any particular mountain bike is how much "travel" it has, which is essentially how much suspension it delivers. The

Diagram of a mountain bike

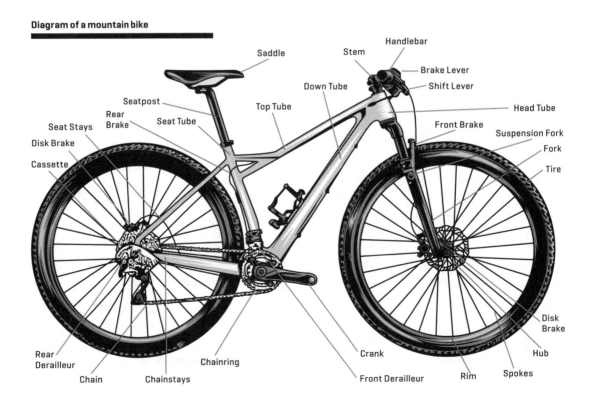

more travel a bike has, the bigger the bumps it can absorb without tossing you about.

See a generic silhouette of a mountain bike on the opposite page.

Here's what you need to know to pick the right one for you.

CROSS-COUNTRY

Cross-country (XC) mountain bikes generally come as either hardtails (no rear suspension) or XC dual suspension (a small amount of rear suspension). They both generally have about 100 to 120 millimeters (4 to 5 inches) of front suspension. They tend to be light and to have a steep head tube angle, which makes the steering quick and responsive. They're very good for climbing, but because they're so nimble and less shock absorbing, it takes more finesse to make them fly down the mountain. If you're going to race XC, this is the bike to get.

TRAIL/ALL MOUNTAIN

These are the "all-arounders" in the crowd. They tend to be a bit heavier than cross-country bikes, but these days, they're still pretty light. They

have slacker head tube angles, which makes the bikes steadier when you're ripping one of them downhill. They generally have about 120 to 160 millimeters (5 to 6 inches) of travel and excel at handling aggressive terrain (rough with many obstacles to ride over). Most trail bikes would be more bike than you'd need or want for a typical XC race, though you could certainly toe the line on one—especially if the course conditions are very technical. They are best suited for fun riding and all-day adventures, when you want a bike that's light enough to pedal up the mountain and plush enough to rail the trip back down. They are also great for racing "Enduro," a type of race where only the mostly downhill sections are timed, but you have to pedal between segments within a certain amount of time. Trail bikes are sometimes called Enduro bikes.

DOWNHILL

These are bomber bikes. Sometimes also referred to as "freeride" mountain bikes, they have tons of travel—180 to 200 millimeters (7 to 8 inches). They feature a slack seat tube angle, a very low seat, and a slack head tube

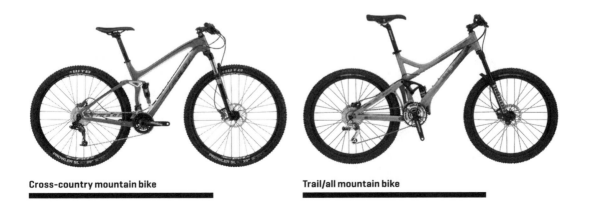

Cross-country mountain bike

Trail/all mountain bike

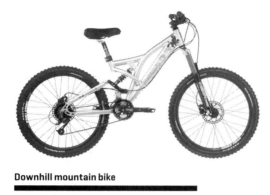

Downhill mountain bike

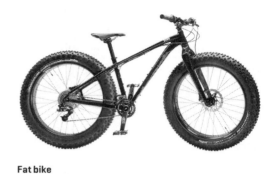

Fat bike

angle. As a result, your center of gravity is low and you're super stable, enabling you to shred over ridiculously difficult terrain. These steeds are heavy and often come equipped with very few gears, because you rarely want to pedal one to the top of anything. Instead, you take a shuttle or, if you're at a ski area, a chairlift to the top and ride back down.

FAT BIKES

These cartoonishly proportioned bikes are characterized by their enormous 3- to 4-inch monster-truck-ish tires that look like they belong on something with an engine rather than two pedals and a chain. Fat bikes used to be a very small niche of the market, reserved for those who wanted to ride on the snowpack in long-winter climes like Alaska, Minnesota, and other mountain states. Their popularity has been surging in recent years, however, as more people hop aboard to explore all the places these big wheels will take them. There are even fat-bike races. Though you can indeed race them, they are not super fast. They tend to be quite a bit heavier and to turn more slowly than even the burliest mountain bike. But speed isn't the point. The massive volume of the tires allows you to run ludicrously low pressure, so you can float over snow, sand, mud, rocks, wet roots, and other terrain that would stop a skinnier tire in its tracks. All that said, unless you're interested in extreme exploration or live where there's good snowpack (they're not good in powder), it's not a bike you would use much.

CYCLOCROSS AND GRAVEL BIKES

At first glance, cyclocross and their closest kin, "gravel" bikes, resemble road bikes. Look more closely, however, and you'll see subtle differences that make these bikes pedal more smoothly and handle confidently over terrain that's choppier than your typical two-lane country road. As the popularity of these bikes rises, so too does their overall quality and versatility. So it's conceivable that, depending on your riding goals, one of these could be the only bike you need. While these bikes are largely interchangeable, there are important differences that significantly affect their handling and performance.

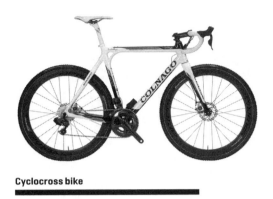

Cyclocross bike

Below is a generic silhouette of a cyclocross/gravel bike.

Here's what you need to know to pick the right one for you.

CYCLOCROSS

Cyclocross bikes—or simply "'cross" bikes, as they are called—are designed to be used in a particular type of racing. Cyclocross races are off-road circuit-style races (a short closed-lap style) held in parks and fields that generally serve up an array of technical challenges, like off camber (sloped) turns, sandpits, tree roots, gravel, deep mud, and barriers and other obstacles that require the rider to quickly dismount, carry or run alongside their bike, and remount to continue racing.

As you might imagine, it takes a good amount of bike handling and some tough equipment to stand up to the challenge. 'Cross bikes step up to the challenge with a slightly longer head tube

Diagram of a cyclocross bike

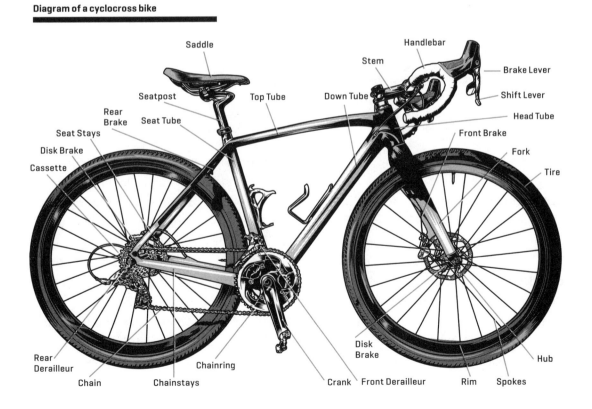

Big Wheels

Mountain bikes also are designed for different wheel sizes. Some use 29-inch-diameter wheels, while others take 27.5-inch wheels. (There are also 26-inchers, but they are quickly becoming extinct.) Which size is best is a source of endless debate in the industry. When making the choice, it's again a matter of what and how you ride (sense a trend here?). Bigger wheels steamroll over tough, technical terrain and are fast on the wide-open fire roads. However, they are a bit trickier to maneuver through tight, twisty turns, and because they're large, it takes a bit more work to put them in motion, though they stay in motion very well once you're rolling. Smaller hoops let you weave more quickly through the tight stuff and are easier to get rolling quickly and toss around (manipulate quickly) on the trail. For that reason, some manufacturers still stand by 29ers for XC riding and default to the smaller wheels for all-terrain and downhill adventures. This debate likely won't be resolved anytime soon. But many manufacturers are settling into 27.5 as the main wheel size they offer.

that raises the handlebar position to improve stability and control. They generally have forks and chainstays that leave more room for wide tires. This design helps prevent mud from collecting on the bike and snagging on the wheels and tires. Traditional 'cross bike geometry features a higher bottom bracket to allow lots of pedal clearance on uneven ground, but that feature makes the bike challenging to remount (because it's higher) and generally makes it trickier to maneuver through tight terrain. More and more 'cross bikes, however, are being designed with lower bottom brackets, which improves their cornering and stability. Because they're made to be ridden on tough terrain, the gearing is lower (easier) than typical road bike gearing.

GRAVEL BIKE

This is a very new category, and honestly, if you walk into a bike shop and ask for a gravel bike, you risk bewildered stares or maybe even laughter, because not everyone agrees that a gravel-specific bike is necessary. While it is true that people have been riding their bikes on unpaved roads for as long as there have been bikes, road bikes have evolved to be so featherlight and pavement oriented. Many really don't hold up very well over dirt, flint, crushed limestone, mud, and the fist-sized chunks of gravel you might find on the more than 1.4 million miles of unpaved roads in the United States—which, incidentally, is 34 percent of the 4.1 million miles of roads in our infrastructure.

There's also been rising enthusiasm for races, particularly long-distance endurance events, or "gravel grinders," that take riders over 50, 100, 200, even 300-plus miles of this type of tough terrain. A 'cross bike, especially one with a low bottom bracket, certainly will do the trick. Some manufacturers are going the extra mile by crafting special bikes that have longer wheelbases; slackened, slightly taller head tubes; and low bottom brackets for added comfort, stability, and handling over many miles of rugged

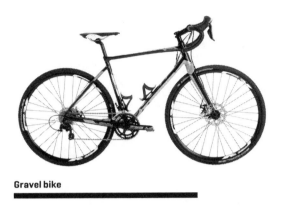

Gravel bike

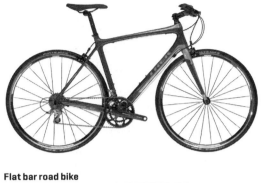

Flat bar road bike

road. Gravel bikes (as well as more and more 'cross bikes) generally come outfitted with disc brakes, which provide optimum braking power in poor conditions and don't get packed with mud, as well as full cable housing to protect the shifting and braking cables from the conditions.

HYBRID BIKES

A little bit road and a little bit off-road, hybrids feature medium-sized tires that let you roll reasonably quickly on pavement, yet provide stability on moderately rough terrain like dirt roads or cinder paths. The position is more upright than aero, so they make comfortable commuting bikes and good all-around exercise bikes. The main thing to consider before buying a hybrid is whether you're thinking about buying a hybrid because you actually want what the type offers or because you can't decide what kind of bike you want. The former is a great reason, but choosing a hybrid for the latter reason will likely leave you with a bad case of buyer's remorse, because it means you probably actually want another type of bike. Shop around until you're sure.

If you truly do want the hybrid for its features, here's what you need to know to pick the right one.

FLAT BAR ROAD BIKE

Some riders are turned off by the low, curved race-style handlebars found on traditional road bikes. So manufacturers responded by outfitting their otherwise sporty road bikes with flat bars for the comfort and control that these cyclists crave. These bikes are plenty fast and fun and definitely worth considering if you aren't particularly concerned about being aerodynamic or keeping up with a pack. The downside of a flat handlebar is that it limits your hand positions. (There are three or four different places to rest your hands on a curved bar, giving your upper body a break from being in the same position mile after mile.) If you go with this option, consider purchasing ergonomic grips, which are shaped to fit the shape of your hands and/or bar end handgrips that add a bit of variety for your hands.

CRUISER

Go to any beach town in America and you'll see lots of big, colorful fat-tired cruisers. Although they aren't very much like hybrids in terms of their design, they're included in the category because they are built to be utilitarian rather than aggressive. This style of bike is becoming increasingly popular as more cities unveil bike-sharing programs that allow you to rent cruiser-style bikes as an alternative means of transportation. The real beauty of cruisers is their wide seats and high handlebars that let you sit straight up and eat an ice cream cone while cruising along (not while riding in traffic, of course).

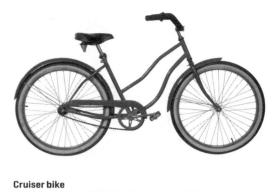

Cruiser bike

WOMEN'S SPECIFIC BIKES

And last, but by no means least, is "women's specific." The funny thing about this category is that it really shouldn't be a category in and of itself because women ride bikes in *all* categories—road, mountain, and 'cross. So there is no single type of bike that is specifically and solely a "woman's bike." Bikes, like attire, are made to fit body type. Just as some women can wear and look fabulous in men's jeans, others look better in pants cut for the female form. And very honestly, sometimes a woman just wants a pretty dress—and there's absolutely nothing wrong with being drawn to a bike because it's pretty. Yes, it has to match your needs and anatomy, but if the tipping point is the cut and color, have at it!

In the end, that's really what women's specific design (WSD) comes down to: making

adjustments that will help women feel good on and about their bikes. Straight up, some WSD bikes are nothing more than smaller, prettier versions of their male-directed counterparts, which is perfectly fine if they work for you. Many have important detailing, like women's specific saddles for our wider pelvis and our specific soft tissues, shorter brake levers for our smaller hands, and other components that make it easier and more comfortable for women to ride. Other WSD bikes are engineered from the ground up to have geometry better suited to a typical woman's frame and proportions and to work with the way women tend to ride—i.e., using their lower bodies more than their upper bodies.

If you are of average height—5 feet 4 inches—or smaller, women's specific bikes are definitely worth considering whether or not you care about pretty colors and feminine design. That's because it's hard to find bikes that suit your size, says frame builder Anna Schwinn. "It's a bell curve, with the average woman sitting at the top of the curve—that's where stuff stops fitting, which means for about half of all women, finding a regular bike that fits them is going to be a challenge. That's not an insignificant number of women."

If you have a petite upper body and are into mountain biking, women's specific geometry is very much worth a look. "Women often don't have the same upper body mass as men, so they don't have enough weight on the front wheel for the bike to corner and perform properly," says Ross Rushin, assistant mountain bike brand manager at Trek. Women's specific bikes are often adjusted for this, with a slightly slackened head tube angle and a steepening of the seat tube angle to bring the rider's weight a bit forward, distributing her body over the bike in a balanced way that allows for optimal handling.

A true—and compelling—story to drive home that point: I have a teammate who is a monster mountain bike racer. Great downhiller. Incredible bike handler. Trail savvy. Super fit. The works. She's also pretty small—5 feet 2 inches, with not a lot of upper body mass. Well, 1 year after about 15 years of racing men's or "unisex" bikes, she got a WSD mountain bike and proceeded to wipe out going into her first hard turn on the thing. She was frustrated and angry and saying all sorts of unprintable things about the bike. But then something happened. As she continued to ride the bike, she started to get a feel for it. She relaxed and let the bike flow rather than try to muscle it through corners like she'd been doing for all those years. And guess what? The bike went where it was

supposed to, with less energy required to power it. And she and that fat bike lived happily ever after.

I've noticed the same thing both on the road and off. Though I ride and race very comfortably on non–women's specific bikes, I can feel the greater ease of riding a bike made with good WSD geometry, despite the fact that I am a pretty muscular woman with more upper body mass than many. I also appreciate having brake levers that I can more easily reach; a suspension that is fully active under my sub-130-pound frame; a saddle that doesn't mash, smash, or dig into me in uncomfortable ways; and many other features of women's specific bikes.

Bicycling magazine's female readers also appear to vary in their preferences: Some love WSD. Others say, "Eh, not for me." In our 2014 women's cycling survey, 46 percent said they prefer women's specific design, about 24 percent said they like unisex bikes, and 30 percent expressed no preference. It all comes down to the bike and the rider. With that, here's a look at all the ways these bikes can be different and what that means to you.

FRAME

Women's specific design starts with the frame. As mentioned earlier, it might simply be a smaller version of the manufacturer's standard frame for that model, or it might have completely different geometry. Either way, you want a bike that fits your body. You should have a comfortable amount of stand-over clearance so you can get on and off the bike with ease, and you shouldn't feel too stretched out or hunched up when your hands are on the bars. Proper fit depends on the following characteristics.

SIZE: Small people—men and women—need small frames, and finding them can be a challenge. Since more women than men are small, it does tend to be more of a woman's issue. That's a fact Amy Miskiewicz knows all too well. When she first got into cycling in 1999, there was nothing on any bike shop floor that fit her 5-foot-tall body with its extremely short torso. "I finally found this nice used Trek 2200 aluminum woman's bike that was *tiny*. It even had 650 [smaller than the standard diameter] wheels. I was very happy on that bike on the road for a long time." Then she wanted to try cyclocross. Again, nothing in her size. "My local shop took my measurements and it was soon obvious that, despite extensive searching, [finding] an off-the-rack 'cross bike was not possible. I ended up getting a custom Dreesens [a bike made in Pennsylvania] that was worth every penny!" Fortunately, more manufacturers are stepping up and making frames suited for women as small as 4 foot 10.

LENGTH: Many (though, again, not all) women have proportionally shorter upper bodies and arms and longer legs—particularly the upper legs—than men do. If that describes you, you may find yourself too stretched out over a standard bike frame, which can make for a pretty uncomfortable ride, as it forces you to roll your weight forward onto your crotch (ouch) and strains your neck and shoulders (common complaints among women). If you have to push your seat back to accommodate your longer upper legs, it can make matters even worse. WSD remedies this with a shortened top tube, a steepened seat angle, and a shorter stem, all of which reduce your reach to the handlebars. It's important to recognize that this geometry works if you have the body type it is designed for. If you do not, you may end up with a bike that doesn't handle properly for you because your weight won't be distributed correctly. In that case, you may be better off with a small-sized standard frame that is outfitted with "female touches," like shorter cranks (see the opposite page), a women's specific saddle, and maybe narrower handlebars.

SADDLE POSITION: Women need to pay special attention to what's called the seat tube angle, which basically determines how far forward or back you're positioned on the bike. If you do indeed have longer upper legs, the seat tube angle should position you behind the bottom bracket to ensure that your knee is positioned properly over your pedal and you're not sitting too far forward.

This is where it gets a little complicated, however. Smaller bikes tend to have more upright seat tubes to make room for the wheels and avoid what is known as toe overlap, which is when the back of the front wheel clips the tip of the shoe on your forward foot during a slow-speed turn. (In the past, small bikes were more commonly made with smaller wheels.) Sometimes bikes will come outfitted with a seatpost that has more setback to adjust for this.

WEIGHT: Cycling is a power-to-weight sport, meaning that the most successful riders are able to generate more watts per pound of their body weight. Given that, obviously the heavier your bike is, the harder it will be to push up hills and ride over long miles. That's *especially* important for women riders, who tend to be lighter. Ironically (and unfairly), women's specific bikes are too often dressed with midrange wheels and components (see page 30), which end up being heavier. This is changing, but slowly. It is worth paying a bit more for lighter, higher-end components if you like to go fast over hilly terrain.

COMPONENTS AND ACCESSORIES

Beyond the frame, equally important considerations when evaluating a bike are all of its components, which means pretty much everything on the bike aside from the fork and frame. Sometimes the biggest difference between a standard "male" bike and a WSD bike is what type of components the bike is outfitted with. Here's what to look at.

BARS AND GRIPS: Your hands should be placed at about shoulder-width on your handlebars on a road bike. Wider than that, and the bike will feel unwieldy; narrower, and you'll have difficulty steering. Too-wide bars can also lead to neck and shoulder pain because your torso will droop a bit between your shoulders. You should also be able to reach down into the drops comfortably. Women's specific bars are generally a bit narrower

and shallower than men's or unisex models to accomplish this. Your hands will be more than shoulder-width apart on a mountain bike's flat handlebars, but they shouldn't be spaced so widely that you're not comfortably in control.

CRANKS: Bikes are generally outfitted with cranks—the arms the pedals are attached to—of a standard length based on the frame size, which, of course, matches the rider's size. But sometimes shorter riders find standard cranks (which are 172.5 millimeters) too long. When the cranks are too long, it's more difficult to pedal at a brisk cadence and you may feel like you have to push too hard because your knees go up too high to stay on top of the gears (e.g., keep the pedals turning smoothly). Both can result in fatigue, and maybe even knee problems over time. If you have short legs, you may also need shorter cranks, such as 170 millimeters, or even 165 millimeters.

LEVERS: This one's really important. Your shifting and braking levers should be very comfortably within your reach. Standard levers often stick too far out from the bars to fit a woman's smaller hands. Women's bikes come outfitted with smaller levers to address this issue. If you're riding a standard bike, look for adjustable-reach levers that allow you to put them where you need them. And be 100 percent sure you can comfortably reach your brake levers when you're riding in the drops, which is the safest, most stable position for descending as well as where you get the best braking leverage on a road bike.

SPEAKING OF BRAKES: Nearly all mountain bikes, many 'cross bikes, and increasing numbers of road bikes are coming with a pair of disc brakes. Each of these, as the name implies, is a large, cutout disc that sits between two padded calipers near the center of the wheel (the hub). Disc brakes have superior stopping power compared to traditional rim brakes (which use pads to squeeze the wheel's rim for slowing and stopping) in wet and dirty conditions. They also require less force for slowing and stopping. So while they're not really women's specific, many women who have smaller hands really appreciate the performance benefits disc brakes provide.

SADDLE: The number one thing that keeps women from cycling is saddle discomfort, according to cycling ergonomics specialist Andy Pruitt, director of the Boulder Center for Sports Medicine in Colorado. Most new riders don't realize that a bike's saddle can be changed, or that there are women's specific saddles. If the one on your bike isn't immediately comfortable, try others till you find one that is. And don't assume wider is better just because you have wide hips. Whether or not you need a wide or a skinny saddle has nothing to do with the size of your derriere. It's the width of your supporting bones, the sit bones, which should support your weight on the rear of the seat (so minimal pressure is placed on your sensitive tissues). It's common for your saddle needs to change over time. I know a number of women who found that as they got older, they lost a little cushioning down below and needed a saddle with a cutout channel to relieve pressure in that area. (See "Saddle Up," page 44, for detailed directions on fitting your saddle.)

STEM: A proper-length stem will allow you to maintain a slight bend in your arms when you're holding the bars. If you're too stretched out, you can switch to a shorter stem, but be cautious of going too small. A very short stem can make the front end feel twitchy.

SUSPENSION: How well your suspension is tuned to your weight and riding style can make or break your off-road experience. Some women's specific bikes have shocks that are specially tuned for women's typically lighter weight ranges. But that's not necessary for good performance. Just make sure that you check the settings on your shock, so you are getting full travel and optimal performance (see page 115 for more details).

WHEELS: There aren't women's specific wheels per se, but as I mentioned earlier, women tend to be lighter than men, yet their bikes are often outfitted with parts that are just as heavy, if not heavier, which means that a greater portion of the total weight that you're pushing along is made up by the bike. One of the easiest (though not necessarily the cheapest) ways to drop a substantial amount of this weight is to upgrade the wheels. The wheels make up what is known as "rotational weight," which is where you actually want the least weight possible because it's that weight that you need to push into motion and keep in motion. Light wheels increase performance exponentially and are a joy to ride. What's more, John Brown, former manager at Philadelphia-area shop High Road Cycles, who has performed many fits and upgrades for women, says many of them would benefit from custom wheels, because women's typically lighter weight doesn't put as much stress on wheels as men's does. "You can get a lighter wheel for half of what many men would have to pay," he says.

———————

That covers the essentials of women's specific design—for now. But keep your eyes peeled as the sport continues to evolve, because industry experts agree on one thing: Women's specific cycling products are only going to get better

and better. "As more women join and grow in this sport, we just keep getting more and more feedback and a larger volume of research to work with, so we're learning more and more about how women ride and what they need and want," says Erin Sprague, women's product manager at Specialized Bicycle Components. "Women's specific products are one of the biggest growth areas in the industry, and it's only going to get better. There's so much momentum, it's an exciting time in women's cycling."

Get in Gear

The gearing you decide on is a small choice that has a big impact. There are three typical options: standard (often, a double chainring with 53 and 39 teeth up front, paired with a 12-to-25-tooth-range 10-gear cassette), triple (three chainrings, with granny gears, often 50/40/30 or 52/42/30), or the increasingly popular compact (50/36 or 50/34 chainrings).

Bikes are often marketed by how many gears they have, but keep in mind that more is not always better. The cassette and chainrings add significant weight to the bike, so the more gears you have, the heavier the bike may become. Road and 'cross bikes generally come with two or three chainrings in the front and 10 or 11 cogs on the cassette in the back. Mountain bikes come with one to three chainrings and the same number of cogs. Mountain bikes are marketed by their gearing. When you hear someone talk about a 1 x ("one-by"), it means there's just one chainring. A 2 x ("two-by") has double chainrings. Important in off-road riding in particular, fewer chainrings mean less weight and fewer components that can break or malfunction on rough terrain.

On the road, triples can be useful if you ride in a very mountainous area, but they add unnecessary weight if you do not, especially since today's road bikes are relatively light and the gear ranges on most doubles offer good climbing gears. One pet peeve around the *Bicycling* offices is that many women's bikes automatically come with a "triple," when a double would make the bike lighter and easier to pedal up even steep terrain. If having enough climbing gears is a concern, you're better off going with a compact gearing setup.

On the extreme end, there are bikes—particularly mountain bikes—that come with one single gear. They're aptly known as single-speeds and have a pretty large cult following. There are also "fixies," which are track-style bikes with one gear that is fixed to the pedals (no coasting), that are popular in urban areas. Both can be fun to ride (fixies also take a good bit more skill), but I wouldn't make either my first or only bike.

What Bike Should I Buy?

It's the most common question that streams into *Bicycling* magazine headquarters. What bike should I buy? As you've seen, there's a huge array to choose from, and even if you've narrowed it down to "road" or "mountain," you *still* need to winnow down a large selection. Here's a quiz I developed that can help with the decision-making process.

PART I: WHERE WILL YOU RIDE?

1. I want to ride mostly on:

A. Roads in my surrounding area.

B. Cinder paths, parks, rail-to-trail systems, around town.

C. Off-road, mountain bike trails, rough terrain.

2. I expect my bike to:

A. Do one thing (e.g., handle off-road challenges like rocks and roots or roll smoothly on the pavement), and do it well.

B. Be a jack-of-all-trades. I don't know enough about what kind of riding I like to fully commit.

C. Be suited for one kind of riding, but offer a little flexibility in case I want to try something a bit different.

PART I ANSWER KEY

Your answer to Question 1 makes the big bike choice easy. If you chose:

A. *You need a road bike.*

B. *You need a bike with some crossover ability, such as a cyclocross/gravel bike or a hybrid.*

C. *You need a mountain bike.*

Question 2 will help you narrow down your selection within that category. If you chose:

A. *You want a purebred bike that is designed for your singular riding needs. Anything else will fall short.*

B. *Consider a high-quality flat bar road bike or a cyclocross bike. You can also consider a hardtail mountain bike with minimal suspension that can handle small bumps but won't be cumbersome and slow on the pavement, or a commuting bike.*

C. *Same as above. For the best bike, try to be as honest as possible with yourself. Maybe you like the idea of off-road riding, but if there are no trails nearby, the reality is that you won't likely do it very often. Determine where you see yourself riding the most and choose a bike that leans most heavily in that direction.*

PART II: **HOW WILL YOU RIDE?**

1. I want my bike to be:

A. Race ready. I plan on riding with a serious group and may even compete.

B. Comfortable and reliable. I'd like to take it out mostly on weekends for fresh air, exercise, and riding around town. I don't want a clunker, but I don't need top performance.

C. Fast, fun, and durable. I'm a weekend warrior, so I want my bike to stand up to some abuse and still give solid performance.

2. Down the road, I see myself:

A. Staying just as I am. I don't anticipate changing my riding style in the next 2 or 3 years.

B. Improving. I'm a novice now, but I hope to learn and grow enough to take on some simple challenges like longer charity rides or short triathlons.

C. As a serious cyclist, baby. I want to fly up hills and tackle challenging rides.

PART II ANSWER KEY

Within each bike category are various price ranges that determine the quality of the ride a bike will give you. Your answer to Question 1 helps define your price range. If you chose:

A. *Splurge now. High-end bikes can run in the $5,000 to $6,000 range (yes, you read that right; you can even spend twice that for top-of-the line, pro quality). But if you want top performance, it's well worth it. Like any investment, it'll sting a little at the initial impact, but you will be really happy down the road. A bike at this price is unbelievably beautiful on every level and will last a lifetime. If you just can't shell out that kind of change, go for a model built for*

recreational to enthusiast riders—you'll still get a great bike and you can always upgrade the components when you have the cash.

B. *Entry level is the way to go. If you don't have great expectations, a no-frills ride costing $600 to $700 will do you just fine. Don't go bargain basement, however. You still want a bike that runs reliably, is fun to ride, and you can count on to brake and shift smoothly.*

C. *Go recreational to enthusiast. Right now is a great time to buy a bike in this category. In the neighborhood of $900 to $2,000 will get you a whole lot of bike—one that will carry you from dabbling newbie to serious cyclist and beyond. For $2,000 to $4,000, you'll get a dreamy machine you'll love for years.*

Don't make the classic mistake of buying a bike today that you will regret tomorrow. If you're reading this book, chances are you're in this sport for life. Your answer to Question 2 helps ensure you buy a bike that will grow with you. Remember, you want to be happy on this bike for at least 3 years, and longer than that if you're upgrading. If you chose:

A. *Fair enough. Invest in a good-quality bike in the right category at a comfortable price and ride to your heart's content.*

B. *Buy at the top end of your price range. Consider going a little higher if you have any suspicion that you'll be looking to upgrade within 3 years.*

C. *Don't sell yourself short. What's "good enough" now will leave you longing for more in a season (or less). You don't have to take out a second mortgage or buy a pro-level ride, but you should consider going directly to the high-end recreational or enthusiast category.*

(continued)

What Bike Should I Buy? *continued*

PART III: THE HUMAN MACHINE

1. My physical condition is:

A. Great. I'm generally healthy, fit, and flexible.

B. Not bad, but I'm carrying some extra weight and/or have a few general aches and pains.

C. Uh, let's not talk about that. (In truth, there are some serious limitations.)

2. My build is best described as:

A. Leggy and/or pear-shaped.

B. Long-waisted and/or muscular.

C. Petite.

3. When it comes to riding a bike, I'm:

A. Not the most athletic woman on the planet. Truth be told, I'm kind of clumsy. I love riding, but I'm not super skilled.

B. Fairly skilled. I feel comfortable climbing on a bike and pedaling away.

C. Experienced. I consider myself athletic, and I feel confident in my ability.

PART III ANSWER KEY

Generally speaking, how fit or unfit you are shouldn't impact what bike you buy. However, it's no big secret that the bent-over biking position can be a challenge for people who are very inflexible or have existing back pain or other orthopedic issues. For question 1, if you chose:

A. *Any bike (in your size, of course) will fit you just fine.*

B. *You'll likely be fine with any bike you buy. If you have a history of back or neck issues, let the shop know and they'll steer you toward a bike that allows a slightly more relaxed and/or upright position (i.e., the height of the handle-bars is only a little lower than or is even with the saddle).*

C. *You'll probably do best with a more relaxed, upright position. Be upfront about any physical limitations when you're buying your bike. If you have limited mobility due to herniated disks, replaced hips, or excess weight, the salesperson can put you on a bike that will offer comfort in your range of motion. You also can make sure your bike is outfitted with gearing that matches your abilities.*

Your body type helps determine your bike type. Many women can benefit from women's specific bikes. Many also can ride standard frames just fine. For question 2:

A and C. *If you answered either of these, consider giving women's specific a try. These bikes are designed for women who have proportionally longer legs and/or carry their weight lower on their frame. Petite women can now find a nice array of women's bikes in small sizes.*

B. *You will likely fit fine on a standard frame unless you are also short in stature.*

Like cars, every bike offers a different type of ride. Some are highly responsive (not always the best quality for newbies), while others respond only to a firmer touch. How you answered Question 3 will help steer you in the right direction. If you said:

A. *You don't need training wheels, but no matter how fit you are, you should look for a bike that forgives rider error. Tell your bike shop you don't want anything too "nervous" or "twitchy," as some high-end bikes can be.*

B. *You can sacrifice some stability for performance. If you don't have orthopedic issues that require a more relaxed ride, experiment with* some more-aggressive bike setups and see what feels best.

C. If you're athletic and have no physical limitations, look for a sweet setup designed for speed and quick handling.

PART IV: WHO I AM

1. When I make a purchase, I want:

A. The best. I like high-def TVs, the newest-generation smartphones, and high-tech appliances.

B. Value. I don't mind spending a little more for a car with a few nice features, but there's a diminishing point of returns. I don't need pro-level gear.

C. Function. I expect what I buy—my PC, my phone, my TV—to work, but I don't ask a whole lot of it.

2. When I start a new hobby or interest, I typically stick with it like:

A. Gum under a desktop. I'm in it for the ages.

B. Suction cups. Some stick. Some plummet to the floor. The garage is littered with unused skis, golf clubs, and other equipment.

C. Like a celebrity marriage. I love it to death for a few years, then move along to the next thing.

PART IV ANSWER KEY

I put these questions here because many people don't put bicycles in the same category as other major purchases. Maybe because a bicycle is sometimes seen as a toy, its true value as a serious piece of machinery isn't recognized. Your answer to Question 1 will help you put your investment in perspective. If you chose:

A. *Put your new bicycle in the same category as you would a new car or TV. You really do get what you pay for, so go for a high-quality bike in your category.*

B. *When buying a bike, being willing to spend a couple hundred bucks more often means the difference between getting a good bike and a really, really great bike. Keep that in mind if a salesperson steers you toward something slightly out of your price range, but that she believes is a better deal. Most bike shop employees are honest and won't try to sell you more than they think you need.*

C. *You can get a very functional bike for about $500 to $700, but any less and you run the risk of bad shifting, sloppy braking, and general heaviness putting a big damper on your ride. Light, well-performing bikes are simply more fun, which means you'll ride them more, and that's worth a couple hundred bucks any day.*

Your level of investment should match your level of interest over the long term. How you answered Question 2 should be your final price check. If you chose:

A. *No need to second-guess yourself. Leave the bike shop with a new ride and a smile.*

B. *Weigh your options a little. If you're not sure this cycling thing will stick, consider buying a good bike that you can improve upon if you end up really loving it. If you buy a high-quality frame with some mid- to low-end components, you can always upgrade down the road.*

C. *They say you never forget how to ride a bike, and even if you drift away from the sport, you can always come back to it. Buy the bike you love and enjoy it today.*

Ride Before You Buy

Just as you would never buy a car without driving it at least a few miles, you shouldn't buy a bike without tossing a leg over it and going for a ride. Ideally, you should test-ride a few to get a feeling for how different models climb, corner, and handle.

Head to your local bike shop rather than to a big-box store like Walmart. Department store bikes may seem like a bargain, but when it comes to cycling, you really do get what you pay for, and what you get off the floor at Kmart is typically a heavy bike with cheap components that won't be much fun to ride. Your bike shop will also be your go-to source for repairs, ancillary gear, information on places to ride, people to ride with, and much more. If you don't get the service you expect at the first shop you enter, leave and try another. Though most shops are friendly and accommodating to riders of all shapes, sizes, and levels of experience, you'll probably run across a few that seem to give the time of day only to those they deem "real cyclists." No need to give them your hard-earned cash when there are plenty of places that will give you the attention you deserve. We'll talk more about that later.

Materials Matter

What your bike is made from has a huge influence on how it rides and often on how much it costs. The following are the most common bike materials and what they mean to you.

CARBON FIBER: This is a composite material made of tightly woven and hardened thin strands of carbon. Most high-end bikes are made from this material. It's ultra light and very responsive, yet absorbs some of the road chatter for a smooth ride. It's also pricey, so a whole bike made of the stuff doesn't come cheap. You can find some less expensive bikes that use bits of carbon in the fork, handlebars, or other parts of the frame to lighten the weight and improve the ride quality.

ALUMINUM: Aluminum frames are snappy and responsive—great if you love racy performance, which is why many race bikes are made from this material. Because it's relatively inexpensive, many entry-level and recreational- and enthusiast-level road bikes are made of aluminum. It's not quite as light and stiff as carbon fiber, but close. One downside is that it can feel a bit harsh.

TITANIUM: Titanium is strong and light and fairly plush. It's also expensive, which is why it's usually only found in high-end bikes. Aside from being light and responsive, titanium is almost literally bombproof. (I once saw a titanium Litespeed fly off a car going 70 mph and cartwheel like a tumbleweed down the interstate without enduring a single ding. My friend rode it the same day.)

STEEL (ALSO CHROMOLY): This is the most popular frame material because of its strength and versatility. It's a bit too heavy and flexy for top-of-the-line race bikes, but otherwise delivers a silky, wonderful ride.

Try to take out at least three bikes so you can make a real comparison. Put each bike through its paces by taking it up hills, pedaling quickly, and trying to come to a quick stop (safely, of course). Pay special attention to details like how quickly and fluidly the chain moves when you shift and how smoothly it comes to a stop when you squeeze the brakes. These are features that have a profound impact on the quality of your ride and how much you'll enjoy being out on your bike. Women are often quick to say they don't need this or that, but if you love to ride and you plan to ride a lot, treat yourself to the best bike you can afford. It will pay for itself in durability, performance, and sheer enjoyment.

Lots of women (and men as well) don't realize that it's actually their bike that's holding them back from being as fast as they want to be. Even if you never pin on a number, if the highlight of your Saturday ride is being the first in your group to the top of the hill, you're technically a racer, says John Brown. "If you're trying to keep up with people faster than you, then you're racing," he adds. "And if it's your bike that's holding you back, and not you, then that sucks." Sound like a sales pitch? Well, sure. But it's hard to argue with him, because it's true.

Note: This may be obvious, but when test-riding bikes, wear the clothes you plan to ride in. "I once had a customer show up dressed to go to dinner downtown," says Brown. Instead, wear (or bring) the shorts, shoes, and pedals you usually ride with. And take your time. "We have customers who come in with a list of bikes they're interested in, and they might spend just 5 minutes in the shop—the rest of the time they're out riding," he says. "They even bring a lunch." Don't worry about taking up too much of the shop's time: "It's your job to be an educated consumer."

My New Bike!

Jot down what you've gleaned from the "What Bike Should I Buy" test for a snapshot of the bike you should buy.

PART I

My bike type: _____

_____

(e.g., road bike, hybrid)

PART II

My price range: _____

_____

(e.g., $600 to $800, $2,000 to $2,500)

PART III

My setup should be: _____

_____

(e.g., relaxed and a standard frame, somewhat aggressive and women's specific)

PART IV

My components should be: _____

_____

(e.g., mid-range but durable, top of the line)

CHAPTER 3

Fitting a Bike to the Female Form

EVERYONE WHO RIDES A BIKE FOR MORE THAN A FEW MILES here and there should take the time and invest in at least a basic bike fitting. The more you ride, the more important this step is and the more care you should take in dialing everything in just right. Bike fit is by no means an issue only for women. However, it is an especially important issue for women because discomfort is a major barrier to staying in the sport. Steve Hogg, a globally recognized bike fitter, believes that comfort—or, really, the lack thereof—is the number one reason there aren't more women on bikes. They don't ride because it hurts their hands, neck, shoulders, and, perhaps most importantly, their pubic area. And you know what? That all comes down to improper fit.

Fortunately, as more women get serious about the sport, they're realizing that they don't have to put up with pain or shorten their rides or hang up their wheels. Folks like John Brown, former manager at Philadelphia area shop High Road Cycles, are retrofitting bikes a lot more frequently these days to get women comfortable in the saddle for as long as they want to be. Those common complaints of back, neck, or shoulder pain and hand numbness come from straining to reach the handlebars on a bike with a setup that puts the rider's position too long and too low—likely because that's the way many riders think they should be set up based on how pro

Tour riders look on their bikes. "The old way of thinking about bike fit was, 'This is how you set up a bike for aerodynamic performance; you'll get used to it,'" says Brown, who began fitting cyclists about 10 years ago. The new—far better—school of thought is that aero is not always faster in the real world, he says. "You may be able to hold an aggressive position for 10 miles, but after 40 or 50 miles, it won't feel comfortable, and you'll get fatigued," Brown says.

Bike fit also affects how a bike performs. If your weight isn't properly distributed among the contact points on your bike—hands, feet, rear—the bike won't brake, turn, accelerate, and generally handle as well as it could or should. Worst-case scenario, poor bike fit can be a safety hazard, which is an often overlooked reason to make sure you have a good fit.

Entire books have been written on this single topic, because good bike fit is essential for maximum cycling joy. The bottom line is, you shouldn't be uncomfortable. Nothing should feel stretched out, scrunched up, or unnatural. Your bike shop will set you up initially, but as you ride longer distances, you may find little niggles or aches cropping up here and there. Those are almost always signs that something doesn't fit just right. This is where a detailed bike fitting comes in.

As opposed to a basic fitting (where the fitter takes a few measurements, sets you up on your bike, and sends you on your way) during a detailed bike fitting, the fitter will ask you questions—lots of them—about how you ride, where you ride, and how you feel on the bike. He or she will also do a full body assessment, checking your flexibility from head to toe, your range of motion, the size and shape of your feet, your legs' lengths, and myriad other physical characteristics that affect how you sit on and pedal a bike. Then they will make adjustments to your bike and even your pedals and shoes to make you one with the machine. Note that, though a bike fitter might make some suggestions to improve a particular aspect of your measurements, such as hamstring flexibility, the fitting should be done to accommodate what Hogg refers to as your "body language" on the bike, tight hamstrings and all. The bike should be adjusted to fit you, not the other way around. (Obviously, if you do improve your flexibility over time, you'll want to make further adjustments.)

You can go for a detailed fit right out of the gate, but honestly, I have found that it's useful to spend a few weeks on the bike so you can say exactly what you're feeling out on the road. Bike fits are done with your bike on a stationary trainer, which can't simulate the feeling of a ride on the road or especially the trail very well. I've had 3-hour mountain bike fits performed on a trainer, only to have to go back and say, "This isn't working for me on the rocks and roots." So it's best to get a basic fit. Ride and see how it feels. Then go back for more detailed adjustments if need be. If you've not had a professional fitting, you'll be very surprised by what a difference in comfort and performance changes of even a few millimeters can make.

How do you find a good fitter? Word of mouth can be very useful. Ask around your cycling circles and see who the experienced riders recommend. And of course, ask your local shops for recommendations. The fitter you choose should be very experienced, if not certified, in a particular fit system/philosophy. Don't be shy about asking for referrals.

The Fundamentals of Bike Fit

Ideally, every cyclist should get at least a basic bike fitting. Sure, you might already be riding a bike in your garage just fine. That's certainly okay, especially if you're doing mostly recreational, moderate-mileage riding. But I've cringed during many 50- to 100-mile charity rides as cyclists pedaled by with their seats *way* too low, knowing that I'd see them later, at the end of the ride, with their feet up and icepacks on their knees. So, I recommend that everyone who pedals a bike, whether it's 200 miles a week or just down to the coffee shop and back every other Sunday, should understand at least the basics of proper bike fit.

The following are the factors that go into putting you and your bike ride in pain-free harmony.

Proper fit is essential for optimum performance and maximum comfort.

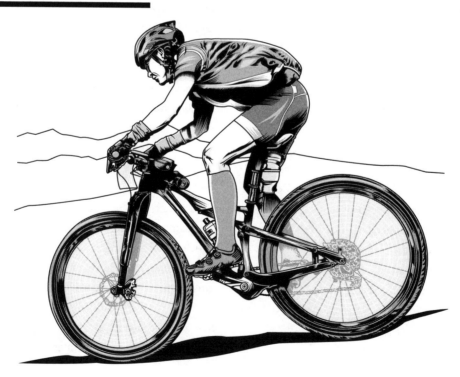

FRAME SIZE

It all starts here. The size of your bike is based on the length of the seat tube. The longer the seat tube is, the longer the top tube and the other tubing sections making up the frame need to be to keep the bike proportional. This is where it can get tricky for women. If you do have proportionally longer legs and a shorter torso, you may find yourself too stretched out to easily reach the handlebars, even if your legs reach the pedals just fine. That's why frames designed with women's specific geometry often have shortened top tubes. Conversely, if you have a long torso and long arms, you'll want a bike with a longer top tube relative to the seat tube. While you can make some adjustments to the saddle and handlebar heights to fine-tune your reach, it's important to have your frame fit as well as possible in the first place.

SEAT HEIGHT

Your seat can be adjusted to be higher or lower. When your leg is fully extended at the bottom of the pedal stroke, there should be a slight bend to the knee (rather than having it locked straight). Your pelvis should stay stable on the saddle, not rock from side to side as you pedal. Seat height is important not just for producing power as you pedal, but also for knee comfort. If the seat is too low, you put undue pressure on your knees, causing pain in the front of the knee. If the seat is too high, you end up overextending and getting nagging aches in the back of the knee. A good way to eyeball whether yours is in the right spot: Sit on the saddle with

the pedals in the 6 o'clock and 12 o'clock positions. The leg in the 6 o'clock position should be fully extended when your heel is on the pedal (it will then have a slight bend when the ball of your foot is on the pedal). For a mountain bike, there should be a little more of a bend in your leg, particularly if you tend to ride over rocky, technical terrain, so set your saddle a little lower.

SADDLE POSITION

You can also adjust your saddle fore and aft, meaning forward or backward. There are many theories about fore–aft positioning, but a good starting point is to position the saddle so that when your feet are in the 3 o'clock and 9 o'clock positions, the front of your forward knee is directly over the ball of your forward foot. When you move your saddle forward or backward, it effectively changes your seat height (by slightly increasing the distance from the saddle to the pedal), so keep that in mind as you make any adjustments. You also want to make sure your saddle is level, not tilting up or down.

HANDLEBAR REACH

You should be able to comfortably reach all the positions on your handlebars while maintaining a slight, comfortable bend in your elbows. Seems simple enough, but there are many women (and men) who can't comfortably reach their drops, so they never ride in that position. Some bikes also come outfitted with fairly long hoods housing the brake levers, which increases the reach since that's where your hands often

(continued on page 44)

Where Does It Hurt?

Pain is your body's way of telling you something's wrong. In the case of bike fit, there are a few well-known culprits that can cause common pedaling aches and pains. This troubleshooting guide will help to quell—and correct—the most common nagging ouches before they become injuries. General aches and pains can be remedied with the fixes below, as well as traditional treatments such as rest, ice, and anti-inflammatories. Don't mess around with sharp pain. That's always a sign that something is wrong and you should see your doc.

WHERE DOES IT HURT?	WHAT'S WRONG	THE FIX
Foot	Hot spots, pain under the ball of your foot, and/or numb toes happen when pressure is concentrated on one small part of the sole of your foot and/or nerves are squeezed between your foot bones. Hot spots can happen to even longtime cyclists who've never had foot pain because the fat pads in our feet shrink over time, leaving the nerves in our feet less protected, says Andy Pruitt.	For burning pain, slide your cleats all the way back; switch to shoes with a stiffer sole; try pedals with wider platforms. For simple numbness, just try loosening your shoes. Or opt for a wider shoe [see page 51]. Note: If you have bunions [common in women], cycling shoes can be painful. Seeing a podiatrist for orthotics can help.
Ankle	Pain in the back of the ankle between the heel and calf is a symptom of Achilles tendonitis. Generally brought on by doing too much [especially climbing] too soon. Having your cleats too far forward, which makes you pedal on your toes, can also strain the Achilles. "It's rarely just cycling, but generally also hiking and running, that causes Achilles problems," says Pruitt. "But you can ease on-the-bike pain with adjustments."	Treat with rest, ice, and anti-inflammatories, so it doesn't become chronic. Move cleats back. Stretch by standing on a step with the ball of your foot on the step and the heel hanging off the edge. Drop the heel as far as possible. Hold 20 seconds. Switch legs. Build up mileage gradually.
Knee	"[This is] cyclists' most common pain, and it hits all riders, from paid pros to fitness enthusiasts, in equal numbers," says Pruitt. "The knee is the victim, but the culprits are the hip above and the foot and ankle below." Incorrect saddle and/or cleat position, weak outer glutes, and doing too much too soon, especially in a big gear, can make your hinges hurt.	Get a professional bike fit. As a rule of thumb, if it hurts in the front of your knee, your saddle is too low. Pain in the back of the knee means it's too high. Spin an easier gear. Strengthen your outer glutes with lateral leg exercises like side lunges and side leg raises. Stretch your quads, iliotibial bands, and hamstrings regularly.

WHERE DOES IT HURT?	WHAT'S WRONG	THE FIX
Hip	Pushing excessively high gears can wreak havoc on your hips, as can tight muscles and weak glutes.	Ride in easier gears and increase your cadence to take pressure off your hips. Follow the glute strengthening advice in the "Knee" section on the opposite page. Stretch your hips (the stretches on page 176 will help).
Back	Often back pain can be blamed on simple fatigue and age-related wear and tear. Other common causes are poor bike fit and inadequate core strength.	Perform plank exercises to strengthen your core. Stretch your hamstrings. Check your bike fit to see that you're not "overreaching" (see Neck below), keeping in mind that over the years you may need to tweak your position to accommodate changes in flexibility.
Hand	Numb, tingly fingers and/or painful wrists are generally caused by placing too much pressure on the nerves in your hand. You may have too much weight on your hands or have your wrists cocked at too extreme an angle.	Check that the nose of your saddle isn't tipped down, shifting your weight too far forward and onto your hands. Hold the bar with your wrists in a neutral position (like the position they're in when you shake hands). Wear lightly padded gloves.
Neck	Poor fit. Too much tension through shoulders and upper back.	The most common culprit is overreaching. When you look at the front wheel with your hands on the hoods, your bars should obstruct your hub. Keep your shoulders down and relaxed when you ride.

go when you ride. Handlebars that are too far away, too close, too high, or too low can leave you with neck, shoulder, back, wrist, and/or hand pain, so it's important to get it right.

You can position your handlebar closer or farther away from you by changing the stem (the piece that connects the handlebars to the bike frame) to one that is longer or shorter. Just be aware that stem length also affects the bike's handling, cautions Brown. A stem that's too long will require an exaggerated amount of upper-body motion to turn the bar. If it's too short, "it might feel like the bike is steering you." You also can adjust your reach by adding spacers between the stem and the head tube. This will raise the handlebars so you don't have to bend as far. Where you place your handlebars also depends on how flexible you are. Don't feel like you must hunker down as low as you can go despite discomfort because the bike came set up in a super "aero," low-handlebar position. Your bike shop can help you get your reach just right.

Also on the topic of handlebars: Check that yours are the proper width. A bar that's too wide "forces you to lean farther forward [to properly place your hands], so it effectively makes the frame longer," Brown says. "Plus, it side-loads your wrists." As mentioned in Chapter 2, women's specific bars are available in sizes that are narrower than standard to remedy this. On the flip side, a bar that is too narrow makes the bike hard to handle and hinders your breathing by preventing your rib cage from fully expanding, so if your bike came with a narrow women's specific bar and you're broad-shouldered, you may need to swap that out. Note: Mountain bikes come with wider bars for increased leverage and better balance and control over rough terrain.

Finally, and importantly, be sure you can reach your brakes and your shifters. Depending on the size of your hands, you may need a road bar with a shallower drop and/or short-reach brake levers so you can easily reach them. Fortunately, many manufacturers are now making brake levers with adjustable reach.

PEDALS AND CLEATS

For years, conventional wisdom held that the pedal axle should line up with the ball of the foot for optimum efficiency, Brown says. If you're using flat platform pedals, it is easy enough to shift your foot around to maintain that basic position. When you use clipless pedals and cleats, it's more important to get the cleat position dialed in for maximum performance as well as comfort. If you experience hot spots in that position, fit experts now believe that moving the cleat back slightly can ease discomfort without decreasing power. Try it yourself: While wearing your cycling shoes, stand up straight and have a friend mark the widest points on either side of your forefoot with a pen (put electrical tape down first). The pedal axle should fall between those marks.

SADDLE UP

When talking women's specific bike fit, no part is more important than the saddle, because all the proper fitting in the world won't make a bit of difference if your seat is a pain in the butt—or vulva, which is exactly what is uncomfortable for too many women with the wrong saddles. Some experts go so far as to say that saddle choice alone can pretty much fix the majority of women's fit issues.

"If you're not using the right saddle, you change your position on the bike to try to reduce the discomfort down there," says Heather Henderson, longtime industry expert. "Most women I see will roll their hips back to relieve the pressure on their crotch, which then makes it harder to reach their bars and then suddenly they have back, neck, and knee pain because they're out of alignment on the bike. They don't need a shorter top tube; they need a proper saddle," she says. Of course that's not true for all women—some do need a frame with different geometry—but it illustrates just how important proper saddle fit is in the overall picture.

What makes saddle selection such a sensitive issue for women? Our anatomy. For one, we have hips that are designed to allow a small human to pass through. That means our hips are generally wider than men's, as are our sit bones—the ends of the pelvic bones that protrude when we sit down. As you might imagine, if you're sitting on a saddle that doesn't support your sit bones, you are sitting directly on your crotch. Women's specific saddles generally flare more in the back to accommodate this anatomical difference and place your butt where it belongs.

While the rear of the saddle supports your sit bones, the nose allows you to control the bike with your legs and supports *some* of your body weight. This, too, is an important factor in female saddle fit. Women are like snowflakes—no two are exactly alike. Some of us have pronounced labia. Others have less. Some women's very sensitive tissues, like the clitoris, are more exposed to pressure, while in others, they're better protected. All of that greatly impacts what kind of saddle will work best for you. It's also why American pioneering bike builder Georgena Terry introduced women's saddles with nose cutaways to relieve pressure on genital soft tissues—she got it decades ago.

Your vulva should not be smooshed, go numb, or chafe. So once you're certain that your sit bones are properly planted at the rear of the saddle and that your reach to the handlebars is comfortable, see how you feel down there. If both your fit and positioning are right but you're feeling too much pressure on your girl parts, look for a saddle with a more forgiving nose, such as one with a groove or cutaway section.

There are dozens of different saddles out there, so try as many as you need to until you find one that is just right.

Here's what to look for in shape, size, and cushioning.

SHAPE: Different shapes abound to suit many body types and bicycle uses. As mentioned earlier, the sit bones—officially called the ischial tuberosities—of women are generally more widely spaced than those of men; that's why women's specific saddles are wider. But don't assume you need the widest seat in the shop because you're a woman. Sex aside, a seat that's too wide will chafe and rub, while one that's too narrow will make you feel like you're straddling a banister. The profiles of seats vary as well: Viewed from the front, some are flatter with squarish sides, while others curve steadily and are more rounded. Some companies offer dedicated models for triathlon (with more thickly padded noses for forward positioning) or mountain biking (with thicker padding overall and a rugged cover). A few saddle manufacturers even supply shops with special pads for measuring your sit-bone width to help take the guesswork out of picking the right seat.

SHELL AND CUTOUT DESIGN: The foundation of the saddle is a hard shell made from injected-molded plastic and sometimes other materials like carbon fiber. The shell determines how the seat flexes and gives under a rider's weight. Many shells now incorporate holes, slots, or grooves in the nose section to help lessen pressure and provide additional comfort. "Saddles with a cutout in the nose work best for about 80 percent of riders by shifting pressure away from soft tissue and toward the ischial tuberosities," says Andy Pruitt, who's done extensive research on saddles as the director of Colorado's Boulder Center for Sports Medicine.

"Solid-nose saddles still work best for some, particularly cyclists who naturally sit crooked on their seats," he says.

PADDING: This is what gives a saddle its squish. Foams and gels alike are molded onto the shell, with the thickness and density of the padding varying in different models. More padding doesn't mean more comfort. "If your bike fits properly overall, the seat can be pretty damn hard," says Pruitt. "Some padding is needed to help disperse that focused pressure point over a slightly bigger area. But when you sit on overly thick padding, it can deform and migrate to places where you don't want pressure, like between the sit bones," he says. And sinking into a squishy saddle actually increases pressure on your crotch, so stick with moderate cushioning.

One important note for new riders: Even the most satisfying seat may leave your tush a little tender after your first few long rides. This will disappear after a couple of weeks in the saddle. As you ride more, your butt muscles will become denser (firm butt = good thing!) and will support you pain-free even for long rides. To minimize this problem until then, start with 30- or 45-minute rides and gradually extend that to give your butt time to "break in" to the sport.

CHAPTER 4

Essentials, Accessories, and Bling

LIKE BIKES THEMSELVES, BICYCLING GEAR, CLOTHING, AND accessories come in women's specific incarnations that are—you guessed it—often controversial and more than a bit confusing. Everyone agrees that women benefit from certain women's specific gear, especially in the clothing department. But not everyone agrees on what that should look or fit like.

A recent survey done by *Bicycling* magazine on the topic illustrates the point perfectly. When asked about women's specific attire, particularly the color pink, more than a few women fired away. "I want more choices, and my preferences are apparently not the best sellers," lamented one. "My bike shop sells gloves with *rhinestones* on them—and they sell. When I find jerseys that actually fit, they are often designed for women who see themselves as 6-year-old girls (glitter! and that was on Castelli!). Pink is for party dresses. Rhinestones are for nightclubs."

That response made me laugh because, though I certainly respect her point of view, I love pink; I dump glitter in my embrocation, and if I could BeDazzle every piece of cycling gear I own, I would. I'm not ashamed of it, nor do I think it makes me any less of a serious cyclist or that any woman who likes butterflies and flower prints should be taken less seriously because of her tastes.

So after dozens of conversations with racers, riders, and women's clothing and gear manufacturers, I've reached the unsurprising conclusion that women want choice. Just as the same woman who shops at Ann Taylor may not be interested in what Urban Outfitters has to offer, not all women who ride a bike want the same "look." The manufacturers? They just make what they hope will sell, making more of what does and less of what does not—simple economics.

Butterflies and rhinestones aside, women's cycling gear has never been better. Manufacturers big and small have been listening to what *all* kinds of women want and have been responding with options in all shapes and sizes and prints and patterns and plains. So if you don't like what you find from one source, keep shopping around. You most certainly will find women's cycling gear that fits and excites you. And of course, as with bikes, there are times when you don't need women's specific simply because you're a woman.

Here's a guide to all the cycling essentials—from jerseys to saddle bags, that you need—as well as a bunch of stuff you'll love, just because. Plus I've added a few words on when you might want to go women's specific (or not).

A note on prices for cycling attire: If you've never shopped for cycling clothes, you're in for some sticker shock. They tend to be more expensive than you would expect because they're made of synthetic fibers that wick sweat, block wind and sun, and stay put without bunching, billowing, or chafing. Good-quality cycling clothing can greatly enhance your riding enjoyment and last for many years.

Attire and Accessories

Cycling attire is often referred to as a "cycling kit." I've heard heated—and amusing ultimately—arguments among some very serious dudes about what a "proper kit" consists of. At the most basic, it's a jersey and a pair of shorts (that's my standard, and I'm sticking to it). At its most complete, it's a jersey, shorts, socks, gloves, a helmet, shoes, and glasses. You'll be happiest, safest, and most comfortable with the whole shebang (and maybe an additional item or two), and yes, all of the above come in women's specific options.

HELMET

Nonnegotiable. You've gotta have a helmet. No matter how seasoned or skilled you are, a dog can still run out in the road and send you tumbling to the ground. Put a lid on your head and keep your brain safe from harm's way. Today's helmets are light, stylish, and extremely well ventilated. Any helmet sold in the United States must meet the US Consumer Product Safety Commission standard (you'll see a CPSC sticker somewhere on the inside), so any helmet will absorb impact and buffer your brain in a bad crash. Pricier helmets tend to be lighter, more stylish, and have better ventilation to keep your head cooler.

SHOULD YOU GO WOMEN'S SPECIFIC? Women's specific helmets often come in pretty colors and have special features like a "ponytail port," a special space for your tethered mane to exit from the back. Look for a helmet with a locking retention system that allows you to get a snug, comfortable fit. The helmet should fit level on your head, sitting right above your eyebrows in the front. Adjust the side straps so they form a V around your ears and tighten them so the straps connect snugly under your chin, allowing just enough room for two fingers to slip through. The helmet should stay put when you shake your head.

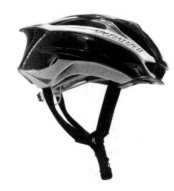

Today's helmets come in many shapes, sizes, and colors. Find one you love and wear it always.

JERSEY

True story. Riding out in Emporia, Kansas, for a long endurance event known as the Dirty Kanza 200 a few years ago, I met a fellow editor who was there with his wife, who, he told me, was recently employed by a cycling clothing company as a "perfect medium" for sizing its women's cycling attire. I thought that was kind of funny. Then he told me how she had tried on clothing made for the former "perfect medium," and, well, it hadn't really fit her.

Like buying blue jeans, buying cycling jerseys (and shorts, see page 50) that fit "just so" can be an exercise in patience. Every manufacturer has different fits per size—and even different cuts within each size—that determine how the jersey will fall on your figure. In general, you will be choosing from:

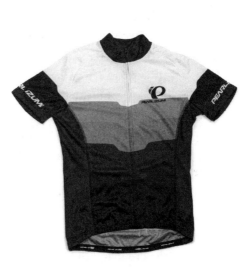

Bike jerseys do more than look good. They provide functions like ventilation, sweat wicking, and storage space for your goods while you ride.

RACE/PRO CUT: Think small and probably pretty skinny. These cuts tend to be based on a European professional fit. Expect the sizes to run small and also to not accommodate too much muscle. If you're very fit, but have muscular shoulders and arms, a pro cut may be too tight in those areas, which is important to note because most size charts won't tell you the size of the armholes.

CLUB/CLASSIC CUT: This is your traditional cycling jersey, which is to say that it will be form fitting, but is designed to fit more typically proportioned riders and recreational racers.

SHOULD YOU GO WOMEN'S SPECIFIC? On top of (or sometimes instead of) the other choices, you may also decide on a women's specific. What defines "women's cut" depends upon the manufacturer. Nearly all women's cycling jerseys have a slightly nipped waist for a more feminine curve. Some will also have a slightly flared waistline to sit better on a woman's curvy hips, which is great if you have curvy hips, but looks and feels off if you don't. Other features include more room in the bust, and sometimes a shorter length, which, again, is great if you have a short torso, but not so much if you don't. Try before you buy.

And a note on sizing. Be prepared to set aside your preconceived notions of what size you *should* be. Cycling clothing sizes are all over the map, and since they're made to fit snugly (to stay in place and not slide up, fall down, or flap in the breeze), a too-small size, purchased because damn it you're a medium, will not fit, will be unflattering, and ultimately will waste your hard-earned cash. Better just to try on a few different sizes and styles, buy what fits, and cut out the tags if you don't like seeing the size.

No matter what cut you choose, spring for a cycling jersey. You can't beat the comfort and convenience of having pockets in the back for stashing your stuff, a zipper in the front for cooling off, and a specially tailored fit that keeps all the material in place when you're hunkered down in the riding position.

SHORTS AND BIBS

Cycling shorts provide extra padding (called a chamois) where you need it most, under your bum and tender nether regions. They come in two different styles: Regular shorts with elastic waistbands and bib shorts that have suspender-like shoulder straps. Most men love bibs because they don't have elastic digging into their belly (which, since it's where most men gain weight, may be a bit softer than the rest of them). Women tend to be mixed on bibs because the straps have to travel over the breasts, which can be awkward (some models have straps that clip together between the breasts). More importantly, they're a pain to get out of when you need to pee because you have to take your whole jersey off. There *are* some bibs that have snaps and "drop tails" and other features that make answering the calls of nature easier, but you have to shop around.

Cycling shorts are constructed using panels to help contour the fit just right in all the cycling positions. The more panels—high-end shorts have 8 to 10—the better the fit. *Very important for women:* Check the leg bands. This is a deal maker or breaker for many women. The leg bands should have light gripping that keeps the shorts in place on your legs, but should not be so tight that they make your thighs feel (or look) like sausages in casings. This is a pet

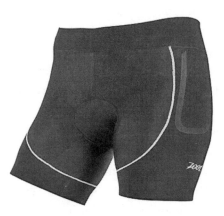

Women's specific cycling shorts now come in many lengths to fit and flatter every rider's figure.

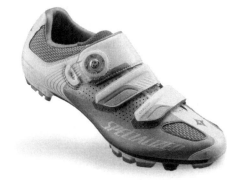

If you're going to be riding paths and trails, mountain bike shoes with a walking tread are the way to go.

peeve of many women riders, and something you won't know until you slip into the shorts. For colder-weather riding you can buy full-length tights or knickers (capri-length tights) that keep your knees from getting cold. (Most riders keep their knees covered until the temperature is at least 65°F; warm knees are less likely to fall prey to aches and pains.)

SHOULD YOU GO WOMEN'S SPECIFIC? Women's specific shorts tend to have narrower waists and a more tapered fit above the hips. They also tend to be shorter, as women tend to be shorter. Maybe most importantly, women's specific shorts have a women's specific chamois. A good chamois is layered to provide a healthy dose of padding under your sit bones and less everywhere else. Generally, a women's specific chamois will be slightly wider to accommodate wider sit bones and is often shorter front to back.

Wouldn't be caught dead wearing Lycra in public? There are more than a few companies making women's cycling skirts (with the attached bike shorts hidden beneath) and/or baggy shorts with padded liners, which are not going to be super-high performance on the road, but perform perfectly well on casual and off-road rides (many mountain bikers eschew Lycra).

Oh, and one final tip for the newbies in the room: You don't wear underwear under cycling shorts. They're designed to be worn bareback. Otherwise, you risk chafing, sores, and visible panty lines.

SHOES

If you plan to get clipless pedals, you need cycling shoes, which accommodate cleats that attach to the pedals. If you do not have clipless pedals (see "Pedals," on page 59), I suggest trying them. Many riders find they make their riding experience exponentially better, as they put increased power and efficiency into each and every pedal stroke. In addition to allowing you to attach the cleats (which come with the pedals rather than the shoes), cycling shoes have stiff soles that ensure that all the energy from your pedaling transfers into propelling the bike. Stiff soles also prevent your feet from fatiguing from bending and flexing with every revolution, which can result in arch pain and other foot problems.

The type of shoes you choose depends on the type of riding you do. Mountain bike shoes accept what are known as recessed cleats. These shoes have a normal tread and the cleat sits higher than tread level, so they're easy to walk in—a plus when you have to hike your bike through unrideable sections of a trail or hoof it on a sidewalk after locking up in town. In contrast, most road shoes, especially high-performance road shoes, have flat soles (they're also lighter and stiffer than their mountain kin), so the cleat protrudes from the sole at the ball of your foot, which makes walking in them pretty awkward. It's a good idea to match your shoes to your riding. This quick guide (see below) will help you find the shoe that fits your riding style and needs.

SHOULD YOU GO WOMEN'S SPECIFIC? There are women's specific shoes for both the road and the mountain. Women's specific cycling shoes are typically designed for narrower feet, especially in the heels and ankles, so your feet stay put in the shoes and don't slip around or up and down. They also generally come in smaller sizes. If your feet fit that blueprint, women's specific shoes are the way to go. If your feet are larger

IF YOU	THE SHOE THAT FITS IS
Like to go fast and stay at the head of the pack, and maybe even compete, at least recreationally	A light, high-end road shoe with a stiff sole and secure closure, a shoe that transfers all your energy into the pedals
Like mountain biking, off-road riding, gravel exploration, and taking your bike anywhere the pavement isn't	A mountain bike model with recessed cleats, a snug yet comfortable fit, and a secure hold on your feet
Are primarily a commuter or enjoy taking your bike on tours where you stop and take photos and enjoy a coffee in towns you pass through	An off-road shoe or even a more casual all-around shoe with cleats; some manufacturers, such as Pearl Izumi, make shoes that are designed to be comfortable for hiking and walking in as well as riding
Are primarily a triathlete	A road shoe (unless you do off-road triathlon, of course) with a quick and easy fastening mechanism, or even a tri-specific shoe
Are a casual group rider who likes charity rides, centuries, and Saturday morning shop spins	A midrange road shoe for its greater comfort due to a slightly more forgiving sole than what's on superstiff race models; and you won't miss out on performance

and wider? Go with whatever works. Cycling shoes should be snug, but not constricting. Your toes should not bump up against the front or the sides. Your heels shouldn't slip up and down. Your feet should not feel squeezed. The best way to describe what a good pair of cycling shoes feels like is to say they're invisible—you don't think about them once they're on.

Keep in mind that if you spend long days in the saddle, especially during the hot summer months, you can expect your feet to swell. So the rules for buying any kind of shoe apply to cycling shoes, too: Shop when your feet are at their biggest (at the end of the day), and choose a shoe that has plenty of adjustability so you can tighten and loosen them as your feet swell and shrink.

GLOVES

Everyone puts on gloves when it's cold. But cycling gloves are a good idea no matter the time of year or temperature because they absorb bumps and vibration from the road for increased hand comfort. They also protect your palms in case you fall. They're not a must-have (you'll see plenty of riders spinning around without them), but definitely are a should-have. You can buy both fingerless (for warm-weather riding) and full-fingered gloves. If you plan on doing a lot of winter riding, invest in lobster gloves (mitten-glove hybrids that bundle together your first and second and your third and fourth fingers for added warmth). They're super toasty and can keep your fingers from freezing in even sub-20°F temps.

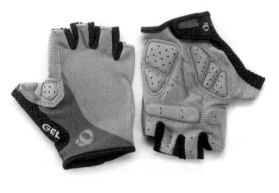

Padded cycling gloves can prevent you from getting sore, fatigued hands while you ride, as well as protect your palms should you take a spill.

SHOULD YOU GO WOMEN'S SPECIFIC? Women's cycling gloves generally have shorter fingers and are narrower across the top to better fit a woman's hand. They also come in an assortment of stylish colors, because gloves are somewhat of a fashion statement in the sport. However, if you have larger hands, you can still find plenty of sharp mitts in the men's department.

GLASSES

You've got to protect those baby blues (or greens or browns or hazels), and there's a dizzying array of cycling-specific shades that will not only block dangerous UV rays and make it easier to see on brilliant sunny days but also protect your eyes from bugs, kicked-up cinders, and other flying debris. Look for glasses with rubberized nose and ear grips to keep them firmly in place on your face, as well as some form of ventilation to prevent fogging.

High-end shades come with photochromic lenses that change their tint to match the light

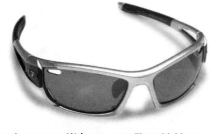

Wear glasses even if it's not sunny. They shield your eyes from bugs and debris that can kick up from the road.

conditions. Or choose a pair with interchangeable lenses so you can have light lenses for overcast days, dark ones for cloudless rides, and so forth. If you're a mountain biker who rides on tree-shaded trails or a commuter who rides in dim light or the dark, pick up a pair with clear lenses to provide protection without diminishing your already compromised vision. Once you get into it, it's actually amazing how matching your lenses to the lighting can improve the clarity of your vision, which is pretty important when you're cruising along at 10 to 20 mph—and possibly twice that downhill. Sports optometrist Don Teig explains how to match the lenses to the conditions (see the chart below).

Polarized lenses, which are designed to direct scattered light rays into one plane to reduce glare, can help prevent squinting in harsh sunlight, but probably aren't the best choice for cycling. Besides reducing glare, they also "flatten" the terrain, and both effects can cause you to miss important road hazards like slick oil or water spots that would otherwise stand out. They also make it difficult to read the screen on a cycling computer.

SHOULD YOU GO WOMEN'S SPECIFIC? Only if you have a particularly small face. Otherwise just choose a style that stays put, provides lens options, and flatters your features.

SOCKS

Unless you're a triathlete, you've gotta wear cycling socks. And even if you are, you should wear them when you're just riding your bike. They protect your feet and your pricey cycling shoes. Look for a pair made from a synthetic like Coolmax or natural wicking fibers like merino wool to keep your feet dry and comfy. Cycling socks come in many lengths, from knee-high to crew cut. Let personal style be

IF THE AMBIENT LIGHT IS	CHOOSE THIS COLOR LENS
Hazy, but light (e.g., early morning)	Yellow, to brighten and clarify
Hazy and overcast	Vermilion (bright red), to brighten
Overcast, but not hazy	Clear and antireflective, for protection
Partly sunny	Light gray, for protection without dimming
Very sunny	Dark gray or brown, to reduce visible light

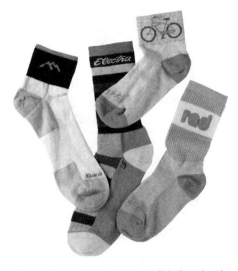

Cycling socks are designed to be stylish, functional, and fun.

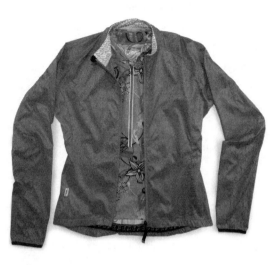

A good cycling jacket can extend your riding season by months.

your guide (but note that knee-high socks are not allowed in some officially sanctioned races—crazy, but true).

SHOULD YOU GO WOMEN'S SPECIFIC? If you have petite feet and/or crave pretty designs. Otherwise, any cycling sock in your size will cover your feet just fine.

JACKETS

Fair-weather pedalers can pass on this piece of cycling attire, but anyone else who rides when it's cool, windy, and/or rainy needs a protective shell. A good-quality cycling jacket will have extra material in the back and longer sleeves than zip-ups designed for daily wear so that you stay fully covered when you're stretched out in the cycling position. Some even have a buttoned-up flap in the back that you can let

down to cover your rear when it starts to rain or the roads are wet.

How much outer protection you need depends on your climate. If you live in one of those regions where the weather changes from sunny to stormy every 10 minutes or so, a lightweight waterproof windbreaker is a must. Ditto if you plan on doing multiday charity rides, when riding in chilly or rainy weather isn't optional. If you plan on riding when the temperatures head south, cold-weather attire is a must. Look for a jacket with a microfiber (fine fleece) lining to keep you warm, wind blocking to protect you from arctic breezes, and other nice features like high collars and fitted cuffs to keep the cool air from going anywhere you don't want it to, especially vulnerable areas like your wrists, neck, and lower back.

SHOULD YOU GO WOMEN'S SPECIFIC? Like jerseys, women's specific jackets are generally nipped in the waist and accommodating in the chest and hips for a woman's curves. Just be sure the arms are long enough. Some women's jackets have narrower shoulders and shorter arms that obviously won't work if that doesn't match your frame.

VEST

Every cyclist should own a vest; often that's all you need to be completely comfortable when it's just a little chilly. Because your upper body is fairly inactive and you generate a lot of "wind" as you ride (since you're slicing through the air), it's easy for your torso to get cold even on a fairly warm spring day. They're also great protection against stiff breezes and during chilly descents. Look for one that has wind and water protection on the front and mesh in the back to prevent you from overheating.

SHOULD YOU GO WOMEN'S SPECIFIC? Having worn *many* vests over the decades, this is one I'd be quick to say yes on. Why? Because you typically wear a vest when it's a bit breezy, and it's annoying (and of course completely non-aero) to have the sides of your vest flapping around as you ride. Women's vests are nipped and tucked to fit closer to your curves.

ARM WARMERS/KNEE WARMERS

To the uninitiated these removable sleeves sometimes feel silly; but once you've worn them, you can't imagine the cycling life without them. Arm warmers mean never worrying

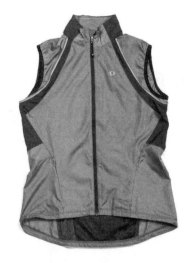

When your core is comfortable, you're comfortable. Keep yours cozy on breezy days with a cycling vest.

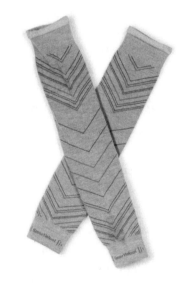

Arm warmers turn a short sleeve jersey into a long sleeve jersey (and vice versa) in a snap.

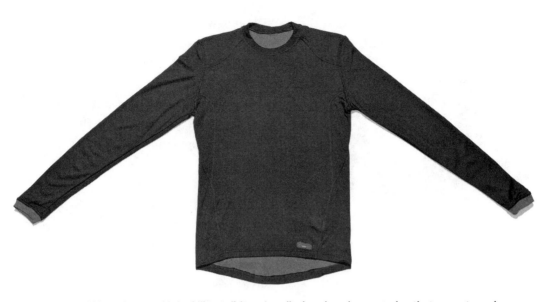

Your torso gets cold fast when you ride in chilly conditions. A quality base layer is a must when the temperatures drop.

about whether you should wear a long- or short-sleeved jersey for a ride that starts at 9:00 a.m. (when it might be 60°F) and ends at 11:00 a.m. (when it can easily be 10°F or 15°F warmer), because you can have the best of both worlds with a pair of portable sleeves.

Unlike arm warmers, which riders tend to pull on and off and stuff in their pockets and use (or not use) throughout a ride, knee warmers generally stay put once you have them on. Unless you're a *really* good bike handler, you're not going to be peeling them off on the fly, and they're a bit bulky for back pockets. They *are* really handy for extending your cycling wardrobe into three, maybe even four, seasons without investing in knickers, however.

SHOULD YOU GO WOMEN'S SPECIFIC? I know more than a few women for whom even the smallest unisex arm warmers sag and slip. So if you're small, absolutely. They also come in a stunning array of colors and designs (men's, too, actually). Though knee warmers don't generally pose the same problems, you can't go wrong with women's specific hinge covers if you're particularly petite.

BASE LAYER

Most riders think of base layers as cool- and cold-weather apparel, which is legit. When the temperatures dip, you need a nice base layer under that jersey to wick away sweat and help keep you warm. But a light base layer can also help keep you cool by pulling perspiration off your skin when it's hot. Is it completely necessary? Not really. Will it make your riding experience more comfortable in all conditions? You bet.

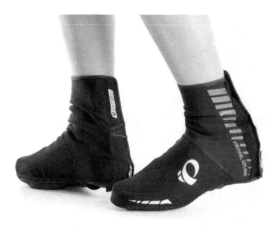

Nothing wrecks a ride faster than cold, wet feet. Booties keep the elements out so your toes stay toasty.

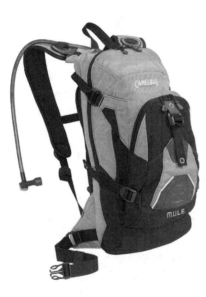

Riding off road where you'll be miles away from water, snacks, and repair tools? Carry a pack and have it all on your back.

SHOULD YOU GO WOMEN'S SPECIFIC? Certainly not necessary, but women's specific base layers are detailed to hug the female frame, which can make for a closer, comfier, less obtrusive fit, if you're of that build. If not, the bottom of the base layer may flare out more around the hips than you'd like.

BOOTIES

Cycling shoes are well ventilated to keep your feet cool. Great for the summer, not so much during colder months. For cold-weather riding, invest in a pair of booties—covers that slip over your cycling shoes and provide an added layer of insulation while still allowing you to clip in to your pedals. You also can buy lightweight rain booties to keep your feet dry in soggy riding conditions. You can even buy mini booties or toe warmers that slip over just the front of your shoes.

SHOULD YOU GO WOMEN'S SPECIFIC? If you have women's specific shoes, sure, they'll likely be a better fit. But truly not necessary.

HYDRATION PACK

These are small backpacks that typically hold 50 to 100 ounces of water. Many also feature pockets for assorted odds and ends, like car keys, food, tools, a cell phone, and anything else you might want to cart along for a day of riding. They are an excellent way to carry water on mountain bike rides, when you're often in remote places where it's not so easy to refill a water bottle. Most road riders don't use them, with the exception of long-distance cyclists and those on multiday tours, both of whom need to carry lots of stuff and may end up riding for long stretches where there's nowhere to stop and refill a bottle.

SHOULD YOU GO WOMEN'S SPECIFIC? Yes, if you have a short torso and/or larger boobs—and especially if you have both! Riders with short torsos find that some standard packs are too long and either hit the back of their helmet or extend too far down their back, blocking access to their jersey pockets. Women's packs are often smaller, which avoid those problems. The chest strap on women's packs (if there is one at all) generally has some vertical adjustment so it can be set at a position that doesn't unduly smoosh their breasts.

Gotta-Have-It Gear

I didn't have my first flat tire until after college, which is a darn good thing because I never carried a single tool or tube and wouldn't have known what to do with them even if I had. I'm not even sure if I ever thought about whether bicycle tires could go flat. Then, once I started riding lighter bikes with lighter wheels and, yes, lighter tires, I became familiar with all of the above. Unfortunately, that first time, I still had no tube, no tools, no clue, and no cell phone. It was a very long 7-mile trek back home, and my butt was sore for weeks from kicking myself.

Don't get a sore butt from kicking yourself. Outfit your bike with the gear you need for the most basic roadside maintenance (and find out how to use—see "Fast Flat Fixes" on page 293). While you're at it, check out a few hot bike

accessories on the following pages that can make your riding more fun, as well.

PEDALS

Midrange to high-end bikes generally don't come with pedals, or if they do, they're just a pair of throwaway flats to get you through until you can put your "real" pedals on the thing. That's not to say that flat pedals aren't legitimate. They are. But, if you're planning on rides of longer than, say, 5 or 10 miles, I think clipless is the way to go. Why? Because they hold your feet securely to the pedals, so all the power generated by your spinning legs goes directly into moving you forward. You save energy while going farther faster. You can use toe clips with straps that hold your feet on your pedals, but you might find them uncomfortable, and possibly even harder to get your feet in and out of than clipless pedals (which you detach from by turning your heel toward the outer side and pulling up). I think that once you go clipless, you'll never go back. (We'll talk more about how to ride with clipless pedals later.)

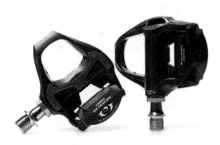

Clipless pedals maximize the power transfer in every pedal stroke.

As I mentioned when discussing cycling shoes, clipless pedals come with cleats that attach to the bottoms of your cycling shoes. So the components of the whole system—pedals, cleats, and shoes—have to be compatible. If you own mountain bike shoes, for instance, you need clipless pedals that are compatible with off-road shoes' treaded soles and recessed cleats. If you have flat-soled road shoes, you need to ride with road pedals.

What pedal system you use is a personal decision, and no one system is "best." These are the key features that will help you choose among them.

EXIT/ENTRY: You can choose between double-sided pedals, meaning you can clip in and out regardless of which side of the pedal your foot falls on, or single-sided pedals, which often have a larger pedal platform. Ultimately, you will get used to either type, but if you'll be doing the type of riding where you need to clip in and out regularly and quickly, double-sided might be your best bet.

FLOAT: Even when you are "locked" in to your pedals, most pedal systems offer at least a small degree of wiggle room, called float, which is the amount of sideways rotation your foot has before your cleat clicks out, releasing you from the pedal. Float is important for maintaining knee health because it allows your feet to fall into whatever position that allows your knees to track correctly and to swivel slightly as you ride without twisting and torquing your joints. Most people pedal best with about 4 to 6 degrees of float. But if your feet turn outward

or inward, or you have other biomechanical issues, you may need to go with a brand that provides more float.

TENSION: This refers to how tightly the cleats attach to the pedals. Most pedals have adjustable tension that allows you to lock yourself in more securely or loosen up so you have an "easy out." Look for pedals that have an adjustable release, especially if you're new to clipless pedals or you know you'll be needing to get in and out often and quickly.

BOTTLE CAGE AND WATER BOTTLE

Most bikes come equipped with two water bottle mounts, meaning places on the frame where you can easily attach cages that will hold bottles. The cages themselves, however, come separately, as do the water bottles that go in them. If you'll be riding over rough terrain, opt for side-pull cages, which are less likely to allow your bottles to pop out if you hit a big bump.

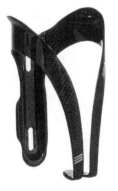

If you ride on rough roads, look for a wrap-around water bottle cage that prevents your bottle from ejecting when you hit a big bump.

SADDLEBAG

This is a small bag that straps on the rails beneath your seat for carrying spare tubes (see below), cash, and whatever else you need to carry with you. It's a great upfront investment, because you can pack it with your emergency items, nestle it under your saddle, and forget about it until you need it.

FIX-IT KIT

Even with the advent of tubeless tires (see page 116), flats still happen. And when they do you need to fix them (see "Fast Flat Fixes," page 293, for a how-to). You'll need:

INNER TUBE: Get yourself a few spares and carry one with you at all times. They come in different sizes for the different-sized wheels, so check the sidewall of your tires for the correct dimensions (the bike shop staff should be

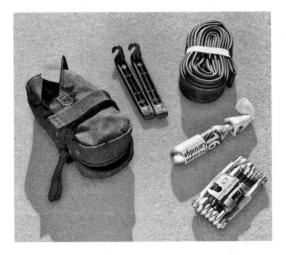

Always carry the tools you need to fix a flat and tighten loose bolts ... just in case. A saddlebag keeps them tucked neatly away for when you need them.

able to tell at a glance what you need). Tubes have one of two different types of inflation valve, Presta or Schrader. Presta valves are slimmer, easier to inflate, and standard on most road bikes. Go with those. Schrader valves are thicker and heavier, so many cyclists avoid them.

TIRE LEVERS: Bike tires fit snugly on their rims, so you'll need tire levers to pry them off to change inner tubes. They're light, cheap, and usually come in sets of three.

PATCH KIT: These small kits can be a lifesaver if you only carry one spare tube and are unlucky enough to have two flats in one day. You can choose between "glueless" patches that you use by simply peeling off the backing and sticking them to the tube like an adhesive bandage or patches that come with a small tube of glue that you use to make the patch stick on the tube. Obviously, glueless patches are quicker and easier to apply, but they really don't last as long or work as well as regular patches, which adhere forever and leave your tire as good as new.

PUMP OR CO_2 CARTRIDGE: You'll need an air source to pump up your tire when the flat is fixed. You have several options: a mini-pump, CO_2 cartridges, or a combination CO_2-and-pump system. A mini-pump will easily fit in a pocket or saddlebag, but be warned, it takes a million little strokes to inflate your tire (and you'll need to top off the tire with a floor pump when you get home). CO_2 cartridges are small metal containers of compressed air that you attach to a special device to unleash the air into your tire. They're amazingly quick. But since they're good for only one use, if you have more flats than cartridges, you're stuck, and because you toss the empty cartridge, some people consider them less than ecological. Because CO_2 leaks out of tires rather quickly, you'll also need to top off at home. That's why I like a CO_2 mini-pump. It's a mini-pump with a CO_2 cartridge attached, so your bases are fully covered. It's also small enough to stuff into a saddlebag.

Also consider carrying:

MULTI-TOOL: Multi-tools are the Swiss Army knives of cycling—they can have almost any number of screwdrivers, Allen wrenches, bottle openers, chain tools, and more, all wrapped up in a portable package. I've used mine about five times in all the years I've been riding, but I was very happy I had it each of those times.

DUCT TAPE: Tear off a few inches of duct tape, roll it around a golf tee or small pencil, and carry it with you. I once used a strip to fasten down a dangling water bottle cage when one of the bolts came loose (and then went missing).

LOCK

A bike lock is optional depending on where you're riding and how you'll be using your bike. Recreational riders who only leave their bikes unattended (usually with the rest of their friends' bikes) for short stretches to grab coffee or water refills often don't fuss over bike locks. Urban commuters carry one wherever they go. Look for a sturdy lock with enough cable to secure your bike frame to a bike rack, signpost, small tree, or other street fixture. If you ride in a city where bikes are targeted by

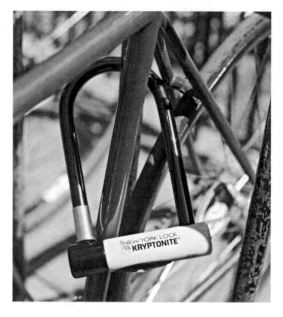

There are many types of locks to choose from. If you're in a high-risk area for bike theft, a sturdy lock like a U-lock is your safest bet.

thieves, carry two locks, such as a chain to secure the frame and back wheel to a rack and a U-lock (a lock literally shaped like a U with a removable bar across the top) to lock the front wheel to the frame.

COMPUTER

You don't need a cycling computer—basically a very sophisticated odometer for your bike—but you will most likely want one because it will tell you all the cool stuff you want to know, like how fast you're pedaling, how far you went, what your average and maximum speeds were, how long you rode, and so on. Fancy models even gauge your altitude, tell you how many feet you've

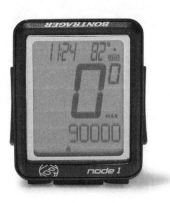

It's fun to use a cycling computer to see how far and fast you've gone and to watch those numbers improve over time.

climbed, and read the outside temperature. GPS-enabled units like Garmins even allow you to download rides and get turn-by-turn directions complete with maps. Many, like Garmins, are also compatible with heart rate monitors and power meters (more on those in the training section) and allow you to program training zones and turn your computer into a virtual coach.

You can also opt for a more basic cycling computer that uses a magnetic sensor attached to a wheel spoke to send data to a unit mounted on your bars, but they don't tell you quite as much information and take more time to set up. The beauty of a GPS-enabled unit is that although they cost a bit more, they're pretty much ready to go right out of the box and provide all the data any rider could ever need.

Some riders opt to forgo computers entirely and just use their mobile phones for ride recording. That's a viable option if you simply want to record your rides, but not so great if you want to actually see the ride as it happens. Mobile phone apps like Strava and MapMyRide let you record your ride stats with the press of a button (more on those, too, in the training section), but unless you have a weatherproof handlebar mount for your phone (which is a bit dicey, even if you do), you won't be able to see what you're doing in real time. These apps also drain the battery fairly quickly. If you have any designs on using your ride data for guidance, training, or even real-time motivation, spring for a handlebar-mounted computer. You won't regret it.

CHAPTER 5

The Cycling Lifestyle: Take Time to Make Time

IF YOU'RE HOLDING THIS BOOK, CHANCES ARE CYCLING IS more to you than an occasional activity, it's part of your life—maybe even a way of life. Like golfers, runners, rock climbers, and other sports enthusiasts, cyclists are, well, cyclists. We love to ride and ride whenever we can. The problem for many of us is that there never seems to be enough time.

And let's face it, cycling does take time. Even the most casual ride to the coffee shop generally takes 2 hours, sometimes more. When you factor in changing clothes, filling bottles, pumping up tires, and the like, even a short ride will take an hour. It's all time very well spent, but it's still time out of what is likely a busy day. Though it's a broad generalization, women also have a tendency to feel guilty about taking time for themselves amidst the demands of career and caregiving and other professional, social, and family obligations. But it can—and should—be done. Taking time to ride with friends (or alone, with your thoughts) will make you a happier, healthier, and more productive partner, employee, mom, and all those other roles you play! It just takes a little creativity and shuffling of priorities.

When I asked a group of accomplished, competitive women cyclists how they manage to fit in training time (which for some of these ladies can exceed 20 hours a week!) while also holding down full-time jobs and raising kids, they all said the same thing: You've got to let some stuff go. I fully agree. The house isn't a disaster, but it's lived-in. Sometimes dishes go unwashed. Sometimes laundry goes unsorted. There are a few weeds in the flowerbeds. And that's okay. All that stuff gets done . . . in time. Here are a few other bits of their best advice.

Plan It Out

Think of time in chunks and schedule the big stuff, and then let the little stuff find its way in. Be realistic about demands on your time and look [at the] long term, not just day-by-day or week-by-week. Maybe during prime riding season the house is a bit unkempt, but during the off-season you take some time to prepare the house for the next season. Cut out little things that waste your energy and time. Spend your precious time on what's most important and those things you most enjoy.

—CHERYL SORNSON, mountain bike and cyclocross racer for Rare Disease Cycling, National Ultra Endurance Women's Open Champion 2008

Make It a Family Affair

I'm a big believer in taking the kids along. That means accessories! I do most of my riding now with the two kids either on the front and back of the bike or both in tow in the bike trailer. If I can't ride for whatever reason, I run with them in the jogger. When I was racing full-time with my first newborn, I had to travel with two essentials: my hardworking breast pump and my harder-working husband. I would pump milk as close to the event as possible, feeding Nico on one side while pumping on the other. You just do what you have to do to get it done.

—MARLA STREB, Luna Women's Mountain Bike Team member and former single-speed world champion

Enlist Support

You can make a lot of excuses for not training and racing once you have kids—too tired, too busy, not enough time, and so on. But I believe that I'm a better mom and wife in the end because training allows me to take a little time to myself each day, stay healthy, and be a role model to my daughter! It just takes commitment and making it a priority while respecting the demands of family life. Recognize that you can't do it on your own and reach out for the support of others—

spouse, parents, in-laws, and babysitters. With motivation, commitment, support, and creativity, you can race and train without sacrificing all your family time."

—DANELLE KABUSH, two-time Xterra World Champion with Luna Xterra

Make Them Part of the Team

Kids like being the cheering committee for "Team Mom and Dad." Each kid has their own cowbell and we tell them how much it helps us when they cheer. Logistically, my husband and I pick designated 'cross series, looking for same-day races that are close in time rather than spread out. We bring a trainer and a backpack full of toys—one parent warms up while kids play in the dirt. The few races I've done without the kids in tow just weren't the same.

—PENNY PISANESCHI COLLINS, former Webcor Club cyclocross racer

Finding the Right Time

For many riders, consistently finding time to ride boils down to finding the right time to ride—the time of day when they have the fewest interruptions and potential disruptions. Consider the pros and cons of the morning, midday, and evening hours.

DAWN PATROL

Many of my friends tell me that if they don't pull "dawn patrol" or ride at "first bird," they don't ride. It takes some discipline, but this is the time that consistently tops the list when cyclists explain how they squeeze more rides into their week. E-mails, texts, and calls from people who need things from you build up as the day wears on. Life doesn't pitch many curveballs at 6:00 or 7:00 a.m. So by getting out the door early, you avoid those distractions. As a bonus, you also avoid a lot of traffic, and in the summer, the scorching heat of the day. By the time you get to work, your workout is done, and the day is yours. All these benefits may be why research consistently shows that morning exercisers stick to their routines better than those who try to fit it in at other times of the day.

The biggest obstacle to a rise-and-ride plan is that "rise" part. It's amazing how many excuses you can dream up while your head is resting on a soft pillow. Make it hard to talk yourself out of riding by placing all of your clothes in a neat pile directly in your line of sight from said pillow before you go to bed. Also prepare your water bottles and have them in the fridge ready to go. If you go to the trouble to pave the way the night before, you'll be far less likely to let yourself down come morning.

LUNCH BREAK

All across the valley where I live, small pods of cyclists gather outside their workplace doors at high noon to ride during their lunch hour. This is an excellent option if you can swing it. It takes a little preparation. You have to find a place to ride. Local parks are a great option if you're in the city. Or maybe you can find some back roads to string together a 10- or 15-mile loop if you work in a more suburban or rural setting. You also need to pack your stuff and be a quick-change artist in the office restroom. But once you try it, you'll be hooked. This midday "brain shower," as a friend of mine calls it, improves your mood, refreshes your energy, and boosts your productivity for the rest of the day. You can just grab a healthy lunch (or bring one with you) to eat at your desk after you ride.

Assuming that you don't have a barrier, like a boss who will breathe fire if you're away from your desk for more than 45 minutes, the most common midday riding quandary is post-ride cleanup. If your office building has a shower facility and locker room (many do), you're in luck. But truthfully, you don't necessarily need a shower, even after a sweaty ride. A quick toweling down and cleaning up with some baby wipes will leave you feeling fresh in a snap. As for your hair, a little gel or mousse and a blast with a hair dryer (pack a mini one in your duffle bag) will help lift it back in place.

EVENING SPIN

There's no better way to release the stress of the day than to ride away from it. During the workweek, this is also the time of day when most rides organized by your local bike shop or cycling club hit the road. So you'll have the added motivation of meeting up with people and being able to enjoy the company of others at the end of your day.

The barriers here are fairly obvious. While post-work is undoubtedly one of the most popular times to work out (just try to get on any gym treadmill at 6:00 p.m.), it's also a popular time for baseball practice, Scout gatherings, school board meetings, and a host of other extracurricular and community activities. Your best bet is to schedule your evening rides as you would any other meeting. Put it on the calendar and commit to it. And get creative. You don't really have to stand there (or sit in your car) during Brianna's dance class or soccer scrimmage. Throw your bike in the car and use her practice time to get some exercise of your own.

CONSIDER COMMUTING

Before people rode bikes for exercise and fun, they rode them as transportation. In light of rising fuel costs and global climate change, many are discovering that getting there by bike saves money and emissions, and comes with a side benefit of getting in shape. You'll find an entire chapter on using your bike to get from point A to point B and all those points in between on page 268.

USE YOUR WEEKENDS

To get better at cycling, it helps to ride at least 3 or 4 days a week. The weekend is your chance to seize 2 of them without the time constraints of work. They're also the times when you're most likely to find shop rides, club rides, charity rides, and friends who are available to spin along on a long, rambling ride.

Get up early, and you can sail around for 2 blissful hours and still get back in time to have breakfast with the family. Even if you have other obligations, you can usually squeeze in a

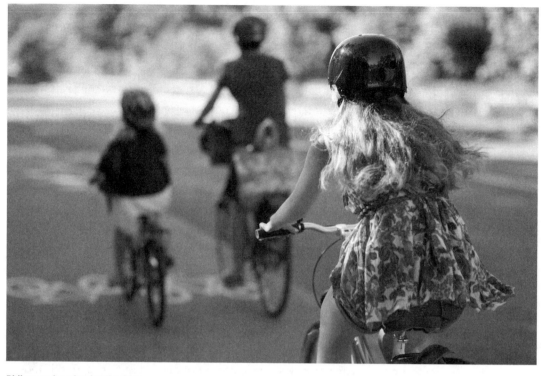

Riding can be a fun family affair.

ride around them. Friends of mine ride to their kids' soccer games (of course, one parent has to be available to drive the kids there), family dinners, and other functions. You'll be surprised by how many opportunities there are to do some really great rides once you start looking.

Light a Fire Under Yourself

Sometimes prioritizing riding takes a little extra motivation. Even people who love to ride can sometimes let it fall by the wayside as other obligations push it to the bottom of the to-do list. One easy way to put it back on top is to sign up for a charity ride, a race, or even a cycling vacation. Having a cycling event on the calendar will fire up your motivation to get in great riding shape so you can enjoy the experience. After all, nothing gets you on your bike like knowing you have a 100-mile ride to do in 3 months.

Riding for a cause can further inspire you to get out and ride because you're pedaling for a greater good. No matter what cause is nearest and dearest to your heart, you're sure to find a ride for it. I've pedaled thousands of miles over the years to raise money for research on an HIV vaccine, multiple sclerosis, diabetes, heart disease, pediatric terminal illnesses, and cancer. Riding for worthy causes also reminds you that it's a privilege to have a healthy body that is able to ride a bike. (You'll find more worthy charity rides on page 273.)

Local bike clubs are great sources of information on races, rides, and organized cycling events throughout the year. You can also check out Web sites like Active.com and BikeReg.com to find events in your area.

Plug In to the Scene

The more you immerse yourself in the cycling scene, the more people you'll have to ride with and the more you'll want to ride. Women's cycling especially is a growing social scene complete with women's bike bashes, festivals, clinics, and rides.

The Internet is your friend here. Search online for cycling groups in your area. Check out the Web sites of your local shops (many offer women's clinics and rides). Click over to Active.com to see all the rides going on within 150 miles of you. All it takes is doing a few rides to become part of the cycling scene, and before you know it you'll have all sorts of Facebook friends wearing helmets in their profile pictures, as well as a community with whom you can grow and enjoy the sport for years to come.

Cecilia Murgo summed it up best when she told me how one ride with a cycling friend broke ground for a bright future she never imagined.

I caught the riding bug when my best friend, who is an avid road cyclist, persuaded me to buy a road bike. I had started running and working out to lose weight for my upcoming 30th birthday and he convinced me that cycling was the way to go.

Thankfully I listened, because buying my bike is one of the best things I have ever done for myself. It's not only good for me physically— I've started to lose more weight and am smaller than I have been in my life, and I also quit smoking cold turkey after smoking for 15 years—but also it feeds my soul and allows me time to focus on myself and push myself in ways I never thought I could. In the short time that I have been riding, I've met and been embraced by our local cycling community (which still needs more ladies) and have been able to learn from some great riders. With some convincing I signed up for my first race in upstate New York, which motivated me to spend the winter training my heart out. I am excited for this upcoming season and all the adventures that lie ahead.

Now *that's* the true cycling lifestyle.

PART III

SKILLS, DRILLS, AND RULES OF THE ROAD

You never forget how to ride a bike. Everyone's heard the saying. And for the most part it's true, if you define riding as sitting on the seat and staying upright while pedaling down the road. What is also true is that many people have never really learned how to ride a bike past those very fundamentals, which, though essential, won't get you very far as a "cyclist."

In fact, for many cyclists (men and women), getting into and trying to improve in the sport can be an exercise in frustration because nobody has taken the time to teach them how to ride since they were 8 years old. And a lot has changed since then! Take Suzanne Kornutiak, who got a bit more than she bargained for on her maiden voyage as an adult cyclist in her mid-30s.

"Growing up in the country, the only way I could get around was by bike. So once I could drive, I stubbornly swore I'd never ride a bicycle again . . . until I met Alaina, who lives and breathes bikes and is also a cross-country national champ, through a mutual friend. We hit it off and she inspired me to put down my workaholic ways and go ride with her. I bought a road bike shortly thereafter and immediately announced to my husband, Chuck, that I was taking it on a 30-mile shop ride the following day, clipped in, of course, despite the fact that I hadn't been on a bike in roughly 20 years.

"God bless Chuck and Alaina, who took turns pedaling next to me, explaining that no, I could not stop pedaling while shifting, and telling me that I needed to unclip my shoe prior to coming to a stop. I fell over twice, scratched my new bike and my knee, and nearly threw up from exhaustion when I got home. But I was so proud of my 26 miles! That was 6 years ago. I've since gotten a nicer road bike, two mountain bikes, and a 'cross bike, rode my first century about a year ago, and even did a few cross-country races. Chuck calls me Frankenbike, and

Alaina continues to be one of my best friends. Cycling has improved my fitness level, provided an outlet for all kinds of stress, and introduced me to some fantastic people. I can't imagine *not* riding, and only wish I'd started sooner."

Skilled and patient friends combined with steadfast stick-to-itiveness will get you far over the course of a few years. However, there's an easier way to learn everything from the fundamentals of shifting, braking, and pedaling to the finer points of riding in pacelines and packs: Read all about it. Practice. Then come back and read some more. I've found that it's easier to understand written directions for more nuanced skills like cornering once you have a few miles under your belt because you have a better understanding of how the bike rides and reacts in general, so the directions simply make more sense.

Though none of these skills is unique to female riders, my experience has been that women tend to be more hesitant than men to learn trial-by-fire style and are less likely to just jump into a group ride and learn on the fly. This is particularly the case when the groups they are jumping into are predominantly male and perhaps don't appear to be 100 percent welcoming. It's not that women can't learn that way, of course. It's just that they're less inclined to.

The following section will take you from tossing a leg over your saddle (there's actually a preferred method for getting on a bike), to confident clipped-in pedaling, to handling your bike through traffic and adverse weather conditions, to mixing it up in your local criterium race. Just keep reading for all you need to know to head out on the road and enjoy every type of ride.

CHAPTER 6

You and the Machine

"OKAY, DON'T LAUGH, BUT WHICH ONE OF THESE LEVERS shifts which way?"

"I know this is a dumb question, but what gear am I supposed to ride in?"

"Why am I never in the right gear?"

These are just a handful of the questions I get all the time from bashful riders who want to join the fun to be had on their local bike shop or charity ride, but can't get the hang of how everything works on their bike well enough to feel confident that a) they'll be able to keep up and b) they won't embarrass themselves.

Fact is, the first bikes didn't even have gears. There was simply a chain around a pair of cogs that made the wheels go 'round when you pedaled. Then someone—likely someone living in, oh, anywhere but the dead-flat fields of Kansas—decided it would be nice if we had a few gears so we didn't have to get off and walk up hills that are really steep. Gears and shifting have been assisting—and confounding—riders ever since.

Seriously. Tour de France stages have been won and lost because of mis-shifts and dropped chains (explained later in this chapter), so while shifting confusion may be most common among new riders, cyclists at all levels benefit from time spent working on the finer points of skills like shifting, as well as braking and even pedaling.

"I had to learn all of those things—and then some—the hard way," recalls Victoria Pink, who has since completed two Ironman races and competes in both cyclocross and mountain bike races. "I bought my first road bike for $200 over 10 years ago. It was a Cannondale with down tube shifters [years ago, shifter levers were mounted near the top of the down tube]. I was determined to show up on the first group ride of the year, which is the Tri-Wisconsin ride in early April. It was cold and the only warm workout pants I owned were yoga pants with flared legs. The pants would surely get caught in the chain, so I tied the right leg with a hook-and-loop tie. I feel every ounce the newbie as we gather and prepare for the ride and roll out of town. Of course I fall behind immediately as we hit the first hill. Local pro and Olympian Brent Emery comes up behind me and offers advice and a helping hand—literally. For the next 30 miles, he has his hand on my back, helping to push me up hills, telling me how to use my shifters and when to shift, all while snot is dripping from my nose and I am trying to swallow my embarrassment. The next day I baked some cookies and took them to his shop in appreciation for all the advice."

You can bake some sweets for your bike shop's owner if you'd like, but we're here to make sure you don't need to. The following are the fundamentals and finer points of becoming one with your machine. As you'll see, though none of these issues is particularly women's specific, we do have some special consider-ations in these areas. Smaller hands, for instance, can present shifting and braking challenges that can—and should—be addressed. Here's what you need to know.

Climbing Aboard and Rolling Out

This might sound silly, but there's a right way and, let's say, a not quite as right way (because, really, there's not a wrong way) to get on your bike. Mounting a bike is one of those skills that nobody ever bothers telling you how to do and you may never really learn, until you see some-one smirking your way as you kick your foot over the top tube the "wrong" way. So without further ado, here is how to swing a leg over a saddle like a pro.

Stand on the left side of the bike. Why? Because this is the opposite side of the drive-train. By starting here, you won't inadver-tently bump up against the chain and get a telltale "newbie" black chain mark on your leg (which, incidentally, I still get all the time). Place your hands on the handlebars and lean the bike toward you slightly. Extend your right leg back and swing it over the saddle and then down along the opposite side of the top tube.

Straddle the top tube with both feet flat on the ground. Using one foot, turn your pedals backward and place the pedal for your domi-nant foot forward and slightly above the hori-zontal position. (Your dominant foot is simply the one you feel most comfortable starting to pedal with, usually on the same side as your dominant hand.)

Squeeze and hold the brake levers and put your dominant foot on the leading pedal. This is the ready position. Look over your shoulder for traffic, pedestrians, and other cyclists moving toward you (a good habit to get into). Then release the brakes and push down with your lead foot as you simultaneously push yourself off the ground with the other foot, lifting yourself up and onto the saddle. Finally, place your other foot on the opposite pedal and start pedaling, sliding your sit bones to the back of the saddle as you start rolling.

Getting into Gear

When I first started riding, I had this notion that shifting into an easier gear was a sign of weakness, that I shouldn't have to shift if I was strong enough. I figured that if I was riding to get fit, cycling should feel like work all the time. Fortunately, it didn't take long before I discovered the error of my ways. Now I coach new riders to do what the best of the best coached me to do: Wear out those shifters.

Gears are designed to allow you to pedal uphill, downhill, over flat land, and into a strong headwind without killing yourself, exhausting your legs, or spinning your wheels like a caffeinated hamster. Cycling is an aerobic activity, not resistance training. So, while you will feel your leg muscles burn as you work your way up a particularly steep hill or as you sprint hard and fast, you should usually feel nothing

Be a Steady Scanner

Scanning for oncoming traffic while you're moving—particularly without inadvertently weaving all over the road or into said traffic while doing it—is an essential skill, and one that takes practice. I know plenty of veteran riders who still swerve precariously into the lane when they glance over their shoulders to check for cars. Practice scanning without veering by riding along one of the white lines in a parking lot. Some riders find it is easiest to keep from turning their whole torso as they glance over their shoulder by dropping the hand on the same side from the bar as they do it. Practice to see what technique works best for you. You'll find more rules of riding the road in Chapter 9.

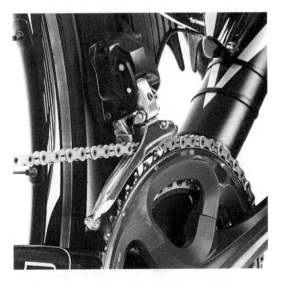

The more gears you have, the easier it is to tackle every type of terrain. Use them all liberally.

but moderate pressure on your legs as you pedal. To achieve this, you need to shift early and often, especially if you live in a place that is undulating or hilly.

Here's how it works: As you saw in Chapter 2, most bikes have a series of gears (generally about 10 of them) on the rear wheel on what is called a "cassette." The biggest gear on the cassette (the one closet to your wheel) makes pedaling the easiest. The smallest one puts you in the gear that's the hardest (good for slight downhills), so you can keep pedaling and have a little tension on the chain when you're coasting, which prevents the chain from rattling around. These gears are usually changed with the right-hand shift levers and make relatively small shifts in gear. The mnemonic "right = rear" is a simple way to remember which hand controls both shifting and braking in the rear. So, say you're pedaling along and the road starts to go up an incline of a degree or two; you should shift down through the stack of gears on the cassette to a lower gear to make pedaling easier. Conversely, if the road tips downward and makes you start pedaling too fast, you would shift up to a higher gear. You also use these gears to accelerate as the pace gets hot. Note: The chain has to be moving as you shift, so you need to keep pedaling.

At the front of the drivechain are the chainrings, which encircle the right-side crank arm that holds your right pedal. Most bikes have two or three chainrings (though mountain bikes increasingly come with just one, doing away with this type of shifting). These gears are controlled with your left-hand shifter lever and make more dramatic gear changes. So if you're rolling along and the road or path suddenly pitches steeply upward, you should shift your chain from the big chainring to the smallest one to pedal more easily up the grade. So on the rear cassette, the smaller the gear in use is, the harder the pedaling, but in the front, it's the opposite, with the smaller one making your pedaling easier.

Also know this: You are not locked in to the gears your bike comes with. You can change the sizes of the gears in both front and rear for ones that suit your riding style and terrain. Like Kelly Szymczyk learned when she first relocated to the rolling hills of Pennsylvania. "I was fit, but on even some short moderate hills, like [an incline of] 7 to 8 percent for $^2/_{10}$ of a mile, I thought I was going to topple over!" As she glanced around and saw some much larger riders cheerfully spinning their way over the crests, it dawned on her that gears might play a role. "I started asking everyone what gears they had. First I bought a new cassette, switching from an 11-to-23 [tooth range] to a 12-to-27; then this past fall I put on a compact, which has smaller, easier to pedal front chainrings. Big help!"

Shifting is as much an art as a science. But once you "get it," you'll have it for good. Here are a few tips to help make yours smooth, silent, and seamless.

EASE UP A BIT. Your chain will move with greater ease from gear to gear if there's less pressure on it. That's particularly true for front derailleur (left-hand) shifts, which require the chain to move up or down between chainrings of significantly different sizes. When making these shifts especially, ease off the pressure on the pedals slightly to let the chain move freely. Also, try to make these shifts ahead of when you need them rather than waiting until you're grinding up a vertical pitch. It's harder to execute a clean shift when there's a ton of pressure on the pedals. Rear (right-hand) shifts are subtler and not as finicky, but still move more fluidly when you lighten their burden by easing up a hair on the pressure.

ANTICIPATE THE SHIFT. This is a golden rule for smooth shifting, and it requires you use your eyes as much as your legs. When you see that the terrain is going to change, start shifting before you absolutely need to. Shifting when you're mashing down on your pedals trying to stay upright is a clunky affair. Remember, you want to be able to back off the force on your pedals to allow the chain to move smoothly. You can't do that under pressure. Anticipate the shift for impending situations, such as punchy climbing, sprinting, tight cornering, and—one many forget—stopping. If you come to a stop in the high gear you've been hammering along the flats in, it'll be tough to get going again when you can proceed. Make it easier on yourself by shifting down as you come to a stop sign or traffic signal.

KEEP YOUR CADENCE. Cadence is the rhythm of your pedal stroke, or how many revolutions per minute (rpm) your pedals are turning. The sweet spot for most cyclists is about 90, give or take 10. You don't have to count right now

(we'll get into that when we talk training), but focus on keeping your leg turnover brisk. That is, you don't want to be pushing down slowly on your pedals, but rather spinning your wheels in a brisk, comfortable rhythm. When you feel that brisk cadence start to slow, shift to an easier gear. When you feel it speed up too much, shift to a harder gear.

MAINTAIN A SMOOTH CHAINLINE. Pedaling along with your chain stretched at an extreme angle is hard on your drivetrain and wears out your chain and gears prematurely. So if you're on your biggest (outermost) chainring in the front as well as the biggest gear (closest to the wheel) in the back, the pedaling may not be silky smooth as your chain tries to work under the tension. Generally, if you find yourself pedaling at those extremes for an extended time, it's a sign that you should shift onto another chainring (in this case to the smaller one) to smooth it out.

AVOID DROPPED CHAINS AND SUICIDE SHIFTS. During one of my first triathlons, I was charging up a low-grade climb when I made a hard right and encountered a steep rise. I tried to throw my chain onto the smaller chainring— only to throw it completely past it and off the rings entirely, in what a friend of mine later called a suicide shift. Bikes cease to make forward progress without a chain, so as you might imagine, I promptly toppled over. Easing up on the chain pressure as you shift can help avert such accidents. But occasionally, whether because the bike is out of tune or you're forced into a sudden awkward shift, the chain can come off toward either the outside or inside of the bike.

Don't panic. Continue turning the pedals very slowly and lightly as you move the shifter in the direction opposite to the way the chain fell—so toward the bike if it fell to the outside and vice versa. If the chain is caught up on the derailleur, try taking one or two gentle backward pedal strokes to free it and try again. That will often get a dropped chain back on the chainrings (and ultimately in the gear you want) without having to climb off the bike and fix it by hand. I won't lie, however. Sometimes you're stuck and need to get off and put the chain on by hand. It's messy business, but thankfully doesn't happen often.

Slowing and Stopping

No doubt about it, once you get going, you're going to eventually need to come to a stop and modulate some speed here and there—especially when you're riding with others. By learning to brake skillfully, you can not only avoid accidents, but also improve efficiency and save energy for when you need it. *Bicycling* once asked Alex Stieda, the first North American to wear the yellow jersey in the Tour de France, how he worked his brakes in a pack of that size and intensity. Here is what he said—good advice for all.

FINGERS READY. Anytime there's a wheel in front of you (i.e., you're drafting), rest your fingers on the brake levers. This way, you'll be able to brake quickly—and feather the brakes gently—and minor slowdowns won't develop into emergency-stop situations while your hands find the brakes.

KEEP IT EQUAL. In the vast majority of braking situations, you want to apply pressure evenly to each brake lever so that both tires share the load. This helps maintain stability and control. Practice on a grass field, sprinting up to speed, then slowing as fast as you can without skidding. You'll need to modulate finger pressure on each brake lever, much like antilock brakes on a car, to stop individual tires from skidding.

Note: These rules change a little when you're mountain biking, because there are times when you don't want to touch the front brake and others when that's the only one you want to use; we'll cover that in Chapter 10.

TURN SMART. Always brake before a turn. As you near the curve, apply equal pressure to the brakes to reach a manageable speed, and then release the levers before you begin the turn to let your speed carry you through. Braking in a turn wreaks havoc on momentum, but if it's necessary for safety, then use the rear brake only—remember "right = rear" to keep them straight in your mind. Skidding the rear may raise your heart rate, but it will allow you to steer out of trouble. When you lock up the front wheel, control is lost. [More on this in the next chapter.]

SHIFT YOUR WEIGHT. As you squeeze the brakes, your bike slows down but your body keeps going, sending your weight forward over the front wheel. This can make it difficult to steer. Counter this effect by pressing your weight toward the back of the saddle as you squeeze the brake levers. Shifting your weight backward is especially important when you're stopping on a decline. Some riders don't like to go downhill in their drops (the lowest part of the handlebar on road bikes) because you pick up speed in that low, aerodynamic position, but it's the safest position for descending. Your weight is back and low and you have good leverage to pull the brakes and brace your body in the proper position. The best way to get used to the feel of this simultaneous weight shift and brake pull is by practicing emergency stops (below), in which you exaggerate both motions, giving you an excellent feel for the physics of braking.

LEARN TO STOP HARD. When you master the emergency stop, you'll have greater overall stopping confidence because you'll know this move is there when you need it. For more braking power, put your hands in the drops. Then, for added stability, push your weight all the way back behind the saddle by shifting your butt and straightening your arms. Practice on the grass, with a goal of not skidding. Remember: Fresh brake pads greatly improve stopping performance—replace them regularly, consulting with your bike shop if you're not sure when.

After you master these, you'll be able to anticipate situations, a key skill for every cyclist from beginner to Tour de France champion. When you anticipate that the rider in front of you is going to swerve, for example, you won't have to overreact by slamming on the brakes. In many scenarios, continuing to pedal while braking lightly will get you out of trouble. The overall effect: You won't be a yo-yo, that person

Adjust Your Reach

This is where women's specific bars and levers can be important. If the levers are so far forward that you can't ride with your fingers lightly wrapped around them, you can't possibly feather the brakes with any finesse. Look into women's specific levers or ask your bike shop mechanic if yours are adjustable. Many are, and you may be able to pull the levers closer to the bars with simple turns of some screws.

who brakes hard and then accelerates to regain momentum, wasting energy in the process.

Smooth Pedaling

Your goal is to pedal in smooth, silky circles, applying even pressure on the pedals throughout the pedal stroke, rather than jamming down on the pedals like you're mashing grapes. To accomplish this, push down on the pedal with the ball of your foot, then pull your foot back through the bottom of the stroke, then pull up and around. Again, think brisk, aiming for about 90 rpm. Your speed will naturally slow on climbs and quicken on descents.

Once you've got smooth pedaling down, you can hone it to squeeze out every watt of power throughout the stroke with a light ankling technique. This technique, explains Todd Carver, cofounder and director of fit at Retül University in Boulder, Colorado, allows you to churn

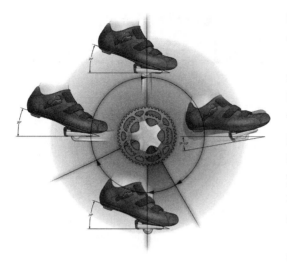

Your ankle is an important player in a strong pedal stroke. The action is similar to scraping a bit of mud off the bottom of your shoe.

out the same amount of power at a heart rate as many as 5 beats per minute lower. In other words, it saves energy, especially when you're hammering away on flat terrain at your threshold intensity. Here's how it's done.

ENSURE PROPER SADDLE POSITION: Proper bike fit, especially saddle height and fore–aft position, is a prerequisite for a smooth pedal stroke. Without it, says Carver, you won't be even remotely as efficient as you could be. "If your saddle is too high, you're not going to be able to drive your heel effectively," he says. "If it's too low, you'll have knee pain." In the right position (knee over the ball of your foot when the pedal is at 3 o'clock and slightly bent when the pedal is at 6 o'clock), you'll maximize your energy output and also be able to adapt your ankling

technique to different terrains, cadences, and effort levels.

CHECK HIP-KNEE-ANKLE ALIGNMENT: Viewed from the front, your hip, knee, and ankle should line up throughout the pedal stroke. "You don't want knee wobble," says Carver. "Just think pistons, straight up and down." If you can't correct this, or if you experience knee pain when you try to restrict lateral movement, you may need orthotics or another type of biomechanical adjustment.

ZONE 1: Known as the power phase, the portion of the pedal stroke from 12 o'clock to about 5 o'clock is the period of greatest muscle activity. "A lot of people think hamstrings are used only on the upstroke," says Carver, "but a good cyclist uses a lot of hamstring in the downstroke, because it extends the hip." The key to accessing the large muscles in the back of your leg is to drop your heel as you come over the top of the stroke, says Carver. "At 12 o'clock, your toes should be pointed down about 20 degrees, but as you come over the top, start dropping that heel so that it's parallel to the ground, or even 10 degrees past parallel, by the time you get to 3 o'clock." The biggest mistake Carver sees in novice riders: not dropping the heel enough in Zone 1.

ZONE 2: Using the same muscles as in the power phase but to a lesser degree, this phase acts as a transition to the backstroke. "As you enter Zone 2, think about firing the calf muscles to point your toes," Carver says. As you come through the bottom of the stroke, the toes should be pointed down 20 degrees. "This ankling technique transfers some of the energy developed in Zone 1 by the bigger muscles to the crank," Carver says. He uses the advice popularized by Greg LeMond: "Act like you're scraping mud off the bottom of your shoe."

ZONE 3: Even though you feel like you're pulling your foot through the back of the stroke, you're not. "When you look at even the best cyclists, they're losing power on the upstroke," says Carver. "The pedal is actually pushing your leg up, so the goal is to lose as little power as possible and get that foot out of the way." One fun way to improve the efficiency of your upstroke is to do more mountain biking. "The terrain keeps you honest," Carver says. "If you're focusing only on the downstroke, you'll lose traction and fall off your bike in steep sections." As for other exercises, Carver advises against single-leg pedal drills—"for recreation-level riders, they injure more people than they help"—but recommends hamstring- and glute-strengthening lifts, as well as squats, "done correctly, in a squat rack with someone showing you how."

ZONE 4: As you enter the second half of the upstroke phase, think about initiating your downstroke. "Many riders don't initiate early enough," says Carver, who often sees riders wait until 3 o'clock—but they should be starting before 12 o'clock. A tip: As you begin to come across the top of the stroke, think about pushing your knee forward, toward the bar. But only your knee, says Carver: "Your pelvis should remain a stable platform, not sinking down and not moving forward."

Clipping In

If you have clipless pedals, learning to clip in is a rite of passage among cyclists. For one, it requires a financial commitment of buying special shoes and pedals. More importantly, it attaches you quite literally to your bike. This is a good—no, a great—thing because it exponentially increases your pedaling efficiency, letting you generate power as you pull up as well as when you push down. Clipless pedals can reduce the risk of injury by keeping your foot in the optimal position on the pedal. And for most riders, they are far more comfortable (and often safer) than toe clips that strap your foot to the pedal. Still. Being clipped in makes some pretty nervous.

One *Bicycling* magazine reader said, "It freaks me out when I feel I cannot clip off my bike—like I'm trapped, doomed to have an unpleasant stopping experience." "Trapped" and "doomed." Heavy language. It really doesn't have to be that way. Many clipless pedal systems are highly adjustable and can be set so the spring action takes very little pressure to release and free you from the pedal. That said, 100 percent honestly, you will very likely topple over once or twice during your learning curve with clipless pedals. Everyone does. It's a bit embarrassing, but a right of passage that doesn't last very long before you get the hang of it. But it is important to practice in a safe place like a parking lot to get the hang of it before motoring down the road.

SET UP

Follow your pedal manufacturer's instructions to set your cleat tension so entry and exit are as easy as they can be. Some brands and models have no release-tension adjustability, so ask before you buy. If you're unsure about anything, stick around the shop and have them assist you with the setup. The shop also can install the cleats to the bottoms of your shoes with special thread-locking grease that will help keep the screws—and hence the cleats—from coming loose, as well as help you position your cleats correctly so your pedaling position and alignment are correct.

STEP IN

Once they're set up, practice getting in and out of your pedals. Prop yourself up on your bike where you can hold on to a stable surface like a railing or wall, and then step in to the pedal by positioning the cleat at the pedal and pressing down until you hear the telltale "click" of the attachment being made. Now clip in with the other foot and pedal backward to get the feeling of being clipped in. If that's too difficult, you can simply stand over your bike and, with one foot on the ground, clip in with the other.

TWIST OUT

Now practice releasing your foot from the pedal by twisting your heel toward the outside, away from the bike. Switch sides. Then step in and twist out again and again until it feels natural.

CRUISE

When you feel comfortable clipping in and out, go for a spin around your neighborhood or on a patch of grass. Practice clipping in and out as you roll.

STOP

Try coming to a complete stop, as if you were riding in traffic. As you slow to a stop, clip one foot out and drop it to the ground just as you normally would. Not feeling that confident yet? Stop next to a tree or telephone pole so you can grab it if you have to.

RIDE

Once you feel comfortable clipping in and out as you cruise your neighborhood and stop on a dime, show up at the next group ride looking like an old pro.

CHAPTER 7

Climbing, Descending, and Cornering

THE EARTH IS NOT FLAT. INSTEAD, IT UNDULATES, WITH STEEP ups and sweeping downs, and twists and turns along the way. This is the fun part of riding—all the amazing terrain you can cover, the sense of accomplishment when you turn those final hard-fought revolutions over the crest of a monster climb, and the feeling of flying as you coast down the other side.

The more varied the terrain you ride, the more skill it takes to smoothly negotiate it. No matter how long you've been riding, you can always hone your technique and become a better climber, descender, and bike handler. Though none of these skills is particularly women's specific, this is where it's important to both have a bike that fits your frame and to be properly fitted on that bike.

Weight distribution hugely affects how well your bike tracks through turns, how the tires stick to the ground when you climb and descend, and generally how the bike responds to your input. Your weight should be pretty evenly distributed between the front and back of the bike, with about 60 percent over the saddle and 40 percent on

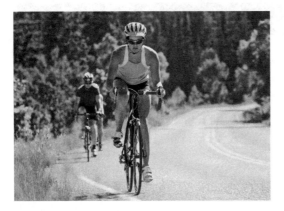

Conquering climbs is one of the most satisfying elements of cycling.

the bars. Since many women carry much of their weight in their lower body, this is why some women's specific designs have altered geometry that steepens the seat tube angle, shifting the rider's weight more forward to put an appropriate amount of weight on the front wheel for optimal steering control.

These are also skills that are learned over time. So be patient with yourself. Even cyclists who have been riding for decades still struggle with them. But just one or two tips can go a long way toward improving your experience. Here's what you need to know.

Going Up the Mountain

Like a towering alpine pass, hills create divisions among cyclists. There are those who love a good climb, and those who will ride 10 miles out of their way to avoid one. Growing up riding in a part of Pennsylvania where the only flat land is the quarter-mile stretch that takes you

to the next hill, I couldn't really avoid climbs. But I didn't exactly relish them either. When I first started doing group rides and races, I actually sort of dreaded them, mostly because I was a bit scared of them.

That changed one summer in West Virginia. I was racing the Twenty-Four Hours of Canaan, which, as it sounds, is a mountain bike race where teams ride around a course, from noon on Saturday till noon on Sunday, amassing as many laps as humanly possible. The course was rugged, with many punchy climbs and one long monster—Salamander Hill, I think it was called—that stretched for a mile or two up the mountain. I was dreading it, knowing I'd be grinding up it multiple times throughout the race. I'd just started the race, and already in my head was a flurry of self-defeating thoughts about how much it was going to suck, but then I pedaled by a spectator who was sitting roadside with his bike. He smiled at me and said, "Enjoy the climb. It's a beauty."

He wasn't being snarky or sarcastic, but completely sincere, almost reverent. It was a lightbulb moment. To me, climbs were obstacles to be conquered, not experiences to be enjoyed. So I relaxed, lifted my head up, put a smile on my face, and discovered that he was right. It was a beauty of a climb. Today, 17 years later, I love climbing. That's actually when I settle in and relax. It helps that I'm now much more fit than I was all those years ago, but using proper technique and having a good attitude have also made a huge difference. Here's how to ascend any mountain or hill with greater ease, including some tips from pro rider Alex Stieda and pro coach Andy Applegate of Carmichael Training Systems.

RIDE WITHIN YOURSELF

As with any test of endurance, it's important to pace yourself when you climb. That means riding within yourself, not charging after faster riders or pushing so hard that you're gasping from the get-go. It's easy to go into the red (way above your lactate threshold, where your muscles start to work anaerobically) on a climb. When you do, your breathing rate skyrockets, your legs begin to feel dead, and eventually you'll pop, unable to continue at even a fraction of your pace. But when you ride within your ability, you will not only reach the top faster, but also increase your fitness so you can go harder the next time.

How hard should you go? You could calculate your threshold heart rate (see "Heart Rate Monitor," page 144), but the simple perceived-exertion method is surprisingly accurate: On a scale of 1 (easy) to 10 (max effort), climbing at 8 should feel just under control. Over that, you'll cross your threshold and begin to fall apart.

MEDITATE UPHILL

Strap on a heart rate monitor and sit on your sofa. Check your heart rate. Now clench your fists and grit your teeth—I bet your heart rate jumps a few beats. When you're climbing a long hill, you want to direct all your energy to your legs, not your face. To stay relaxed, Applegate swears by "Qigong climbing," a kind of moving meditation. As you approach the climb, think light thoughts—clouds, birds, angels. While climbing, progressively relax your body from the top down, starting with your eyes, then your mouth, jaw, shoulders, chest, back, arms,

and hands. "You want your upper body so still that if someone were to watch you from the waist up, they wouldn't be able to tell if you were climbing or casually riding along," says Applegate. Also, stay light on the pedals and keep your legs moving rhythmically. The goal is to erase every ounce of unnecessary tension. "You'll feel better, ride smoother, and have more energy to keep riding strong after you've crested the climb," says Applegate.

PEDAL WITH PURPOSE

On climbs, drop your heel slightly to initiate the pedal stroke; push with your whole foot. Pull up on your heel at the bottom of the stroke, much like a running motion.

ASSUME THE POWER POSITION

To pull maximum air into your lungs, keep your back straight and your chest open. Position your hands on the brake hoods and relax your arms so your elbows sit wider than your hips. Women generally are of shorter stature and are proportionally more muscular in the lower body than in the upper body. Practically speaking, this means that your turbochargers are located under bun no. 1 and bun no. 2. Tap into those turbines by sliding back on the saddle to fully engage your glutes, which will generate more force over the top of the pedal stroke and help keep your heels down as you pull back around the bottom of the revolution. If you're on the taller side, however, slide forward, positioning your hips so they come close to lining up with the bottom bracket, to generate maximum muscle force. On long climbs, I'll intentionally slide forward and back on the saddle to engage different muscle groups and keep myself fresher all the way to the top.

KEEP THOSE PEDALS SPINNING

Your cadence will naturally slow a bit, but don't let it come to a crawl. A general rule is the bigger the rider, the more important it is to sit and spin. On an extended climb, the pro peloton's larger climbers pedal seated in a relatively small gear and at a high cadence. Lighter riders tend to be in and out of the saddle, pushing a bigger gear at a slightly lower cadence. But this too is a personal preference. Even seated, I prefer to push a larger gear a little more slowly because that seems to work best with my muscle fiber composition and keeps my heart rate in check.

A conversation I had with Chrissie Wellington (who jams a monster gear) confirmed that suspicion. During an interview, she put it like this: "It's a misconception that you need to spin a smaller gear at a higher cadence on the bike. You don't. Doing that actually raises your heart rate and makes you more tired, which doesn't serve you very well in long-distance racing. Cranking it down and pushing a bigger gear lets me lower my heart rate. It's what feels natural to me and enables me to go the fastest I can go."

Sounds reasonable to me, and advice my experience confirms, despite being told to quicken my cadence over the years. My take: Try both and see where you find your sweet spot. In general, you likely want to keep that cadence at or above 70 rpm, even if you go bigger.

BREATHE

Avoid gasping for air. Instead, "belly breathe" using your diaphragm. Find your rhythm, both by breathing steadily and by maintaining a steady pedal cadence. On especially long and/or hard climbs, try timing your breathing to your pedal strokes, inhaling for three pedal strokes and then exhaling for two pedal strokes (when the going gets hard, that might change to inhaling for two and exhaling for one). This technique keeps your breathing controlled and quiets and focuses your mind.

GET UP AND GO

Seated climbing is technically the most efficient because it uses fewer muscles and less energy. When you stand, you put more weight on your leg muscles, so they have to work harder, which uses about 10 percent more energy and sends your heart rate about 5 to 10 percent higher. But there comes a time when you need to get out of the saddle to keep momentum going. How often you stand is a matter of personal preference. When you feel like you need to stand, click into the next larger gear and stand when one foot reaches the top of the pedal stroke (2 o'clock) to minimize momentum loss. Shift your hips forward, but keep most of your weight back and over the bottom bracket. (Leaning too far forward puts excess weight on the front wheel, causing the back wheel to spin out and slow you down.) Gently pull on the handlebars to generate more power as you push down on the pedals—right arm pull, right foot push; left arm pull, left foot push—so you feel like you're running on the pedals, allowing the bike to rock gently, but not excessively, from side to side. When you're ready to sit back down, downshift and smoothly sit down at the top of a pedal stroke.

USE THE FORCE

Most climbs have a pitch that allows you to mostly spin your way up. But occasionally you find yourself facing a wall, which is a climb of 10 percent or higher. There are two ways to tackle these vertical assaults: One is to shift your weight *way* back, hold the top of the handlebars close to the stem, and pull back on the bars with both hands as you power through each pedal stroke. The other is to stand up and use your body weight to push the pedals down and around. The key is to keep all your energy focused on forward momentum. You'll inevitably see some riders who "tack" or "paperboy" up steep climbs, zigzagging across the route. That lessens the grade by cutting across the hill rather than going straight up it, but it lengthens the climb and is more dangerous on a road ride because you're bobbing and weaving in front of other riders and traffic.

If all else fails, walk. Seriously. Cycling snobs may gasp and cluck their tongues at the very word, but we've all been there. It doesn't feel great. But it's not the end of the world, either. Just make sure you come back again (and maybe again), until you can conquer that climb.

WORK THE TERRAIN

Most climbs don't have a constant grade. When you reach a flatter section, shift into an easier gear and spin at a faster cadence to let your legs recover. As you approach a short, steeper section, you may want to shift into a harder gear and get out of the saddle. As the terrain levels out, you can sit down and go back to your easier gear and higher cadence.

FINISH STRONG

When you finally reach the crest of the climb, pedal faster. Many riders slow to a crawl as they near the top because the hard work is behind them. With all your momentum gone, it's that much harder to get going again. Instead, keep pedaling, trying to pick up speed, until you feel gravity start to pull you over the other side.

LIGHTEN UP

Gravity sucks—literally. And the heavier you and your bike are, the more force it takes to fight it. For that reason, cycling is referred to as a power-to-weight sport. That's also why cyclists often go to great pains to buy the lightest carbon fiber bikes, wheels, and gear they can. Heck, you'll see pros start tossing unnecessary bottles off their bikes before a big climb, because bottles of water weigh you down.

Of course, most of us could save money by foregoing the expensive carbon gear and shed a few pounds off our human frames. The single best measure of your cycling performance is your power-to-weight ratio: the maximum power output measured in watts that you can sustain for an extended period of time, generally 30 minutes or more.

Expert coach Joe Friel, creator of the Training Bible series (and somewhat of a cycling scientist) has calculated that successful elite women cyclists

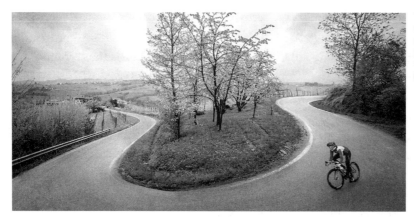

The reward for working your way up the mountain is coming back down. Always look where you want to go. Your bike will follow.

have 1.9 to 2.2 pounds of body weight per inch of height. (This isn't an exact measure of power-to-weight ratio, but it's close, and it doesn't require an expensive power meter to figure out.) By comparison, top male riders generally carry in the range of 2.1 to 2.4 pounds per inch.

For elite climbing specialists, those numbers drop, because weight becomes more of a consideration as the pull of gravity increases up those 10 percent grades. Pro climbing specialists in the female peloton carry about 1.8 or less pounds per inch. Top elite male climbers generally have less than 2 pounds of body weight per inch of height. That means a 5-foot-5-inch-tall woman should tip the scales at 117 and a 5-foot-10 man would need to weigh 140 pounds—yeah, *really* light. But again, we're talking pro Tour-caliber cyclists.

Coming Down the Mountain

Kelly Szymczyk had been a Spinning instructor for a dozen years, but buying a road bike didn't make her take a shine to riding outside. "My husband would ride, but frankly I was scared. There's that bike-handling thing you don't have to do indoors. We weren't in the most bike-friendly place in Alabama. I had little kids. I was tired—and full of excuses." When her husband's job was transferred and they relocated to Pennsylvania, with its wide-open, cycling-friendly country roads, at the end of 2009, she was determined to give it another go. "No excuses anymore!"

She wasted no time and joined the Harrisburg Bicycle Club first thing. "I didn't know the roads and I wanted to meet people to ride with," she says. Once she got the right gearing and learned to climb, she started seeking bigger, longer climbs, only to encounter a more daunting obstacle—descents.

Her first big one was Kings Gap, a gradual 5 to 6 percent climb that ascends for 4 miles. Once over the top, she pointed her bike down the mountain and started freaking out. "It was switchback-y and there was some gravel on the shoulders. I rode my brakes so hard all the way down, I was smelling rubber," she recalls. "The whole thing was very uncomfortable. My shoulders were so tensed up, I felt like my traps were hanging off my ears! My hands were completely cramped up and beet red by the time I got to the bottom."

Though she's gotten more comfortable since then, Kelly still doesn't like to descend with her hands in the drops, and she still takes her time. "I'm a very cautious descender, but getting more comfortable with it. I feather the brakes more and I am learning to relax and enjoy the air as I go down." Relaxing is good, because it's the stuff you do when you're nervous and tense that actually makes descending more dangerous.

That said, fear helps keep us alive, and it's natural to be afraid when you're pushing 30, 40, maybe 50 mph on two wheels. Descending also doesn't come naturally. Your first instincts (like, *Brake—hard!*) can send you to the ground instead of just slowing you down. It takes finesse and confidence, both of which are built with practice. "There are even some pros who don't descend correctly," says Stieda, "because they're either nervous or don't practice it enough." Here's what to do.

PRACTICE THE PROPER POSITION

Start with a short, straight downhill you can descend with no brakes to practice riding in the proper descending position—a key element in making it to the bottom both safely and quickly. "New riders often sit bolt upright because they don't like how they speed up when they're in the drops," says Applegate. "But that's a very unstable position, because your weight is too high and generally too far forward."

Instead, place your hands in the drops and shift your rear end back, which keeps your weight evenly distributed on the bike. "This position lowers your center of gravity, keeps the rear wheel firmly on the ground, and makes the bike more predictable and stable," says Applegate. "It also gives you more leverage with the brakes."

USE A HIGH GEAR

Depending on the pitch of the descent, you may need to pedal, or you might choose to coast all the way down. Either way, use a high gear. A little tension in the chain helps you control the bike.

STAY RELAXED

Start at the top of your body and let go of tension. Keep breathing, open your mouth to unclench your jaw, drop your shoulders, bend your elbows, release your death grip on the bar, uncurl your toes, and let your feet lie flat on the bottoms of your shoes.

SCAN AHEAD

The most important law of safe descending (and cornering, which we'll discuss next) is to look where you want the bike to go. The bike will follow your head and eye. When going through corners on a descent, "flatten the curve" by starting wide (without crossing the yellow line, of course), cutting through the apex of the turn, and exiting wide. Keep your eyes on the exit, which will help you carve a smooth, steady line all the way through. Looking ahead will also give you time to react to any potential dangers, like gravel and potholes.

SCRUB SPEED

Control your speed by feathering the brakes rather than grabbing fistfuls of them. Be *very* careful when braking in turns. When you brake, your bike stands up and goes straight—the opposite of what you want it to do to negotiate a turn. For controlled slowing, gently squeeze both levers equally in 2- to 3-second pulses. Constantly riding the brakes on big descents can make rims overheat, which can cause a tire blowout. Feather your brakes ahead of time so you're going at a comfortable speed when you get to a turn.

Be sure to brake with both hands. Hitting the front brake too hard makes the bike very difficult to handle and may even send you over the handlebars. Hitting just the back brake will cause the rear wheel to skid out, but won't stop you very well. Use both evenly to slow the bike while still keeping it under control.

You can also "pull your parachute" somewhat and use your body as a brake to slow down on long descents. Simply make yourself big, so you catch all the wind you can (if you have a jacket on, you actually will look like a parachute from behind when you do this). You can even stand up on the pedals (though keeping your weight on the back) to increase the resistance. It's an easy way to slow down without braking.

LEAN IN TO TURNS

Steer by leaning your bike, not your body. Extend your outside knee and press heavily into that pedal as you approach the turn to keep pressure on your tires. Drop the other knee to the inside, which will automatically shift your hips and shoulders into the turn and the direction you want to go. The faster and sharper the turn, the more you'll lean the bike. This action is similar to downhill skiing: The lower body angulates into the turn while the upper body remains upright. To exit the turn, gently straighten the bike.

Carve Through Corners

The shortest distance between point A and point B is a straight line, which you rarely find when you're out on a bicycle. More often, you encounter swooping curves, hairpins, and every type of angle. Corners and curves are some of what makes the sport so fun. But they definitely add an element of danger when taken at speed, which is why so many riders get hung up in them.

However, mastering corners is a huge advantage that will give you a leg up in races and even on competitive group rides. And it's just plain fun, as *Bicycling* pro columnist Stieda told us with this great anecdote:

"As a pro cyclist, I worked to improve my cornering skills. During a stage of the Tour of Britain, I remembered there was a turn 400 meters before the line. I attacked early, railed the corner, and opened a gap. I raised my arms in victory at the finish, only to be told that this

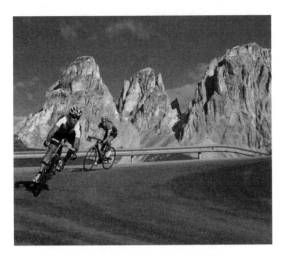

The key to cornering is that your torso stays mostly upright while you lean into the turn with your lower body and the bike.

gesture was against the rules. I was relegated to last in the break, but relished the fact that my strategy had worked," he says. Once you feel the power and control of a properly carved turn, there is nothing better. It takes practice, so be patient. Find an empty parking lot and mark off a corner with water bottles or cones. Here are some of his and other pros' tips.

STAY LOOSE

You corner with your whole body—hips, feet, hands, torso. If you tense up and get rigid, you'll end up straightening your arms and pushing the bike to the outside. At best you'll be fighting your bike through the turn. At worst, you're going down. As you approach a turn, consciously relax your hands and arms, so you have a firm, but not tight grip on the bars and your upper body feels loose.

APPLY PRESSURE

Feather the brakes as you approach the corner, squeezing the levers just enough to caress the rims. You should barely feel your weight going into your bars. If your weight shifts forward, you're squeezing too hard. Again, braking makes your bike sit up and straighten out— neither will help you negotiate a turn. The goal is to brake enough before the turn so that you can lean and coast through it with minimal, if any, braking, and then pedal out of the turn. Weight distribution is critical: To keep from sliding out, weight the front wheel by putting your hands in the drops of the handlebars with your elbows bent. Next, exert pressure with your outside hand and foot, creating angulation like you would in a ski turn. Don't try to pedal in a corner.

Note: Here's where mountain biking rules are a bit different because of the tires and terrain. When you're on the dirt, you can carry your speed longer, brake later (and harder), and whip your bike through the turn with your hips and torso, allowing the back wheel to drift a little. You wouldn't do that on a road bike.

LEAN THE MACHINE

Release the brakes and start the turn by leaning the bike—not your body—into the turn. To do this, push lightly with your inside hand; some call this counter-steering. If the turn is tight or your speed increases, lean the bike farther in, and vice versa. Once you have that down, you can progress to an advanced, über-pro move called "ankling," which helps you keep even more speed in corners. As you go into the corner—outside foot down and weighted, inside foot up, body leaning in—bend your ankles sideways toward the inside of the corner. The move slightly repositions your body and weight to better drive your bike around the corner. That's an advanced move, so try it on a flat road before using it on any descents.

START OUTSIDE; AIM INSIDE

As mentioned earlier, you want to flatten the curve as much as possible, creating what is in essence a straighter line through it. To carve a smooth arc through the apex of the turn, start at the outside of the corner, near the center line of the road (but not crossing or even touching it). Aim toward the inside of the turn, then exit as far to the outside as possible. Do not cross any yellow line.

KEEP LOOKING

Look in the direction you want to go. This will help you maintain a smooth line. Pay attention to what some pros call your "third eye" (your navel). That, too, should be "looking" in the direction you want to go in, as it ensures that your hips and torso are carrying you through the turn.

MAKE YOUR EXIT

As you come out of the turn, gradually straighten the bike until it's upright, then start to pedal again. Your goal is to slow down going in and accelerate out of every turn.

MIND THE RAIN AND OTHER SLIPPERY THINGS

Painted lines, manhole covers, and oily pavement become slippery in wet conditions. Wet roads exaggerate everything you do: Braking while the bike is leaning will cause you to skid more easily, and sudden turning can make your wheels slip. So slow down. Same thing with grit and gravel and other loose debris on the road. Respect the terrain and the surface and adjust your speed accordingly.

DRILL THOSE SKILLS

Coaches like Carl Cantrell of Alamogordo, New Mexico, ask their racers to practice cornering drills, much like swimmers practice their pull and kick and runners do strides. The idea is to make the right motions automatic, so there's no thinking required when you approach the real thing. Here's what he recommends.

CIRCLES. Put your bike in a low gear and ride in slow left-hand circles, gradually picking up speed and bringing the circle tighter and tighter until you feel the rear wheel break traction. That's your tipping point. Get a feel for that point and get comfortable riding within it. Practice in both directions.

FIGURE EIGHTS. Once you've got circles down, move on to figure eights, which are perfect practice for real-life riding because you have to change directions quickly to maintain control. This is where you should really feel countersteering at work.

CHAPTER 8

Pacelines, Packs, and Group Riding

CYCLING IS A SOCIAL SPORT, AND CYCLISTS BY AND LARGE travel in pelotons or packs. The reasons for this go beyond making small talk down the road, however. Like geese in echelon flight, cyclists can travel farther and faster when in a wind-cheating formation like a paceline (with all riders in a tight single- or double-file line, taking turns at being in the front pulling the others along) or peloton. Drafting, as it's called, lets you use 30 percent less effort when you tuck yourself into the air current coming off a rider in front of you.

The irony here is that this same energy-saving arrangement can be absolutely nerve-racking for some riders, because you're literally inches away from one another's wheels. It's also most certainly not a women's specific issue. Plenty of men find themselves struggling to fit in seamlessly when it's time to ride in formation, especially pacelines, which are governed by many unspoken rules you'll never find out about if no one tells you.

Take Vicki Ford, who encountered a paceline during her first big ride and hated it. "I kept thinking, 'I don't want to screw up the person behind me and I'm afraid of running into the person in front of me.' I would try and get up to the rear tire of the rider in front of me and just freak out worrying I'd crash. They didn't give me a lot of advice." She's made it her goal to master pacelining, but it hasn't happened thus far.

Then there was Matt Cook, who also was completely unnerved by riding in such close proximity to others. He got dropped over and over (and over) on many group rides because he was simply too freaked out to stay in a paceline. "I had a terrible time with it. I'm a big guy, so I make a good draft, but when I'd pull off the front, the riders would whizz by and I got dropped about 75 percent of the time. I couldn't accelerate to close the gap. Sometimes it was tough to even hold the draft. I'd get dropped on the bridges and when the group was hit with a crosswind."

Fortunately Matt fell in with a group of advice-sharing, sage riders. "There were 20 to 25 people in the local group, and I got a lot of schooling about soft pedaling versus coasting, keeping off the brakes, how to shift to maintain my speed and cadence, and how to look at the grass to find where the wind is coming from so I can tuck in on the correct side to get a good draft and keep the line."

Join the Pack

Matt clearly got some good schooling because he stuck with it and shed more than 15 pounds in the process. I won't lie. Group riding can be tricky business no matter how long you've been riding, and it's even harder if you only do it occasionally and/or with unfamiliar riders. But there are some tricks of the trade that can lessen the learning curve and help you feel more comfortable with your place in any pack, peloton, or paceline. Here's what you need to know.

UNDERSTAND THE EXPECTATIONS

Group rides are a bit like snowflakes in that no two are exactly alike, though all are similar. Most have a certain "way" about them. Sometimes that way is expressed outright: "We roll at an average 16.8 mph, double paceline, no one is dropped." Others are a bit more organic, depending upon who shows up. Some will always ride in an organized paceline. Other packs are pretty loose, falling into a line when it makes sense, breaking up and chitchatting when space allows. If it's not clear, you can always ask the riders in the lead; they'll let you know. Ultimately, remember, it's your responsibility to know the expectations of the group you're joining. If they're a "no drop" ride, then you know that even if you fall off the back, someone will wait—and you'll have to wait if others drift off. If it's not, then the pack will move at the majority speed and the stragglers will be left behind to fend for themselves.

Once you find your group, the number one rule is to ride predictably. Even if the group is casual, it's important that the riders around you be able to anticipate your actions. That means riding in a straight line (and holding your line), keeping a fairly steady pace, and not making any sudden stops or swerves without alerting the rest of the riders.

RELAX

Your bike always handles better when it's not held in a death grip. So take a deep breath and relax your shoulders and arms. Keep a little bend in your elbows. Smile. Once you relax and get the hang of it, being swept along with a group of cyclists is fun. You can go faster using less energy, and it just plain feels cool to zip along at speeds you simply couldn't sustain by your lonesome.

When the pack forms a paceline:

START SLOWLY

If you're new to paceline riding, get comfortable by starting slowly and positioning yourself a bit farther back than directly behind the rear wheel in front of you. You can enjoy huge drafting benefits from even 2 feet away. So start there, but don't drift *too* far back. You'll lose the draft and break the rhythm of the line. Remember, relax and stay loose. As you get more comfortable, move in a bit closer. Ideally, you want to be just about a foot (or less, if you're *really* comfortable) away from the back wheel in front of you. You may also feel more comfortable riding a few inches to one side or the other of the wheel in front of you, as that will give you a little more reaction time should that rider do something unpredictable. Once you get about a wheel length away from the rider in front of you, you'll start to enjoy the benefits of drafting.

KEEP THE PACE

The number one mistake riders make is picking up speed when they get to the front, notes Ray Ignosh, a former USA Cycling expert coach based in Lehigh Valley, Pennsylvania. "Some riders just want to show off; others are well-intentioned—they just aren't in tune with their effort and feel like they're supposed to take a pull, so they pull." As you're riding through the line, pay attention to the group's average speed and effort. When you get to the front, do your best to maintain those levels. The goal is to keep the pack together, not blow it apart or shell riders off the back.

DON'T STARE

Focusing on the wheel directly in front of you is a natural instinct when riding in a line, but it gives you zero time to react should something go awry. It's like driving in heavy traffic. You don't stare at the car directly in front of you. You look down the road to see what traffic is doing. The same rule applies here. "Keep your head up and check about 10 meters down the road," says Ignosh. "Look through holes in the leading rider—over the shoulder, under the arm,

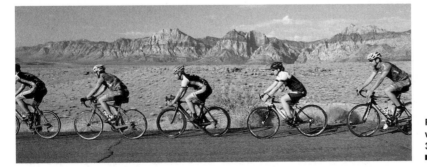

Pacelines let you get where you're going with 30 percent less effort.

or through the legs—and ride proactively instead of reactively. This will help keep the line moving smoothly."

WATCH YOUR FRONT WHEEL

Do not overlap your front wheel with the wheel you're following. If that rider has to swerve suddenly to miss an obstacle and hits you, you'll be the one to hit the pavement when her wheel taps into you.

MICROADJUST

It's nearly impossible for everyone to put forth equal amounts of effort, especially on undulating terrain. You need to make adjustments along the way to prevent what Ignosh calls the Slinky effect, where the line alternately bunches together and becomes strung out, with big gaps. "It's better to make two small undercorrections than one big overcorrection," he says. "Again, think of it like driving: You don't slam on the brakes, then hit the gas; you moderate your speed." To do that in a paceline, try one of these techniques:

SOFT PEDAL: If you feel like you're getting sucked into the rider in front of you, take a light pedal stroke or two where you barely press down on the pedals to adjust your speed accordingly.

AIR BRAKE: An easy (and safe) way to trim speed is to sit up and catch some wind. It'll slow you down a notch without disrupting the rhythm of the line.

FEATHER BRAKES: Gently squeeze the brakes while continuing to pedal. You can scrub speed while shifting up or down as needed to alter your pace.

SHARE AND SHARE ALIKE

Don't feel like you have to sit up there and pull everyone along for 30 miles. Pacelines work best when the lead riders limit themselves to ½-mile pulls because it keeps everyone fresh. So limit your pulls to a few minutes to stay fresh and give other riders a chance.

PULL OFF; PULL THROUGH

When the rider at the front is ready for a break, she checks behind for oncoming cars, then drifts to the left and allows the pack to pull forward. She then drifts back, taking her place at the end of the train. Sometimes it's helpful to point left or flick your elbow as you're ready to pull off so the rider behind you is fully aware of your intentions.

Be careful to keep your speed relatively constant and decelerate just slightly as you drift to the back of the line. "New riders often slow down too much, then they have to accelerate too hard to catch the line and eventually pop off the back," says Andy Applegate at Carmichael Training Systems in Asheville, North Carolina. "Keep pedaling at a moderately fast pace, so people aren't whipping by you. Be sure to stay close enough to the line, so you're still catching a draft as they are going by; it will help you maintain contact. Then start sneaking over as the last rider goes by."

CLIMB WITH CARE

It's hard to keep a paceline together when the road tilts up. It's wise to give the rider in front of you a little more space when climbing, because she may slow down or stand up.

Standing is particularly troublesome because there's a tendency for your bike to drift back (and potentially into the wheel behind you) when you stand. If you do need to get out of the saddle, shift up a gear so you don't drift back when you stand, and if you're in a close group, announce "Standing!" before you get up.

CALL OUT CARS AND OTHER HAZARDS

Communication is key to safe, happy group riding. The riders in front call out oncoming hazards like potholes, gravel, roadkill, cars pulling out of driveways, and so on by pointing down and calling out, "Gravel!" "Hole!" etc. They should also call out turns and stop signs well in advance so the pack can prepare. The caboose in the back alerts the pack to approaching cars (unless, of course, you're on a heavily trafficked road) by calling out, "Car back!" Everyone is responsible for keeping the pack together. If you see someone falling back, call, "Sit up" or "Soft pedal."

If you get a flat tire or develop another problem that forces you to stop quickly, don't panic. Just yell out, "Stopping!" and try to keep your forward momentum going as best you can as the other riders scurry around you.

EAT AND DRINK IN THE BACK

Save your drinking, eating, and nose blowing for the back of the line, where your sudden movements won't disrupt the flow of motion.

CONSERVE YOUR ENERGY

If you feel tired, sit out a few turns until you're ready to take another pull. Simply open a spot for riders to rejoin the line in front of you, or come to the front and immediately pull off and drift to the back. You'll do the pack a favor by staying with them rather than working yourself into the red and falling off the back, which makes the group slow down to let you catch up.

DO THE DOUBLE

If your group is large (say, more than a half-dozen riders), it makes sense to ride two-by-two in a double paceline. (Though do first check that your state allows cyclists to ride two abreast.) Different rules apply, depending on the group. Sometimes the echelon is in constant rotation, with the inside line moving faster than the outside line. In this case, if you are the front rider on the inside, you start drifting left as soon as the rider in front of you has moved left and drifted a bike length back. Then you drift back and the next front rider drifts to the left-hand line. This is pretty tricky to pull off, and it tends to be more erratic and punchy than other formations, so weaker riders often get shelled off

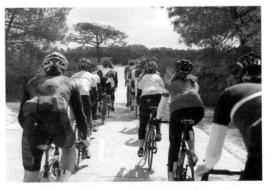

When you've got a big group, it's wise to double up. Cars need to go wider to pass, but the passing distance required is shorter than if you're all strung out single file.

Group Dynamics 101

Got all the ins and outs of pack riding etiquette? Sit in for a moment, take this quiz, and see.

1. It's your turn at the front. You gracefully slide into position, then . . .

A. Accelerate to drag the line with you.

B. Maintain the average pace of the group.

C. Adjust your speed to accommodate all levels of effort within the pack.

2. Midpack riders are not expected to point out hazards or announce traffic.

TRUE Only the lead and rearmost riders can see what's going on from ahead and behind.

FALSE It is every rider's responsibility to relay messages through the pack—whether from front to back or vice versa.

3. If you don't feel up to taking a pull . . .

A. Ride near the back. You'll do the pack a favor by conserving energy.

B. Suck it up. You made a commitment to the group and it's your turn to pull.

C. Do your best to stay as close as possible to the lead rider.

4. When rising from the saddle on a climb . . .

A. Do it quickly while pedaling harder to keep the pace.

B. Decelerate to give yourself room, then put all your power into the pedals.

C. Shift up a gear first, to adjust for a slower cadence, then pedal smoothly.

5. It is common courtesy for the group to accommodate every rider who shows up.

TRUE Everyone is there with the same goal— to enjoy a nice day on two wheels. All skill levels should be tolerated.

FALSE The group has a set pace and it's up to you to ask questions to determine if it's the right fit for you.

---

the back. In the easier technique, the front riders both pull to their respective outsides and the riders behind pull through, allowing them to drift back. When riding in this formation, take care to stay even with the rider at your side. Riding a little bit faster or ahead of them is called "half wheeling" and considered bad form.

MIND INTERSECTIONS

Intersections pose unique problems for cyclists riding in a pack. In some cases, when there's little traffic and a cohesive group, you can treat the pack as one vehicle and all cross together (as in the case of stop signs). In the case of traffic lights, however, it's never okay to blow the light just because the front half of the pack made it through and you don't want to get dropped. In that case, the lead group should simply soft pedal until the light changes and the rest of the riders have pulled through and caught back up. It's a nice gesture to yell, "Clear" when going through an inter-

6. You're coming up on fresh, buggy roadkill. You should . . .

A. Point to the deceased or call out its presence, then shift your line in advance.

B. Swoop around it as you get close.

C. Do nothing. Interrupting the flow of the ride is a no-no.

7. At an intersection, it is not the lead rider's sole responsibility to get the group through safely.

TRUE Though everyone is riding as one group, each individual must look out for his or her own safety.

FALSE Whoever is at the front of the pack at the time calls the shots for everyone else.

8. Your eyes should always be focused . . .

A. On the rider directly in front of you.

B. Around or beyond the riders ahead of you.

C. On the ground, where potholes, glass, gravel, and other debris lurk.

9. If a few riders fall off the back or get hung up at a stoplight, the lead pack should . . .

A. Pull over and wait for them to catch up.

B. Keep the pace; everyone knows the route.

C. Soft pedal until they rejoin the group.

10. In a paceline, your front wheel starts to overlap the rear wheel of the rider in front of you. You . . .

A. Call out "Wheel overlap!" to give the rider fair warning.

B. Speed up until half of your front wheel overlaps his or her rear wheel.

C. Drift back into position; the rider ahead of you should maintain his or her line and cadence.

D. Slap yourself for half-wheeling and humbly excuse yourself to the back of the pack.

ANSWERS: 1. B; 2. False; 3. A; 4. C; 5. False; 6. A; 7. True; 8. B; 9. C; 10. C

section to let riders behind you know that no cars are coming (or yell, "Car left" or "Car right" if there are oncoming vehicles in either direction), but ultimately *every rider is responsible to look left and right and be sure the coast is clear* as they ride through an intersection of any kind.

PICK YOUR PACELINE

On big group rides, the pack will generally splinter into smaller packs and pacelines. So if you find yourself in one that is disintegrating into a Darwinian survival-of-the-fittest hammerfest where riders are ratcheting up the pace every time they take the lead and spitting riders off the back like so much litter, and you don't feel like playing along, simply drift back and find another group to join. By the same token, if the pack you're in is poking along and you're feeling frisky, don't feel bad about bidding them adieu and finding a faster flock. The goal is to have fun out there, so find yours.

CHAPTER 9

Life on the Road

I GENERALLY TRY TO AVOID SWEEPING GENERALIZATIONS when it comes to gender. But sometimes the facts are just the facts. Women are less inclined to participate in activities they feel are risky. Yes, there are exceptions. There always are. But there's a reason that there are far more men racing motorcycles, dirt jumping, skateboarding, mountain biking, and bike racing, even just riding bikes regularly. We can debate all day whether it's a matter of nature (preservation of the species and all), nurture (how we're brought up), societal, or a cocktail of all of the above, but the numbers are the numbers.

Women still lag behind men in our sport, especially in areas where they feel it's not safe. New York City, for instance, lags behind San Francisco, Portland, Oregon, and Washington, DC, in the proportion of riders who are female. Many cities, like New York, are working hard to lay down miles of protected bike lanes and paths to encourage more people—especially women—to ride. In the meantime, let's talk about the realities of risk and how to stay safe out there on the road.

Cycling is getting safer all the time. According to research compiled by Rutgers researchers, fatalities per 10 million bike trips plummeted 65 percent between 1977 and 2009, from 5.1 to 1.8 fatalities per 10 million trips. Those are pretty good odds.

What's more, states are increasingly enacting "3-foot or 4-foot laws" requiring motorists to stay a certain distance away from a rider when they pass and other legislation designed to help cyclists share the road with less risk.

Finally, though you can't control motorists, you *can* control how you ride, which goes a long way to keeping you safe. It's also important to note that most cycling accidents aren't because of cars. They're simply accidents. Cyclists bumping into each other. Cyclists overcooking corners. You know, the stuff accidents are made of. While it's true that if you ride long enough, you're bound to fall down at some point, it generally doesn't result in more than scrapes and minor injuries. Like most accidents in life, cycling wrecks are also largely preventable. Here's how to ride smart and safe.

Share the Road

You've seen the road signs: a car and a cyclist peacefully sharing the pavement. Those signs generally serve as reminders to motorists, but cyclists need to take heed too. When you ride on the roads, you need to follow the rules of the road, same as you would if you were behind the wheel. First and foremost, that means riding in the same direction as traffic (so on the right-hand side in the United States).

Some riders mistakenly believe they'll be safer if they can see oncoming cars. Nothing could be further from the truth. Riding against traffic is dangerous and a leading cause of bike-related accidents. Why? Physics. Let's say you're riding along at 15 mph and oncoming traffic is flowing at 45 mph. The combined speed that you and any given car are approaching each other is 60 mph. That leaves very little reaction time for either of you should something go awry (like you swerve to miss a pothole). Now turn yourself around and ride the right way with the flow of traffic. Cars are now approaching you at just 30 mph. Drivers have more time to see you and maneuver around you. You're also a more predictable part of traffic flow. Statistically speaking, getting struck from behind when you're riding with the flow of traffic makes up a small percentage of bike accidents. When you ride predictably, cars can accommodate you.

So you know to ride on the right. But how far to the right? That depends. If there's a bike lane, that's your best bet (though realize that sometimes you'll need to leave the lane to avoid obstacles like parked cars). If there's no designated bike lane, ride on the shoulder to allow cars to pass freely with a good bit of buffer room. If there is not much shoulder, you should ride a bit more *into* the lane rather than trying to squeeze onto 2 inches of pavement. Think of it this way: If you cram yourself onto the edge of the road, 1) cars will squeak by you too close for comfort, and 2) you leave yourself no bailout room should you need to move to miss an obstacle. By riding a bit more in the lane, you have a little bail-out room on the right and you're making cars perform a clean pass around you, which results in there being more space between you.

This isn't too difficult on country or low-traffic roads. Riding in the city or on more turbulent streets takes a bit more finesse. These tips will help you flow with heavier traffic.

TAKE THE LANE

Ride well into the lane when traffic is stop-and-go. You can usually move at least as fast as cars in heavy traffic, but if you hug the curb, you're less visible and drivers will be tempted to squeeze by you. Stay far enough in the traffic lane to avoid being struck if doors on parked cars are suddenly opened (an unpleasant type of accident called "being doored"). You might hear some honking from motorists who don't understand why you won't pull to the right to let them pass, but a honk in your ear hurts less than a door in your face.

When you stop at a light, move to the center of your lane. This prevents drivers from edging forward, trapping you between them and the curb. When the light changes, accelerate to your cruising speed before moving right to allow them to pass.

On a road with no shoulder, ride in the right wheel track of motor vehicles to ensure you don't blend into the scenery along the edge of the road. This also gives you 3 to 4 feet of space from the edge of the pavement to let you dodge potholes or deal with wind gusts.

WATCH THE WHEELS

When you see cars stopped at cross streets, watch the front wheels for the first hint of forward movement. If you see any, get ready to brake, and yell to get the driver's attention, because they likely don't see you.

SCAN THE WINDOWS AND MIRRORS

Keeping an eye on the side view mirrors and through the rear windows of parked cars will help you spot someone who might suddenly pull out into your lane or throw open a door. You can also use this method to spot pedestrians about to step out from between cars.

HOLD YOUR LINE

Ride in a straight line past cars that are intermittently parallel parked—don't weave in and out of empty spaces. Drivers might not be ready for you to suddenly reemerge into the traffic lane. When you're in a bike lane and a car is making a right turn in front of your path, do not swerve out to the left and around. Slow down, stay in the lane, wait for the car to turn, then proceed.

GRASP THE BARS

Sure, you may be heading out for a training ride on your tricked-out tri bike, but stay off the aero-bars in traffic. It's just not safe. Similarly, no matter how comfortable you are riding no-handed or otherwise, wrap your thumbs around your handlebars and have full grasp of the bars when riding in traffic. Even very seasoned pros have been known to hit the deck because their hands are jarred off the bar when they hit a bump.

SIGNAL YOUR INTENTIONS

Use hand signals to indicate your intention to turn left or right or let drivers know they should pass. It shows you're aware of their presence and gives them more information. Forget fancy hand and arm signals. Simply point straight out with your right arm when you want to go right, point with your left arm when you want to go left, and place an arm out and down with your palm facing the driver to let them know that you're stopping or slowing.

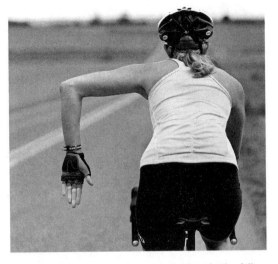

You wouldn't stop and turn in your car without letting fellow drivers know your intentions. Use your signals every time you ride.

LOOK BACK

Sometimes you need to cross through moving traffic to get into a turning lane (which shouldn't happen too often). Maneuver just as you would in a car. Look behind to find a break in the traffic and signal your move. Then move confidently over.

Important note here: Simply glancing back with your hands on the brake hoods may work, but this method often causes the bar to turn in the direction you're looking. This way is better: To look left, move your right hand toward the center of the handlebars near the stem, then drop your left hand off the bar as you turn your head to look back. Keep your upper body relaxed the entire time. Make sure to practice, ideally in an empty parking lot with lines you can follow.

LOOK 'EM IN THE EYE

When possible, make eye contact with drivers. This ensures that they see you. It also reminds them that you're a living, breathing human being, not an annoying obstacle. Smiling and waving goes a long way, too.

RIDE SINGLE FILE WHEN POSSIBLE

Save the double paceline and pack formations for the open roads. When you're in urban areas or on busy roads, single up.

PRACTICE COMMON COURTESY

Finally, be polite. Give cars room as you can. Don't cruise past a line of cars at a stoplight, forcing drivers to pass you again if they had trouble passing you the first time. You may

Danger Zones

Be extra vigilant during these traffic situations, which generate the three most common driver errors resulting in car–bike crashes.

➤ When an oncoming motorist turns left in front of you while you're going straight through an intersection. Drivers often underestimate how fast you're going on a bike. Keep your head up and watch for turn signals and angling front wheels.

➤ When a driver fails to obey a stop sign and pulls out in front of you. Take it easy through all intersections. Better to have to come to a stop than hit a car or be hit by one.

➤ When a vehicle passes you and immediately turns right, across your path. Taking the lane helps prevent this situation. But when you're on the shoulder or in a bike lane, keep an eye out when a car overtakes you close to an intersection. Look for their turn signal and the front wheel changing direction, and give them plenty of buffer room just in case.

occasionally encounter a mad motorist. Resist the urge to engage in a war of finger-flipping and name-calling. It's not a battle you'll win and it doesn't help the next cyclist who comes along. By and large, people are polite if you're polite to them. And if they're not, being polite tends to diffuse jerks more effectively than throwing insults—the verbal equivalent of lighter fluid—on them.

LOOK AND LISTEN

Whether you're out on a country road or in downtown DC, pay attention, just as you would while driving. Use your senses—often you can hear an engine in advance of seeing the car, and see or hear a dog before it chases. Problem sounds include tires squealing, high engine acceleration, and loud music from an open window. Those are all sounds that indicate it might be a good idea to pull over and let the vehicle pass.

CHOOSE LOW-TRAFFIC ROUTES

Seems obvious, but it's worth mentioning. The best roads have few cars, low speed limits, and no blind corners. Often, a slightly longer route with fewer cars will be faster than a shorter, busier one. Also, try to find roads with a shoulder you can ride on.

DON'T DRINK AND RIDE

The worst wrecks I've seen—those that have led to brain injuries and extended hospitalizations—haven't been because of cars, they've been because of booze. National Highway Traffic Safety Administration statistics have consistently pointed to drunken riding as the culprit behind about a quarter of fatal wrecks among riders over age 16. Riding a bike requires balance. Alcohol makes you tipsy. The two don't mix very well.

Beware Common Road Hazards

No matter who you are or where you ride, there are common road hazards you're bound to encounter, like train tracks, potholes, and slippery surfaces. Here's how to negotiate them like a pro. (In fact, all these tips came courtesy of former Olympian and current USA Cycling coach David Brinton, who rides bikes for a living—and as a professional stuntman, he used to get paid to crash them, too.)

GRAVELLY OR CHIP-SEALED ROADS. "It's better to pedal through gravelly roads than to coast," says Brinton. Propulsion provides stability. There is such a thing as too much speed, though. If you start sliding, back off the power (without braking) while staying in the saddle to keep your bike planted.

GRAVELED CORNERS. Road debris gets kicked to the outside of the road, often leaving corners filled with sketchy debris exactly where you want maximum traction. If you can't avoid the gravel, you need to try to go into it in the most stable position possible. Take the turn wide and lean your bike more than normal at the beginning. Straighten the bike as you approach the gravel, then, once on clear road, resume leaning. "It's pretty much the opposite of how I recommend riding corners in normal conditions," says Brinton.

WET ROADS. Be extra cautious during the first 10 minutes of a rainstorm, when oil and dust have floated to the pavement's surface, creating a slick film but haven't yet washed

Hey, Baby!

Whether you're walking down the street or pedaling along a country road, as a woman, you're always vulnerable to the errant catcall. Generally, it's nothing but annoying (and to be fair, men in Lycra are also subjected to verbal assaults by the rude boys—in fact, some of the guys I ride with seem to get harassed far more than I've ever been). As with any jerk encounter, it's best to ignore it. Practice all those anti-bullying tips you learned in school: Look strong and confident, and keep on pedaling. You may even be pleasantly surprised sometimes; I've rolled past stereotypical trouble zones like construction sites and gotten only sincere thumbs-ups and even a few friendly—not lurid—cheers.

away. To turn, exaggerate the normal cornering technique of driving weight into the lowered, outside pedal. This helps your tires grip the road as much as possible.

Painted road lines and metal surfaces (manhole covers, grates, railroad tracks, bridge decks, and expansion joints) get slippery right away and stay treacherous until they completely dry. "The slickest parts of any wet road are the lane markings," says Brinton. To stay safe, cross road lanes at as close to a right angle as you can. If you get forced onto a slick road line, avoid an abrupt reaction. "Clear the line gradually," he advises.

You should always try to cross railroad tracks at as close to perpendicular as possible. That's even more important when they're wet. If possible, cross railroad tracks near the side of the road, as well. It's usually smoother there than in the center, where traffic has worn down the pavement.

POTHOLES. Swerving around potholes makes sense—unless there's traffic or you're surprised by one while riding in the middle of a group. Learn to lightly roll or hop over potholes. Master popping the front wheel over small cracks by pulling up lightly on the bars. Once you can do that, practice popping the rear wheel over the same crack by rising out of the saddle and pulling up with your feet. When you can clear both wheels separately, combine the two maneuvers. With your pedals parallel to the road, pull up on the handlebars while lifting your feet. "For most potholes you don't even need a full bunny hop," says Brinton. "At 25 miles per hour, all you really need to do is take a little bit of your bike weight off the road and your wheels will float right over."

PARALLEL CRACKS. If your wheel gets caught in a large crack running the length of the street, chances are you'll make intimate contact with said street. To cross a parallel crack without getting a flat tire, lean your bike slightly toward the damaged pavement, then pop your front wheel sideways so it clears the crack. If your wheels get caught in the crack, pull directly up on the front wheel, and it will automatically pop out and to the side.

ROADKILL, ROCKS, TRASH. The rule of object avoidance is to look past it, not *at* it. If you lock your peepers on poor deceased Rocky Raccoon, you will soon find yourself careening straight into his decaying carcass, because your bike goes where your eyes focus. Look past obstacles to where you want your wheels to roll. And as a rule of thumb, look about 20 yards up the road, not 5.

COBBLED AND BRICK ROADS. Those yellow bricks might lead you to the Great and Mighty Oz, but first you'll need to pull a bit of wizardry of your own to negotiate them. "Avoid death-gripping the handlebar," says Brinton, "and use your arms as a suspension system for the rest of your body." Push a bigger gear than normal, which will float your butt just above the saddle. Just like in mountain biking, let the bike find its own, natural line through cobbles. On brick roads, slot into the path smoothed out by car tires.

Who Let the Dogs Out?

You may never know who the hell opened the door and let that dog out, but once it's chasing you, it barely matters. If you ride in rural areas, you are bound to encounter a loose canine or two somewhere along the way. The good news is that they're generally friendly. The bad news is, it's hard to tell sometimes, and even a friendly dog is a menace when you're doing 18 mph on a bike and it's bounding your way. Keep these tips in mind should you end up being "hounded" on a ride.

DON'T PANIC. This is the No. 1 rule for safe cycling, and it applies here. Try not to swerve, even if you're riding alone. You don't want to crash yourself out before the dog even gets to you. If you can easily escape the dog by speeding up, do so. But don't try to flee a dog that's coming in close. Fleeing sends a signal to the pooch that he's predator and you're prey. It also encourages the dog to give chase.

ANTICIPATE. Canines are harder to anticipate than cars, but not all pose the same danger. Most run parallel to their target before drifting toward it, but these pups are usually all bark and no bite. The real threat comes from the ones brave or stupid enough to jump right in front of you.

BE THE AGGRESSOR. Dogs are among the few road hazards that can see you. Use this to your advantage. You can't intimidate a pothole or shout at a patch of gravel, but the best way to fend off hounds is to take their aggression and get all Alpha Dog on them. Very often a deep, guttural "GO HOME" will send the dog back to its territory, or at least attract the attention of the owner, who will call for the dog. Spraying the dog in the face with your water bottle (provided it's still within a safe distance and not an obviously aggressive dog) often repels it, too.

SHIELD YOURSELF. Should the dog not retreat and you feel seriously threatened, get off the bike and put it between you and the dog. Follow all the usual rules about aggressive dogs. Don't stare it right in the eyes, but keep an eye on it. Talk as nicely as you can to it. Avoid sudden moves. And stay calm until the dog's owner reels it in or the situation becomes safe (i.e., the dog leaves or help arrives).

PART IV

OFF THE BEATEN PATH

"Breckenridge, Colorado, is where I first decided that I would become a biker chick," Kelly Summers told me with pride as she relayed an awesome story of determination.

My husband and I were in Breck for the Fourth of July. They have a great parade that starts in the morning, so we got there early and set up. About a half hour before the parade starts, we heard lots and lots of cheering. There were hundreds of mountain bikers coming down Main Street. It was the start of the Firecracker 50 mountain bike race. The waves were broken into sections: men 50-plus, men 45 to 50, men 40 to 45, men 35 to 40, men singlespeed. Men. Men. Men. Men. Waves and waves of men. Then at the very end there was this sad little wave of women. Not waves of women. Just one, and there weren't that many. I looked at my husband and said, "We just saw about 500 men in various categories—and by the way, what the hell is a singlespeed?—and this is the women's field? I'm going to start racing mountain bikes!"

He laughed so hard he about fell out of his chair. He thought I was joking. Boy, was he wrong. Once we got back to Illinois, I researched and test rode literally dozens of bikes. Eventually, I bought a full-suspension 29er and that July 21st raced in my first competition—the Palos Meltdown. I raced beginner class and came in dead last. But damn if it wasn't awesome! Fast-forward to today: I am now selling my 29er because I want a 27.5. I have a cyclocross bike and just bought a fat bike 3 days ago. My husband bought a fat bike and also has a singlespeed (clearly, we figured out what that was!).

We have found an amazing community of cyclists in our area that we now call friends. We discuss and obsess about things such as SRAM versus Shimano and SPDs versus Eggbeaters—things that weren't even in our vocabulary a year ago. We are both fitter than we've ever been and have found a new way to stay outside all year-round. I still come in last in races, but I don't care. I'm having a blast! All because I realized that not enough women are in this sport and I wanted to help change that, one woman at a time.

How awesome is that? Kelly's story also illustrates something that is really awesome about cycling: While to the outside world it may look like cycling is a singular sport—and it kind of is, since it's all pursued on two wheels—what makes the sport so unique and engaging to so many is the fact that there are so many ways to engage in and enjoy it. Sure, you can ride on the road. But you can also buy a fat-tired, full-suspension 29er and ride that bike through places you would never, ever dream anyone could ride a bike. You can pick up cyclocross and go charging through sand and mud and gravel and grass. If you're lucky enough to live near a velodrome, you can even saddle up on a whippet-thin bike with no brakes and one giant fixed gear and race around a banked oval for fun and thrills.

The following chapters will introduce you to all the amazing types of riding you can do where the paved road ends. Women's participation in these different types of riding and racing, particularly mountain biking, still lags behind the boys', but it's growing as more women get involved and pull their friends and sisters along for the ride. One survey by Pinkbike.com found that a whopping 90 percent of women who got into mountain biking did so because a friend or partner invited them. In cyclocross, which is the country's fastest-growing cycling sport, the women's fields are growing exponentially. Ditto for ultracross (which is a combination of endurance, cyclocross, and "gravel grinder" riding). Even track-racing licenses are up among women, with national sensations like Sarah Hammer leading the charge.

These days, many riders—of both sexes—are like Kelly and her husband. They own multiple bikes, participate in all sorts of cycling types, and are always on the lookout for new ways to ride and enjoy the ride, even if they aren't particularly expert at all of them.

"What I love is the great variety of riding styles cycling offers," says Anneke Prins. "There's mountain biking, which I'm rubbish at, but it *always* puts a massive smile on my face. I'll be track racing later this year. And of course, there's the road. My bikes have all become my friends. We've shared some awesome times together."

Now it's your turn. Keep reading and let the awesome times roll.

CHAPTER 10

Take to the Trails

"WHEN MY HUSBAND FIRST PICKED UP RIDING, HE CHOSE mountain biking before road biking. Every other ride, he came home with new bruises, scrapes, and bleeders. That gave me pause, and when I started riding, I never thought I'd do mountain biking because I didn't want to come home looking like he did!" recalls Elizabeth Seifert. "But then I started doing really well on the road. I completed my first century and was climbing mountains in Georgia I never thought I could. So I thought maybe I could try mountain biking, too."

Elizabeth checked out a mountain bike demo day at her local trails, where a sales rep put her on a singlespeed mountain bike. "I rode it—and FELL in LOVE. Again! There was the joy of just being in the woods and the simplicity of the singlespeed. It was a new kind of heaven. I bought the bike on the spot. Then later bought another full-suspension bike with gears that I love, as well."

Though some women dive straight into mountain biking of their own accord, many are like Elizabeth: a little wary of stepping into a sport that seems so extreme. Fact is, while there most certainly are *very* extreme versions of mountain biking, riding a bike off-road is only as adrenaline-fueled as you want it to be. I tell people to think of it like skiing: You can cross-country (XC) ski on groomed trails, you can take it nice and easy down a bunny slope, or you can have someone drop you out of a helicopter at the tip of some sheer cliff on top of the world. It's your call. Even if you go out somewhere and find it's beyond your riding ability, you can always get off your bike and walk.

The problem is that unlike road cycling, where you can sort of fake it even if you don't really know what you're doing, being green in mountain biking is glaringly obvious. Heck, just being a little less fit or having slightly less finesse even if you're otherwise in shape and capable can be glaringly obvious depending on the group you're with and the trails you ride. For too many women, the first experience is anything but positive, and sadly, it's sometimes their last. Mountain bike pros—many of whom run women-only clinics to remedy this situation—see it all the time.

"Women typically start mountain biking by riding with a group of guys," says multi-time national champion and Olympic mountain bike racer Lea Davison. "Most of the time, this includes getting dropped, crashing, and just surviving the first experiences." Davison says that, while this does mean that mountain biking attracts an awesome group of hard-core females, there are more women out there who would be excellent riders if their first-ride experiences were more about having fun and building confidence and less about just trying to escape without injury.

Agreed. I spent a lot of time picking myself up off the ground and nursing wounds of all types over the years. Even today, despite having raced my mountain bike around the world for the past 10 years, I'm still learning how to handle the machine so I'm smoother, faster, and more efficient. And yeah, I still hit the ground sometimes; crashing is part of racing. I've also grown to appreciate that even the most well-intentioned man may not be able to give you the best instruction because honestly, they don't know what it feels like to be a woman on a mountain bike. Our weight distribution and general size characteristics can result in a very different ride—hence the rise of women's specific geometry (as discussed in Chapter 2).

Basic Handling

As with any sport, it takes plenty of practice to get really good at mountain biking. But a little basic bike-handling knowledge goes a long, long way in getting you down the trail in one piece and with a smile on your face. Here's what you need to know (including tips from some of my off-road heroes, like Davison, who now run clinics to get more women to put their tires on the dirt).

RELAX

Your bike wants to flow and keep moving forward. Your job is to help it along. At the most basic level, that means riding loose and not fighting it. When you tense up, the bike becomes harder to control. Soften your elbows and knees so your body can easily absorb the stutters and bumps.

LOOK WHERE YOU WANT TO GO

This is a lesson for *all* cycling, but particularly mountain biking, where there can be many obstacles to avoid. Your bike follows your eyes, so focus your attention on where you want to go, not on the tree or whatever other obstacle it is that you're trying to avoid. Also, take a tip from world downhill champion Leigh Donovan and keep your head up so you can look as far down the trail as possible—*not* straight down at the ground in front of your tire, which is a mistake many riders make.

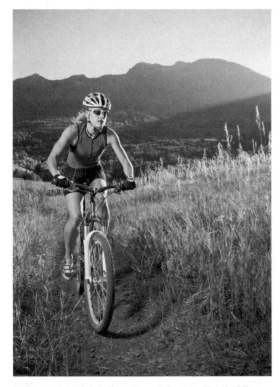

Keep your knees and elbows loosely bent and let the bike flow beneath you when riding off road for a smoother, more enjoyable ride.

"As hard as it is sometimes, you've got to look as far down the trail as possible, especially when you're riding a big downhill. If you only look a few yards in front of your tire, you're not giving yourself time to adjust to the terrain and it's much, much easier to crash that way." Keep your eyes up and take in as much of the trail as you can, looking at the line you want to follow.

STAND UP

Many new women riders struggle with this, Davison says, because women tend to carry their weight lower and have a lower center of gravity, so standing can feel odd and unstable. Riders who are predominately road cyclists struggle with this as well because they're so accustomed to spending the majority of their time firmly planted on their saddle. Getting out of the saddle frequently and moving around on the bike are essential for mountain biking success, and particularly important on descents. "Standing up off the saddle with your pedals level to the ground leaves your body free to maneuver," Davison says. "And your arms and legs can work as natural shock absorbers so you can stay in control."

You'll find that you also have a "strong" or predominant foot, which is the one that feels most natural in the forward position. That's okay, but recognize that this means you'll probably find cornering in one direction easier than another. For instance, if you always ride left foot forward, switchbacks to the right will come more naturally than switchbacks to the left. Advanced riders will actually practice riding with their weaker foot forward until it comes more naturally and they can corner with ease to either side.

WATCH YOUR WEIGHT

And we don't mean the numbers on the scale. Smooth, efficient mountain biking is all about proper weight distribution as you negotiate technical terrain. Your tires need to be properly weighted to keep contact with the ground and to respond to turning and braking. You especially need to weight your front wheel, which is something that men do easily, almost automatically, by virtue of the fact that they have more muscle and therefore more weight in their upper bodies. I washed out in more corners than I care to talk about while following a train of guys through the woods, taking the exact same lines, and simply not being able to hold those lines because my weight was too far back for my front tire to keep traction. Then my friend and four-time national champion Sue Haywood gave me two little words I live by: pushup arms. When riding technical terrain, get your weight a bit forward and bend your elbows out like you're going to do a pushup. It makes a world of difference.

Likewise, there will be times when those tires need to be a little "unweighted" to keep rolling over larger rocks and roots. In general, you want to shift your weight from the front to the back to allow the front wheel to get up and over something, and then immediately shift from the back to the front to give the back wheel room to move. Curbs are a good place to practice this. As you approach the curb, lean your weight back slightly and lightly pull up on the bars to loft the front wheel. Once on the curb, move forward and off the seat to lift the rear wheel, too.

On very steep hills, the same rules apply. When climbing up a steep vertical pitch, you may find your front end losing traction or even popping off the ground. Slide forward on the saddle and lean low over the bars to weight that front wheel. When you're heading down the mountain on a steep decent, push your weight all the way back behind your saddle to keep the rear wheel firmly planted.

BRAKE LATER, HARDER

The same rules of cornering apply on a mountain bike as a road bike, but as mentioned earlier, you can and should play them a little faster and looser in the dirt. You can carry more speed into the corner, hit the rear brake a bit harder, and turn your shoulders and hips through the turn to allow the back wheel to drift a bit. Remember to keep your weight forward on those pushup arms to keep the front tire dug in.

USE YOUR BODY MORE THAN YOUR BARS

Your bike will respond to your weight shifts and leans. So you actually don't turn the bars very much to negotiate the trail, but rather you look and shift your body in the direction you want to go.

COUNT, SING, MEDITATE— JUST DON'T THINK

I might be making a broad-brush generalization, but I honestly think that one of the things that makes mountain biking particularly hard for women is that we think too much. Overthinking leads to hesitancy, which leads to getting bogged down or off line or hitting the dirt. You need to check your head, keep calm, and flow with the rhythm of the ride without overprocessing or fretting over every flick of your tires. The best tip I ever got for that was from Donovan, who recommends counting.

"One of the things that helps me keep calm and hold a rhythm on the bike is counting. I'll just grab a number out of the air and start counting up or down. Like after a crash, I may get on my bike and just start: '33, 34, 35, 36.' It gets me back into focus quickly." If numbers aren't your game, you can pick a favorite song refrain or random mantra, says Donovan. "Everyone plays their own mental games."

DIAL IN YOUR BIKE

I'm firmly convinced that many women think they "suck" at mountain biking when in fact they'd be quite good if their bikes were set up properly. Mountain bikes can be insanely complicated. On any given bike, you can have a front shock, a rear shock, a dropper seatpost lever, a suspension lockout lever, and suspension adjustment levers. Then there's also tire width, tire pressure, and any number of little factors that can have a big influence on how your bike handles. Men aren't necessarily inherently better at this; I think they just have more resources by virtue of being surrounded by other guys talking about suspension settings and tinkering with tire pressure.

In any event, take the time to do a little research and really get to know your bike. What follows are the features to focus on. Don't be shy about asking someone at your bike shop or a more experienced friend to help you. They really make a huge difference.

SUSPENSION PRESSURE (PRELOAD). If the pressure of your bike's shock or fork is too low for your weight, you may bottom out on bumps. If it's too high, the ride will be so rough and bumpy, you'll barely notice that you have any travel; set it just right, and you'll get the most from your suspension. Generally, you use a special pump to put the proper amount of air into a suspension component. The shock pump may have a weight/psi chart right on the side, making it a no-brainer. Otherwise, you can look it up in your owner's manual or online. Remember, you want to set it to "rider" weight, not naked-on-the-scale weight. Riding clothes and shoes, a helmet, tools, and a pack can add a lot of weight to your frame. That's the weight you need to use for your suspension settings.

SUSPENSION SAG. The amount your suspension moves when you initially sit your butt on the saddle is your sag (this obviously applies only to dual suspension bikes, not hardtails). You want your sag to match the type of riding you do. For example, an XC rider wants relatively little sag for efficiency, whereas downhillers and freeriders need more in order to suck up bigger bumps. Your manual will have a list of suggested settings for your style. To set it up, place a zip tie on the bottom of the fork stanchion—the part that travels up and down—and one at the bottom of the shaft of the shock. Set up next to a wall, so you can support yourself as you sit on your bike in a normal riding position—with your feet on the pedals and all your weight on the bike. Carefully get off the bike and measure the amount each zip tie moved from its original spot. This is your sag (typically, it is about one-third of your travel). Adjust it according to your bike's manual.

SUSPENSION COMPRESSION. The time it takes for your suspension to slow a downward force (your body weight pressing down on it) is compression. To dial it in, start with the control knob completely open (counterclockwise), then adjust the compression by turning the knob clockwise. Turn the knob too much and your suspension will take too long to go through all of its travel. Turn it too little and your suspension will bottom out on small bumps. Experiment to find the sweet spot that best matches your riding style and terrain. Many of today's shocks also come with switches that allow you to fine-tune on the fly, letting you opt for a more rigid setup on smooth terrain or a more yielding setup when riding gets rough.

SUSPENSION REBOUND. Rebound is the speed at which the suspension comes back to full travel after it's compressed. Though rebound is a preference thing, in general you want your suspension to rebound as fast as it can without the shock topping out or feeling too springy. Set it slow, and the suspension can't extend back into its travel before you hit the next bump, resulting in a harsh ride. Set it fast, and your bike will bounce like a pogo stick. To adjust, use the clearly marked control on your fork or shock.

TIRE PRESSURE. Confession: For many more years than I care to admit, I ran my tires with about 40 psi in them (i.e., rock hard for my sub-130-pound self), because I really, really didn't want to get a pinch flat during a race. (A pinch flat is when the tire and tube get pinched between an object, like a rock, on the trail and the rim of the wheel. It snakebites, or double punctures the tube.) Sure I bounced all over the trail like a pinball, but it was worth it . . . not really. *Slowly*, I softened up—literally—for a more supple, controlled ride. Today, with tubeless tires, I run about 21 pounds, which some of my fellow racers say is still too high. And they may be right. At times when I let them drift down to 18, my traction in turns is notably better and my tires stay put on the trail, as they absorb the ground's irregularities rather than bounce off it.

How much pressure you run depends on your weight, the size of the tire (bigger tires take lower pressure), whether or not you have tubes (tubes require higher pressure), and the conditions you're riding in. You can go higher for firm, smooth trails than you can on root-heavy, rocky terrain. You can go too low, even with tubeless, however. Too little pressure leaves your tires feeling squirmy and can have you bottoming out (banging against the rim, which is okay once in a while, but not multiple times in a ride).

The best approach is a little trial and error. If you have tubes, start at about 40 psi, depending on your size. Then let out 3 to 5 psi and see if you feel more control. You'll know you've gone too far when you bottom out (not good with tubes) and need to put a bit back or get flats. For tubeless, you can start lower, about 30 psi, again depending on your size, and do the same thing until you reach a point where the tires feel squirmy or too soft, or you're tearing the sidewalls because they're bulging out too much over the rocks. Again, add a bit back.

TIRE PROFILE. Confession, part two: I also paid embarrassingly little attention to the kind of tires I ran with for many years because I simply hadn't ever educated myself about tire selection. This was plain stupid on my part because I had plenty of resources at my disposal and should have known better. Your tires are the only part of your bike that has contact with the ground. How well (or not) they connect with the terrain determines how fast (or not) you roll, how much (or little) traction you get in various conditions, and how well (or not) you stay upright. Tires come in different sizes, tread patterns, and materials to match all sorts of trail conditions and riding situations. Be sure to check the descriptions of any tires you buy to find the ones that best suit the riding you do. You'll be glad you did.

GET STRONG

One look at the painfully skinny arms of Tour de France riders and you know they're not lifting any weight heavier than a salad fork. Mountain biking is a little different. You don't need to start bench-pressing, but some basic strength training (I recommend some exercises in Chapter 15) will help you be a stronger rider and better bike handler. Mountain biking takes a great degree of leg strength, as well as core and upper-body strength and stamina, for powering over obstacles and maneuvering the bike over tough terrain. Women simply don't have as much testosterone or muscle as men, so we need to work a little harder to get and stay strong.

RIDE WITH BETTER RIDERS

If you want to ride better, faster, more skillfully, ride with folks who are better, faster, and more skillful. "You can learn so much by watching and imitating better riders," says Donovan. "Even if you can't pull off all their moves, always try to ride with people who are better than you." But always stay within yourself. If you really feel like you can't ride something, you likely can't—at least not without some concrete instruction and practice—simply because you don't know how yet. Keep watching and learning and practicing, but remember, there's no shame in getting off and walking it when need be.

REMEMBER WHAT YOU'RE RIDING

This is important, especially if you're relatively new and riding with others. Mountain bikes are not all created equal. Unlike road bikes, which will perform pretty similarly within the same price range, mountain bikes are spec'd to perform very specific jobs, like race fast over cross-country trails or bomb down wicked descents. If you have a bike designed to do one, it won't do the other super great, and vice versa.

REBOUND FROM CRASHES

When you're mountain biking, it's a matter of when, not if, you're going to crash, says, oh, everybody who's ever mountain biked. "Everyone crashes," Davison says. "You aren't the only one. There's a lot of crashing going on even at the highest level of the sport." The key, she says, is to make each unexpected dismount a learning experience. Take a moment to visualize what went wrong, and how you'll overcome the obstacle next time. "Then," Davison says, "go back and try it again." Spoken like a true Olympian. If you take a moment, you generally can figure out what went wrong and how to avoid the same type of crash again.

Keep Chilled on the Rocks

Whether it's a rock garden or a loose gravel road, you can't be a mountain biker without encountering at least a few rocks, if not a whole trail full of them. For some, rocks are the fun stuff. For others, they're the sources of sore knees and angry scars. Here's how former downhill pro Chris Kovarik stays smooth on the rough stuff.

DO A LITTLE LIMBO

"Some riders get tense and sit really upright on their bikes when they get into a rocky section," he says. "You want to do the exact opposite. Stay loose. Bend those knees and elbows, and crouch a little lower on your bike. It lowers your center of gravity so you're more stable, and it gives you less distance to fall, so you don't hurt yourself as much if you do."

RATCHET, DON'T HAMMER

"Sometimes you can muscle your way through a jagged, rocky section of trail. But you risk catching a pedal on a high rock and throwing yourself off balance. Instead, ratchet your pedals by taking a partial pedal stroke forward to propel you through the obstacles. Then backpedal for a partial stroke. It'll keep your momentum going forward, but you won't bash your feet."

GET YOUR GRIP

"Large rocks can be ideal riding surfaces because your tires can get lots of grip on their rough surfaces. Maintain momentum going into them and keep your weight slightly back so your rear tire can grab and roll as you pedal over them. Just remember: Some, especially smooth, rocks lose all their grip when it rains. So don't brake on them when they're wet."

PLAY IT SMOOTH AND FAST WHEN IT'S LOOSE

"Loose gravelly rock can be the hardest stuff to ride on. Keep a higher cadence and smooth pedal stroke to float through it. When you're cornering on loose rocks, keep steering to a minimum. Lean your body instead."

1-2-3 Drop-Off!

Little on the trail inspires the same stomach-in-mouth sensation as the drop-off. You're rolling along and suddenly, just like Columbus was warned would happen, the earth falls away.

Your natural fear: Cracking your head as your front wheel plunges straight down and pitches you overboard. But most riders can handle bigger drop-offs than they think, even without high-trick maneuvers like wheelie drops, says lanky former downhill champ Steve Peat.

Overcoming Obstacles

Part of the fun of mountain biking is clearing (riding over cleanly) obstacles like rocks, logs, and roots. Here are some pro tips I've amassed over the years for tackling even the most challenging terrains.

DO THE HOP

Even if you never actually catch air like a cottontail, learning the fundamentals of a bunny hop will help you clear larger obstacles on the trail. As it sounds, a bunny hop is when you lift your front end and then your back end up over a larger barrier like a log or large rock. Performed correctly, the bunny hop can get you up and over even the biggest logs without missing a beat. Here's how it's done.

HIT THE GAS, NOT THE BRAKES. Though talented trials riders can bunny hop from a standstill, the rest of us need some speed. You want to come into it at about 10 mph or at cruising speed, so you have enough momentum to complete the move.

LEVEL THE PEDALS. About 3 feet away from the obstacle, stop pedaling and level your pedals horizontally.

CROUCH AND COMPRESS. Crouch into your bike, shifting your weight into your handlebars and pedals to load the suspension.

THINK FRONT FIRST. After crouching, immediately pull up the front wheel—and only the front wheel; lifting both wheels at once is a common mistake—so that it's just high enough to get over the obstacle.

PUSH FORWARD, AND SUCK UP. As the front wheel comes up, lean your weight forward and, once you see the front wheel clear the obstacle, push the handlebar away and down, and suck your legs up toward your body to bring the back wheel up and over. *Remember to stay off the brakes as you come down on the other side*, unless you want to endo (go end over end over your handlebars) spectacularly.

The most important thing is to practice small first. And practice on something more forgiving than a rock or log—like a built-up dirt pile. This way you can build your confidence without hurting yourself as you learn. And even if you never master hopping large objects (I sure haven't), this type of bike-handling finesse can still help you roll over large logs without going over your bars.

Which Way to the Trailhead?

There are a few Web sites like Trails.com that compile trail systems in any given area. But honestly, the best way to find great places to ride is still word of mouth. Ask at the local bike shop and get linked into a riding group. Mountain bikers are social animals who love to share their favorite trails with each other. Find your pack and you'll have places to ride for life.

Here's the technique he recommends. (Always practice on small stuff like curbs first. Don't drop for the first time off a 2-foot ledge.)

LOOK DOWN, THEN GET BACK

Obviously, you need to know what's on the other side of the drop-off so you don't crash into some unseen obstacle, but that doesn't mean you should lean forward and gape down with saucer-sized eyeballs the whole time. "The biggest thing that'll get you in trouble is not getting your weight back," says Peat. "Take just a quick look down, then move your weight back behind your saddle."

KEEP SPEED

"You don't want to catch major air, but you want to get enough of a launch so your rear tire lands first or at least both tires touch down together. Stay away from the brakes."

STAY LOW, STAY BACK

Quantum physics is tough; riding physics, not so tough. "The farther back your weight is and the lower you are on your bike, the less likely you are to pitch yourself headfirst down a drop-off," says Peat. Stay in the attack position, crouched low with the crank arms horizontal and your weight back.

WATCH YOUR FRONT WHEEL

"It's easy to tip forward, especially on bigger drops. Keep an eye on that front wheel. If it dips, lift on the bars to bring it back up," he says. Landing on your front tire makes it hard to control the landing.

STICK IT BRAKE-FREE

Keep your mitts away from the brake levers as you land. "Stopping your wheels after launching off a drop-off is a sure way to crash, especially if you hit the front brake."

IF YOU NEED TO TAKE IT SLOW . . .

Sometimes you don't have the luxury of speed. The drop-off might be immediately before a tight turn, or maybe obstacles stop your momentum. No worries. With a few adjustments you can take the same drop in slo-mo. Here's how.

APPROACH PERPENDICULARLY. For the best bike control, you want to roll off the drop as close to perpendicular to the edge of the drop as you can. It'll make for a smoother transition off the drop.

PUSH AND DROP. "You need as much weight as possible off the front tire so it can keep rolling at the foot of the drop, rather than pitch you over the bars," says Peat. That means butt back, way back, off and over the saddle. Push the bar forward as you drop down. As your front tire hits the bottom and starts rolling, shift your weight toward the center to help the rear wheel drop and roll.

WAIT TO BRAKE. Again, stay away from the brakes during a drop—especially the front brake. If you need to scrub speed, use no more than a tap of the back brake, but even that's not recommended, says Peat. Otherwise, don't brake until both wheels are on the ground and you're rolling.

CHAPTER 11

Cyclocross Fever

CYCLOCROSS RACING IS A CRAZY—AND CRAZY FUN—MASHUP of mountain bike and road racing. Courses are generally about 1½ to 2 miles long and feature terrain of all sorts, including grass fields, sand pits, wooded trails, pavement, gravel, steep hills, and obstacles or hurdles that require you to quickly dismount and shoulder your bike to hop over them, then remount and race on. You race around the circuit for about 45 minutes as fast as humanly possible. The cyclocross season stretches from September to February, so the weather comes into play as well, with racers often sailing around through mud and sometimes snow. There are generally tons of spectators ringing cowbells and trying to feed you everything from bacon strips to beer as you go whizzing by.

Cyclocross began in the 1900s as a way for European pros to stay in shape and sharpen their bike-handling skills over the winter (running keeps your feet from freezing and it's easier to stay warm when you're pushing harder at slower speeds over rough terrain), and it's now enormously popular here in the States, and getting more so every season. In just 5 years, participation in 'cross grew from 32,000 to 80,000. Though the men's fields are still larger—there can be 150 guys on the line—the women's fields are getting bigger and deeper all the time, more so than in any other type of bike racing. Speaking from experience, I can say that even some of the smaller local races can have 30 women lined up. Larger races can see more than 100 women on the line.

'Cross Is Boss

If you haven't tried 'cross, you should. Whether or not you like racing or competing, 'cross is a great way to get fit and have a blast. It's also extremely accessible. The races are generally held at parks and run all day, with various categories going off from morning to late afternoon. People pack up a grill and a cooler and bring the whole family and make a day of it, cheering on the racers (which usually includes many of their friends) when they're not racing themselves.

Because the races are short, you can jump in one even if you're not super fit or don't have time to train. There will be plenty of women just like yourself out there for a personal challenge. And if you are super fit and have time to train, you can mix it up in the front of the field for a podium spot.

As described in Chapter 2, you can get a specific bike to race cyclocross (they're fun bikes to have for just riding around, too), but you don't need one. Unless you're a pro, you can use a mountain bike. (You may also be able to convert your road bike to make it 'cross friendly, but some road bike frames don't accept tires as wide and knobby as what you'll want to race 'cross.) Some companies, like Liv

(made by Giant), even make women's specific 'cross bikes that feature women's specific geometry and lighter tubing, as well as women's specific accessories like handlebars and saddles.

'Cross 101

My first exposure to 'cross was in Philadelphia, where they were holding Super Cup races (read: high-level racing). I had a borrowed bike that was two sizes too big and I had never so much as seen a 'cross race before, let alone raced one. My friend Dondo signed me up for the A-level race (for pros and elites) because, he said, "you're too fit for the beginner category races." I was the only one not wearing a team-sponsored kit. I was blown off the back right from the gun. I jumped clear over my bike trying to remount it twice. And I got lapped by the leaders. (At one point, I was jumping over barriers as I ran up a steep stretch, and the crowd started to go nuts. I thought they were cheering for me. They were actually roaring for the lead train of women who were about to come blazing by me.) Somehow I managed to not finish last and picked up a bunch of fans along the course who were rooting for me because I was trying so hard and able to laugh at my own lunacy.

My skill set has come a long way since then, though I still don't have a very smooth remount. In any event, I'm living proof that if you can pedal a bike, you can race 'cross. But a little practice hopping on and off your bike can go a long way in increasing your confidence and enjoyment of the sport. If you want to be competitive in 'cross, that kind of practice is a must. Any pro will tell you that a race can be won or lost in those transitions.

"There's nothing more discouraging than losing time because you can't comfortably get off and back on to the saddle," says Adam Myerson, a professional 'cross racer and coach, and founder and president of coaching concern Cycle-Smart, who offered his tips to *Bicycling*. The key to speedy transitions, says Myerson, is conserving your forward momentum. Here's how to do it.

DISMOUNT

Dismount on the left side of your bike to protect your legs from your drivetrain. As you approach an obstacle, slow down and coast. As you coast toward the barrier, have your hands on your hoods, unclip your left foot, and shift your weight onto your left instep. (This is an advanced skill—and the most efficient way to dismount. If you find it too tricky to unclip but maintain contact with the pedal, you can keep this foot clipped in until the end.) When you're ready to dismount, unclip and swing your right leg over the saddle and around the back of the bike, bringing it between the bike and your left leg. Move your right hand to the top tube about 6 inches in front of the seatpost. Coasting with your right foot behind the left, hit the ground with your right. Begin running with the left. Give yourself room to take a few strides before the obstacle.

PORTAGE

Carry a bike in your hands or on your shoulder. If you choose your hands, don't lift your bike so that your saddle goes into your armpit; you may hit the barrier or trip over your pedals. Instead,

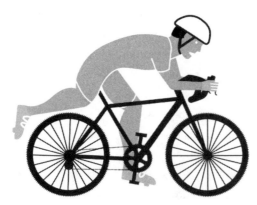

Dismounting on the left side helps you avoid getting hung up in your drivetrain as you get off and run with the bike.

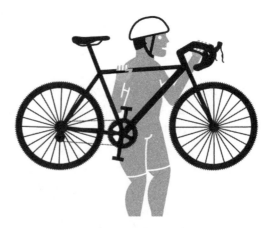

Lift the bike high enough to clear the barriers. Keep it far enough away from your body to avoid bashing into it with your body as you run and hurdle.

place your right hand palm-down on the top tube and keep your elbow between you and your bike. This helps to move the bike a little farther away from your body so you can lift it to shoulder height.

SHOULDER IT

It's easier and faster to shoulder your bike for uphill runs, stairs, and muddy sections. As you dismount, instead of grabbing the top tube, reach through the frame and grasp the down tube near the bottle-cage area. Lift the front of the top tube onto your right shoulder. Then wrap your right arm around the down tube and grab the left drop of your handlebars with your right hand to hold the bike securely.

REMOUNT

"You want to run onto your bike the way a track hurdler steps over a hurdle," Myerson says. "This keeps your momentum moving forward." The remount starts with both hands on the tops or hoods of the handlebars. Running on the left side of the bike, look forward and keep your hips in the area between the cranks and saddle. Push off your left foot, open your hips to the right, and drive your right knee forward over the saddle. "Like the trailing leg of a hurdler, catch the saddle with the inside of your right thigh," Myerson says. Then bring your right foot down onto the pedal. Twist your hips closed and center yourself on the saddle. Start a pedaling motion, find the pedals, and clip in.

TAKE A PRACTICE LAP OR TWO

At a race, take a few practice laps during your warmup to develop a strategy for how to approach barriers and run-ups.

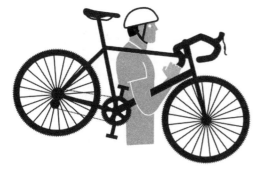

If you're going to be running uphill or for any distance, it's easier to just shoulder the bike. Some cross bikes even have a flattened area on the top tube for added comfort.

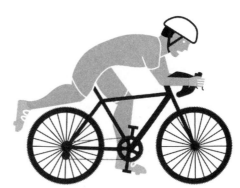

You should have some forward rolling momentum as you remount so it's easier to get back up to speed when you start pedaling again.

The Finer Points

When you really get into 'cross, you'll note that there are lots of details to take into consideration that can make your race even more successful, if not also more fun. Here are a few to note:

TIRES

'Cross racers obsess about their tires. Just as in mountain biking, the kind of tread you run, the tire width, and the pressure all have huge impacts on how well (or not) your bike handles. Generally speaking, for the best traction, you want to have tread that matches the course conditions (the tires will note if they're good for mud, etc.), and you want to run your tire pressure as low as you can without bottoming out on the rims.

FEEDING

Most 'cross racers strip the bottle cages off their bike so it's easier to carry on their shoulder. That means no bottles during the race itself. You don't usually need one for a 40- to 45-minute race. But if it's very hot out, you might find yourself wanting a drink. During hot races, the organizers will set up a feed zone where you can have a friend hand you a bottle. Or, just keep one bottle cage on your bike—a setup that is becoming increasingly common even in the pro ranks.

THE PIT ZONE

'Cross races are often held in such abysmal conditions that people bring a backup bike and wheels to make equipment (if not whole-bike) changes during the race. At big races, you can even have a pit crew, where some very good-natured friend takes your mud-caked bike, hands you your fresh one, and then hoses off the dirty one so you can grab it on the next lap. But that's a whole other level of racing.

TRAINERS

You will see rows and rows of people with bikes set up on trainers, spinning their legs in the parking lot to keep warm and limber for their race. This is good race strategy when it's cold outside, but some coaches argue that it's unproductive when the weather is warm. I generally agree and prefer to warm up by rolling around the venue rather than sitting on a stationary trainer.

CHAPTER 12

Dirt, Gravel, and Cinders Galore

SOME OF THE BEST RIDES BEGIN WHERE THE PAVEMENT ENDS.
There's a childlike joy to be had in taking your bike off the pavement and onto dirt roads and cinder paths. You can really appreciate the simple pleasures of feeling the crunchy gravel under your tires, kicking up dust, and soaking in the scenery on what are often quiet, less-traveled, and incredibly interesting throughways. "Gravel grinding," as it's called, requires some special skills, and if you get serious enough about it, special equipment helps, too.

"Taking skinny tires off-road can turn a regular ride into something far more memorable," agrees Michael Gibbons, a coach at Walton Endurance in Philadelphia. "Plus, you'll improve your handling skills along with your fitness," he says. Seasoned pro racer Alex Stieda agrees.

"Some of my best pro-cycling memories are of the adventure rides the team did during training camps, when we'd explore whatever paved roads, dirt tracks, or trails were available—on our fresh, team-issue road bikes. But we weren't just having fun:

Riding a road bike on dirt can yield huge benefits. Your bike-handling skills will improve by necessity: If you use your front brake in a dirt turn, you will most likely wash out and go down. If you stand up to pedal on a steep climb, your rear wheel can spin out. But with some off-road practice, you'll learn to brake before turning and to apply pedal pressure evenly in smooth circles. Riding on softer ground will also improve your power by forcing you to push against a higher resistance."

Here are some pro tips, courtesy of Alex Stieda, to keep in mind.

PREP YOUR BIKE

To maximize comfort and traction, use the widest tires your frame will permit—at least 25 millimeters. Allow a little space between the tire and the frame in case your wheel goes slightly out of true. Carry at least two spare tubes. A CO_2 cartridge is good only once, so bring a mini-pump, plus a multi-tool and, ideally, a chain tool—and make sure you know how to use them. If you have race wheels, leave them at home. Now isn't the time to break out the aero carbon clinchers. Durable alloy box-section rims dampen vibration and are best suited for these types of rough surfaces.

DRESS SMART

What to wear and carry to wear "just in case" depends largely on where you live and what time of year it is. If you're going out in Florida, you can probably leave a lot of the layers, save maybe a rain cape, at home. Heading out onto some gravel passes in the high mountains? It's not unreasonable to bring a windbreaker, long-finger gloves, arm warmers, and maybe even knee warmers in case you encounter nasty conditions. You can also wear a wind vest with pockets, which will give you another place to store gear. No matter where you ride, it's wise to wear a cycling cap and sunglasses to protect your eyes from dust and debris. You can also consider adding spandex booties to keep kicked-up grit from lodging in your shoes.

FILL YOUR POCKETS

You burn more calories off-road because of the increased demands on your body. Aim to take in about 200 calories an hour. Pack plenty of energy bars and two large water bottles. Put your GPS on your bike if you have one, and carry some cash and a charged cell phone in a plastic bag to keep them dry.

PERFECT YOUR FORM

Practice some shorter dirt rides first. Find a stretch of gravel road and try riding at different speeds in a variety of gears and cadences. Notice how your wheels slide underneath you as you turn or move from one track to the next. Scan the terrain ahead and find the smoothest line to ride. Keep the following technique tips in mind.

LOOK AHEAD. Look where you want to ride and your bike will follow. Don't fixate on ruts and other obstacles.

KEEP CALM AND IN CONTROL. Keep hands, arms, shoulders, and neck relaxed. Visualize the bike bouncing around while your core remains motionless. Bend your elbows slightly more than usual for additional shock absorption.

EXPERIMENT WITH HAND POSITIONS. Move from the brake hoods to the bar top to the drops and find where you feel most comfortable. For extra control when things get really rough, use the drops.

LET THE BIKE FLOW. Hover over the saddle to let the bike flow beneath you (and reduce the impact on your sensitive spots). Peek down at your toes once in a while to make sure they're pointed straight ahead: Where the ankles go, the knees follow, and flailing knees waste energy, send the bike off line, and may even set you up for injury. But don't lock your knees or ankles—that will make the bike harder to control. This is especially important on descents. When you're descending, keep your grip relaxed, float on the balls of your feet, and train your vision as far up the road as possible.

CLIMB LOW. Traction is a fleeting commodity on sketchy roads, especially steep sketchy roads. Stay far enough back on the saddle to keep the rear wheel on the ground while leaning forward enough to prevent the front wheel from popping up. Try to keep your pedal stroke smooth and circular.

BRING A BUDDY

On many adventure rides you start out with a rough plan, but end up spending twice as long as you expected. It's safer—and more fun—to do this kind of ride with at least one other person.

Feeling Sketchy?

Do this simple drill once a week to build your handling skills.

WEEK 1: While riding at an easy pace, carefully steer off the road into the adjoining grass, gravel, or dirt. Maintain the same speed and gearing you had on the road, while staying calm and relaxed. Practice grabbing your bottle and taking a drink. After 1 minute, pull back onto the road and recover for 1 minute. Repeat two more times.

WEEK 2: Increase off-road effort to 3 reps at 2 minutes each.

WEEK 3: Do two sets of 3 reps of 3 minutes off-road.

WEEK 4: Do two sets of 3 reps of 5 minutes off-road.

Ready, Set, Gravel Grind!

Gravel riding has become so popular that you can find races around the country that are on mostly, if not 100 percent, gravel roads. The racing is tough—a mix of road, mountain, and cyclocross—and many cover huge distances. Among the better-known events are the 300-mile Trans Iowa, Nebraska's 150-mile Gravel World Championships, and the 200-mile Dirty Kanza through eastern Kansas, the latter of which I've done and can attest that it's beautiful, engaging, and at times really hard!

Perhaps the biggest appeal of gravel racing is that unlike road racing, which is mostly (wo)mano a (wo)mano, gravel grinders are truly a test of self, as my teammate Stephanie Swan eloquently explains. "I entered my first gravel race, the Hilly Billy Roubaix in West Virginia, thinking it was a non-race. I didn't really expect to do well, I just liked the idea of a mammoth bike adventure—the challenge, the survival, seeing how fast I could go against myself. I survived, and then wanted more. I wanted to see what other gravel races were like, and soon I was doing a series, testing myself—my endurance, my mental strength, my bike skills. I found a community of gravel racers I looked forward to seeing at all the events. Eventually it was less a test of self, but more about finding my friends and allies in this big chaos of dirt, gravel, and sweat, and becoming a stronger force together.

"It feels good in the midst of some very hard riding. You get overcome with a great feeling of appreciation for the other riders you are with. And when the race is finished, the 'event' is far from finished. The party has just begun! There's always food and beer and you are surrounded by so many exhausted people who have just done the same thing as you. There's a great feeling of unity. Whether you win, you DNF [Did Not Finish], or you roll in midpack, you're a card-carrying member of the gravel club. What matters, how you 'win' the party (if not the race), is trying your best, encouraging others when they're having a dark moment, and listening to and sharing your own stories of a day well spent."

The techniques for gravel racing are similar to gravel riding, but exponentially more important the longer the event. *Bicycling* caught up with Dan Hughes, owner of Sunflower Outdoor and Bike Shop in Lawrence, Kansas, and multi-time winner of the Dirty Kanza, to get his pointers for success. As you'd imagine, he had some great tips.

CHOOSE TIRES FOR WHEN YOU'RE TIRED

Ask four gravel riders which tire is best, and you'll get four answers—or more. That's because the right tire choice depends on your location and the type of gravel you'll encounter. The Kanza runs through the Flint Hills, where the gravel tends to be sharp and can shred tires, Hughes says. One competitor he knows dealt with seven flats over the course of the event. But the consensus is that you want a tough tire—not a lightweight racer—that's as fat as you can get to fit your frame (Hughes rides 700 by 32s). "You'll get tired as the day goes on," Hughes says. "And the fat tire will help when you're less careful in picking your line." He also recommends learning how to boot a sliced tire. (See "Fast Flat Fixes," page 293 for a complete how-to; been there, done that.)

RIDE WHAT YOU GOT

A gravel-specific bike is great, but not necessary. "I ride my cyclocross bike with a compact double [chainring] on the front," Hughes says. "And it rarely leaves the big ring." Disc brakes are also nice, but not necessary. Besides tires, the big issues are your contact points—you'll want a comfortable saddle, extra padding on your handlebars, and supportive shoes for long days of pedaling.

PUSH IT

Pushing a bigger gear in rough terrain can keep you from bouncing around and help with overall control. "I push as low of a cadence as I can, high power, and it helps," Hughes says. You might not be able to keep the gearing super low for a couple hundred miles, but avoid high-cadence spinning as much as possible.

USE YOUR HEAD

One of Hughes's worst Kanza experiences came from taking too big a risk on a descent. His front tire sank into a gravel-filled water crossing and he "yard-saled"—that is, he crashed so spectacularly that the contents of his pockets ended up all over the road. "You've got to scan ahead all the time for those deep gravel patches," he says. "You never know if the filled-in water crossing is 6 inches deep or 2 feet deep." Slowing down a bit more than usual on corners and descents might feel counterintuitive in a race, but you need to make it to the finish line if you want to win.

KNOW YOUR NUTRITION

"Where people fail is with nutrition," Hughes says. He recommends practicing eating—and eating lots—on long, hard training rides to prepare for the rigors of a gravel event. "If you haven't done a ride over 120 miles, you don't know how your stomach is going to handle it. If you lock up and can't get food to go in without it coming back out, it's game over." That said, he's been known to stop for pizza at Casey's convenience store on the Kanza route, which probably isn't the best choice for everyone. As a general guideline, nutritionists recommend consuming about 200 calories per hour during long races.

REMEMBER WHY YOU'RE THERE

You're going to flat. You're going to be tired. And it's going to be hard. But come on: You're riding your bike! "Sometimes I remind myself that I want to do this," Hughes says. "Think about it: I get up on Sunday, I don't have any responsibilities—I basically get up and go ride all day. That's pretty awesome." Hmm. Gravel ride, anyone?

CHAPTER 13

Try the Track

I AM FORTUNATE ENOUGH TO LIVE WITHIN 10 MILES OF A world-class velodrome, which, in case you've never seen (or even heard of) one, is an oval track with steeply banked sides that cyclists race on using bikes with fixed gears and no brakes (no kidding). It's called Valley Preferred Cycling Center, or "T-Town," and it opened in 1975. Over the past 40 years, Valley Preferred has hosted multiple Olympic Trials, Track Cycling World Cups, and USA Cycling National Championships, along with countless other major races. Founded by the late cycling aficionado Bob Rodale (a former CEO of *Bicycling*'s parent company), this one-time cornfield has been turned into a home for cycling champions.

It's a giddy good time to ride in. Once a year, they host the Rodale Corporate Challenge, where local businesses (including Rodale and *Bicycling*, along with Red Robin, Air Products, Mack Trucks, and many others) field teams of six riders to face off in Italian pursuit, where teams line up on opposite sides of the track and chase each other. It gives regular non-bike racers a chance to feel the thrill of high-speed competition in a pretty safe way and packs the stands like no other night.

I'm not much of a track racer by build or disposition, but training on the track helps develop strength and speed and is just plain fun, so I'll sneak in there once or twice a season for kicks. Racing on it is as much a mental game as it is physical. It's some of the most exciting women's racing you'll see because it's very aggressive and tactical, sort of like high-speed, hypoxic chess. In an interview with *Bicycling*, four-time world champion and world-record holder Sarah Hammer explained why she finds track racing more exciting than road racing.

"The events are a lot shorter and much more intense, the speed is so much faster than other cycling disciplines, and it can be a lot more aggressive. In one of the best events, the elimination, on every other lap the last person to cross the line gets eliminated. People put their wheels just about anywhere possible to not get eliminated. It's just a mad dash."

My friend Liz, who chased an Olympic track dream for the better part of 2 decades and racked up multiple national championships along the way, waxed so poetically (and intelligently) about the track, I'll let her explain what makes it so special and likely why more women are giving it a go. And you should, too, if you live in the vicinity of 1 of the 30 or so velodomes around the nation.

"Long before I became a track racer, my bike took me to places I'd never been. I've spent vacation time riding and even racing through tropical rainforests.

"But never in a million years did I think a plain cement oval would so aptly capture how I spend my time and the route I would cover weekly, often daily, by bike.

"I'd be lying if I didn't say I've found myself in warm-up a few times, staring at the wheel in front of me, watching my speed tick from 32 to 36 to 40 kph, around turns one, two, three, then four, again, wondering 'How did it come to this?'

"One day, I gave riding a bike with no brakes on a banked cement oval a try. Today, all these years later, here I am . . . still riding in circles, trying to perfect the chemistry that equates to performance and keeps me coming back for more.

"There's a saying in velodrome circles (no pun intended) that there's no hiding on the track. That goes beyond fitness and race preparation to how you carry yourself both on and off the bike. My sports doc calls the track 'racing in a fishbowl,' which isn't far from the truth.

"Unlike the road, where you can wander aimlessly, anonymously for hours—track training is a discipline of accountability. There's structure to the time you spend there. A session typically starts with warm-up before moving on to big gear starts, 2K repeats, a 20-minute tempo effort behind the motor pacing vehicle or reaction drills on the whistle. There's both an art and science to what you do any given day. The outcome depends largely on that mix, how it's applied and how much you commit in the process.

"I love the track because I like the discipline. I always learn something new and it's a challenge. Like the racing—the lessons come at you fast and furious. One minute, you're exhilarated, the next, humbled to the core. There's no hiding on the track.

"There is, however, a lot of socializing, which is another thing I love, and that I think is attractive to many women (and men, too). You train in a group. You race in a group. You go to the track and do your efforts or race, but in between you spend a lot of time on the infield swapping stories, sharing advice, and shooting the breeze. It's a real community."

Get in the Ring

Convinced? Or at least intrigued? Here are a few things to know.

TRACK BIKES ARE HIGHLY SPECIALIZED

Velodromes will often let you ride your road bike on the track when it's not in use, but if you want to try your hand at competing on one, you'll need a track bike. Track bikes are very light and completely minimalist. There are no brakes, no gears, and no freewheel hub. If the wheels are turning, so are the pedals. You control your speed by pushing the pedals and resisting or pushing back on the moving pedals to slow down and stop.

Of course, most casual or simply curious cyclists don't own track bikes. Generally, the track will have its own fleet of bikes that you can borrow or rent to try out. Many will also offer classes that culminate in races.

YOU ARE ONE WITH THE MACHINE

You *must* be fully clipped in or strapped to the pedals to race a track bike because you have zero control if your feet come flying off at high speeds. If you're not accustomed to being clipped in, that's the first step to conquer before checking out the track.

THERE ARE MANY TYPES OF RACES

There are many different types of races in the discipline of track racing, including team races, time trials, match sprints, and pursuits. Here are a few of the most popular events.

SCRATCH RACE. These are your basic, standard races. All the riders line up at the same place and the first one that crosses the line on the final lap wins. Races vary in length, but are generally eight laps and up.

MATCH SPRINT. Riders (generally two) go head-to-head in a three-lap race that barely resembles a race until the final lap. It's definitely one of the more tactical races, as the riders crawl and block each other at near walking pace around the oval until one of them finally makes a move and the race is fully on.

MISS AND OUT. Classic survival of the fittest (and the wiliest). Here, the last rider across the finish line in every lap is eliminated from the race until the field is narrowed down to three riders who sprint for first, second, and third place.

KEIRIN. Popular in Japan, the Keirin is a motorpaced event where riders are paced by a motorcycle for the first few laps. The moto accelerates gradually from about 15 mph to 28 mph before it pulls off the track and the riders sprint for the finish.

POINTS RACE. Points races look chaotic (and kind of are chaotic), but there's definitely a method to the madness. Essentially, there are many races within the main race, which generally covers anywhere from 10 to 40 kilometers, and riders are awarded points for their placement on intermediate sprints. The rider who has racked up the most points at the end wins.

INDIVIDUAL PURSUIT. Two riders start on opposite sides of the track and try to catch each other over the course of 3 kilometers (4 for men). Obviously, if you catch your opponent, you win, but generally it's the rider who records the fastest time for the distance who wins. There are also team pursuits.

TIME TRIAL. As the name implies, the racer just sprints around the track as fast as they can for a given distance—generally 1 kilometer—and the one who clocks the fastest time wins.

PART V

GET FIT, GO FAST!

Cycling feels like flying. That's one of the biggest joys of the sport. Wind in your face, hair blowing in the breeze (from under your helmet, of course), soaking in towering mountains, flowering meadows, and all the surrounding beauty in a way that is best appreciated humming down the road on the saddle of a bike.

No matter whether you're a recreational rider or a budding pro, having the fitness to travel far and wide on two wheels makes the sport more enjoyable. Speaking of enjoyable, it's also just plain fun to be fit and fast for whatever kind of riding you're doing. I asked a wide, diverse group of diehard women cyclists if getting fitter, stronger, and faster on the bike was important to them and why. Their answers pretty much nailed what the following chapters are about.

Going fast is super fun! Especially with a welcoming, friendly field of women who smile big and rip my legs off every week! More fit. More fast. Most important, MORE FUN.

—RACHEL RUBINO

I train because I like to ride fast so I can race faster.

—INSUK DIOVISALVO

I like to feel strong on the bike and get the ride done. I like to go distances and up hills. I don't really care how fast I go, I train to not suffer.

—SAMANTHA LOCKWOOD

I don't race much, but I train and pursue speed because it's fun, and also so I can keep up with the guys.

—ANNA CANNINGTON

I race against myself and try to keep me in shape. I want to keep riding enjoyable. It's not always about getting there the fastest, but enjoying what's on the way.

—SUZANNE SAWYER-BURRIS

I train to maintain my fitness and eat fettuccini Alfredo once a week. . . . The speed is a bonus.

—SARA PANCAKE

No training . . . just going out and enjoying the ride. The key is to push yourself out of your comfort zone occasionally. I am a much stronger and faster cyclist than I was a few years ago just by going out with friends as much as possible.

—**LAURA KELLY**

Fun, fitness, speed. In order of importance.

—**BRANDY KILKENNY**

I race mountain bikes. I train when I can, because I like that feeling of being able to get through the course.

—**HADLEY TAYLOR**

I would like to be faster, but then when I think harder, I think maybe no, I wouldn't. Because I like riding for scenery, and with others who like to stop and smell the roses along the way. Still, I do enjoy being off the front of such group rides.

—**ANN JASPER**

Train, yes. Race, no. I do try to beat my own personal records, but I don't enter formal races. I knew I was getting pretty good when I was able to reach the end of a 100-K ride more than 20 minutes before my husband. He has been faster than me our whole marriage. That was kind of awesome.

—**ROCHELLE MACDONALD**

Racing keeps me goal oriented and always learning more. One problem my coach sees with his female clients is [their] not being able to reach the higher-intensity workouts when on our own. I enjoy the weekly crit practice with the guys who generously help me try to hang on to the fast wheels. It has really helped. I try to show up for races when they offer Masters women categories, even though the fields are small.

—**JENNIFER LACKER**

Keeping up with the guys, enjoying the ride, competing and sometimes just completing a hard ride or event, eating treats, and kicking ass were the most common themes to come up. Interestingly, "getting a bikini body" didn't get a single mention. These women appreciate that fitness and strength are different from being skinny, and though riding can make you lean, the end goal is enjoying being fit and strong for the ride and maybe the race.

The pages that follow are chock-full of advice that will help you accomplish each and every one of those lofty goals. At the heart of this section is learning how to train. The human body is an amazingly adaptable machine that will reward specific training with improved results—most of the time. But training is as much an art as it is a science, and the female body is an even more complex, wonderful machine than its male counterpart, which means women might sometimes want to train a little bit differently than their male peers. You'll learn how to maximize your training time to get the optimal performance from your personal engine.

We'll also address your body off the bike. Strength training and stretching are both controversial topics in the world of cycling training. Women have very different needs than men when it comes to both. It's possible you need more of the former and less of the latter—or at least a different approach. You'll find those answers along with specific resistance training and flexibility routines that cater to the female cyclist.

Finally, let's get a little goal oriented and talk about what it takes to toe the line (and successfully get to the finish) at cycling events, including races—on and off-road—Gran Fondos, and the ever-popular century ride. While many women ride and participate in charity events, far fewer race, which is a shame because racing can boost your confidence, send your fitness through the roof, and add even more fun to your relationship with the sport. Here's what you need to know to get started—and if you already do race, to take it to the next level.

CHAPTER 14

Why and How to Train

MY FRIEND LISA USED TO RACE TRIATHLONS, SO SHE GOT A coach. Then a year or so passed and she stopped doing triathlons. Yet she continued working with her coach, which I found curious. "So you're not racing, but you're still following a plan?" I asked one afternoon over coffee. "Yeah. I found that I really like training—even more so than racing. It keeps me fit and engaged, and I like that I don't have to think about what to do." So Lisa treated her monthly check to her coach the way other people do their gym memberships—as an investment in her health and fitness.

I'd never really thought of it that way before, but it made perfect sense. So often people come into a sport or activity wanting to get fitter, and they do, for a while. But then they stop making progress—and sometimes then just stop altogether. Or at least slow down, because their enthusiasm wanes. That happens less with cycling because it's so social that there are other incentives to stick with it. But it does happen. It's also easy to get a little burned out or bored if you're always riding the same loops at the same pace every time you roll out, even if it's an activity that you love, like cycling.

What's more, training is fun. Yes, it's hard. If you do it right, it's ludicrously hard at times. But there's little that feels as amazing and satisfying when you're done.

Leg-searing, eye-popping, please-God-make-it-stop hill repeats, Tabata sprint sets, and full-throttle 'cross and mountain bike training sessions make me high for hours, sometimes for the better part of a day.

And it's not just my highly active imagination. I've got science on my side. Soon after you throw the amount of effort you're making into turbocharge, your brain steps up to the bar and starts serving you an intoxicating cocktail of soothing chemicals like serotonin, dopamine, norepinephrine, and cannabinoids (that chemical sound familiar?). Research shows that for many people, just three 45-minute interval sessions a week are enough to reduce symptoms of depression as effectively as prescription antidepressants (with far better side effects).

Plus, hard training (and racing, which we'll talk about later) is just really good for you. For one, it boosts levels of growth factors in your brain, helping to create new brain cells and establishing new connections between cells to help you learn. You may feel rock stupid minutes after a 45-minute charge through peanut butter mud, but trust me, you're really developing your inner genius.

Riding hard and fast also puts Father Time in a headlock, keeping you perpetually young—or at least younger. In a 20-year study that began with more than 960 men and women ages 50 and older, Stanford University researchers found that the ones who regularly performed vigorous activity not only were leaner, but also had less than half the mortality rate and started experiencing age-related disability a full 16 years later than those who spent all their time in the slow lane.

Convinced yet? Good. Because in this chapter you'll find everything you need to know about how training works and how to do it, as well as some sample plans to get you started and/or take you to the next level.

How Training Works

In a nutshell, training acclimates your body to doing what you want it to do. If you want to go faster, you need to spend time pushing as hard and fast as you can. If you want to go longer, you need to log saddle time and make the adaptations that lead to better endurance. Want to be stronger on hills or a better sprinter? Well, guess what you need to do? Of course some adaptations will come more easily or naturally for each individual based on body type, musculature, and so on, but we can all improve even our weakest areas with a little work.

To understand how training makes you a stronger and fitter cyclist, here's a little peek at the anatomy of adaptation. Consider your typical Saturday morning coffee shop ride: The pack rolls out at an easy conversational pace. You're spinning along, able to form complete sentences, while your heart rate sits in a comfortable aerobic zone that's about 60 or 65 percent of your maximum heart rate (MHR). At this exertion, your legs use mostly slow-twitch muscle fibers to turn the cranks. These fibers make the energy you need by taking stored fats and some carbohydrates and blasting them with oxygen in the mitochondria, the cells' furnaces. Like windmills, this aerobic energy system uses oxygen to create steady, clean-burning power. The little bit of lactate you're producing is easily cleared and used for energy. The pedaling is painless; your legs are silent.

Then you hit your first hill and the pack amps the effort, everyone gunning to be first to the top. As you crank up the pace, your heart rate soars to 80 or 85 percent of your MHR. Like overloaded fuses, your slow-twitch fibers start fading. They scream for more oxygen to produce more power. But it's for naught. Those endurance fibers need more oxygen than you can provide, so they call in the backup generators—your fast-twitch fibers. These fibers go straight for your glycogen—stored carbs—and blast away without oxygen. This anaerobic system yields pure power, but like burning fossil fuels, it's messy work, dumping waste by-products into the environment that is your body. As lactate builds faster than you can clear and use it, you reach threshold. You've got 30 to 60 minutes at this level of exertion before the by-products of lactate metabolism create an acid bath in your muscle cells and you're forced to dial it down.

Training simply raises the point at which you have to dial it down. Here's how.

MORE POWER IN YOUR PUMP

The average resting heart rate for a typical woman is between 60 and 100 beats per minute. The average for a well-trained woman plummets to 40 to 60 beats per minute. Like your quads and calves, your heart—which is a muscle—gets stronger and can squeeze out more blood with every beat. That way it doesn't have to beat as fast or work as hard to circulate oxygen- and nutrient-rich blood through your system. That's particularly useful when you're punching those pedals in a sprint or grinding up a steep incline.

YOUR NETWORK EXPANDS

All that blood squeezed out per beat will do you no good if your muscles can't soak it in. The more you push your muscles to perform, the more oxygen-rich blood they need to produce energy. So your body forges thousands of new capillaries in your muscles to maximize your circulation. I saw evidence of this phenomenon firsthand at one of the Body Worlds traveling museum exhibits that featured cadavers engaged in sports and other activities to show the miraculous workings of the human body. It's my favorite example of how the body adapts. There was a cyclist standing upright in a glass case. His legs had been stripped of everything but the capillaries, which had been shot full of bright red ink. It looked like a colony of spiders had thrown a rave. His legs were webbed solid with hundreds of thousands of tiny vessels to deliver blood to every inch of his quads, hamstrings, and calves.

YOU MAKE MORE CONNECTIONS

Newbies make improvements in strength and speed fairly quickly. That's because one of the earliest adaptions your body makes to training is waking up sleeping neuromuscular connections. Your body is extremely efficient. So it uses only as many muscle fibers as it needs for you to keep going. Once you start pushing those pedals harder, your brain goes, "Hey, we need more horsepower," and fires up more motor neurons so you can activate more muscle fibers with every single pedal stroke.

What's more, you also maximize your muscle fiber type. We each have two general types of muscle fibers: type I, which are your slow-twitch endurance fibers, and type II, which are your fast-twitch power fibers (and are further split into type IIa and type IIb). We're born with a certain mixture of each, which is why some people are better suited for endurance activities while others are more suited to those requiring speed. But the ratio isn't set in stone. Some of our fibers are switch-hitters that we can coax into behaving more like one or the other depending on our training. In fact, exercise scientists have estimated that about 40 percent of the variance in our fiber types is due to environmental influences (e.g., training), with the rest mostly genetically determined. So even if you weren't born a speed machine, you have a lot of influence over how much you can maximize your power, speed, and sprint.

YOU BURN FAT BETTER

As you recruit and develop more muscle fibers, strengthen your heart, and lay down a thick bed of capillaries, your body ramps up production of aerobic enzymes to extract more oxygen from your blood. Meanwhile, your body expands the energy-generating mitochondria in your cells so they hold more oxygen and make aerobic energy more quickly. Research shows that all of these adaptations increase the amount of oxygen-rich blood you pump out by about 32 ounces per minute while you're cruising down the road. You also increase your ability to use O_2 to the tune of about 10 percent for each minute you ride. In essence, you become a better fat burner. The better you are at burning fat, the longer you can ride without hitting the wall.

GET FITTER FASTER

According to a 2011 study presented at the American College of Sports Medicine Annual Meeting, just 2 weeks of high-intensity intervals improves your aerobic capacity as much as 6 to 8 weeks of endurance training does. Another study, from 2006, found that after 8 weeks of doing high-intensity interval training (HIIT for short), men and women could ride twice as long as they could before the study while maintaining the same pace.

Monitoring Your Efforts

The more specific you get with your training, the better your results will generally be. Most riders spend far too much time riding comfortably hard, in that place where you feel like you're doing something, but you're not pushing your limits. By going much harder sometimes and much easier other times, you make more dramatic improvements. That means monitoring your intensity so you can hit—and stay in—the right intensity zone at the right time.

Some riders like to use speed to measure their output, but honestly, speed doesn't always tell you how hard you're working. If there's a hard headwind, for instance, you may be cranking with all the watts you've got and still be going only 11 mph. Likewise, if there's a stiff breeze at your back, you might be going 23 mph and barely breathing. Better ways of monitoring workload are measuring watts using a power meter, tracking your heart rate with a heart rate monitor, and/or rating your perceived exertion (how hard you feel like you're going based on things like how hard you're breathing—or how easy!). You can use any one or all three. Here's a snapshot of how each works.

RPE: MENTAL MONITORING AND TALK TEST

The most basic training tool you have is your breath. When you're working really hard, you're breathing really hard because your muscles need all the oxygen they can get. It's that simple. To keep tabs on how hard you're breathing, some coaches prescribe a talk test. Can you talk in full sentences? That's easy breathing. When your sentences are clipped and punctuated by your breathing, that's moderate. When you can get out one or two words at most, that's vigorous.

This method is best paired with rate of perceived exertion (RPE). On a scale of 1 to 10, how hard are you working? A 1 is coasting down a wide-open road with a tailwind. A 10 is charging as hard as you can go, legs searing, barely able to see straight, let alone speak. You rate how hard you're riding by ranking your effort on a scale

between the two extremes. Research shows it works just as well as a heart rate monitor or other equipment when you use it properly. The key is that you have to pay attention so you don't inadvertently slack off (or start pushing too hard on an easy day). That's why it works best in conjunction with monitoring your breathing. You don't stop breathing, so it's always there as a reminder to check your efforts.

HEART RATE MONITOR

As you pedal harder, your heart rate increases. Monitoring the number of beats per minute (bpm) with a heart rate monitor will tell you just how hard you're working—to a point. Heart rate can be somewhat fickle, and it can be influenced by dehydration, caffeine, menstruation, rest (or lack thereof), hormones, mood, and weather. There's also a great deal of variation from one rider to the next. You may hit your lactate threshold (LT) at 75 percent of maximum effort or heart rate, while a more seasoned cyclist doesn't bump hers until she reaches 85 percent. So it's important to pair it with your perceived exertion or the reading on a power meter, if you have one (more on that in a bit).

If you've never used a heart rate monitor, it's a two-piece device. The first part is a transmitter that is held against your breastbone right over your heart with a strap that wraps around your torso. The second part is a computer monitor that acts as a cardiovascular dashboard. You mount this computer to your handlebars (or wear it as a watch) and the sensor on your chest picks up the signal from your heart and transmits it to the computer so you can see how many times your heart is thumping per minute. Most models also let you program in your training zone parameters and will beep at you if you fall below or push past your target zone.

If you invest in a heart rate monitor, you'll find instructions for setting your training zones based on your maximum heart rate (MHR), the greatest number of times your heart can pump in 1 minute. There are a couple of ways to find your MHR. One is by using an age-based equation. If you go that route, it's important that you do *not* use the old (and sadly most-often repeated) one: 220 minus your age.

That equation was not designed to be used by an athletic person. It's also notoriously inaccurate among older adults—the ones who may be most reliant on it—because it shows a steady decline that is not necessarily true and possibly underestimates their MHRs by more than 35 bpm. In fact, it may be pretty useless as a measurement tool for older adults. Fortunately, a team of Norwegian scientists analyzed 3,320 men and women ages 19 to 89 to come up with a more accurate formula: 211 minus 64 percent of your age. So a 45-year-old woman would have an MHR of 182 (7 beats higher than the old formula). No formula is without some margin of error, and with this one it's about 10 bpm, so again, check in with how you're feeling rather than going strictly by the data on your screen.

You can also get a more accurate MHR by taking a field test, but because it's hard to push yourself to the max when you're alone, this is best done with a faster friend or a coach, or even during a race. First, warm up thoroughly. Then ride as hard as possible for 10 minutes, pushing like a million dollars is on the line for the final 30 seconds. Then cool down and check your monitor for your MHR. Repeat this test one or two more times (taking rest days in between) to find your true maximum. For the best results, prepare for the field test as you would for a race. You should be well rested, well hydrated, and feeling good going into the tests.

Once you've determined your max, break your heart rate down into training zones to accomplish goals, including endurance training, lactate threshold training, and recovery. Calculate your zones based on your MHR. For instance, a recovery heart rate for a rider with an MHR of 180 bpm would be less than 115 bpm ($180 \times 0.64 = 115$ bpm). There are many different ways to divvy up your training zones. I prefer to keep it simple with five, as described on page 147 (including how they correspond with the breathing/RPE zones described previously).

I should note that monitoring your heart rate can be tricky during training because there's a lag between when you start pushing yourself and your heart rate response. It's meant to be used as a guide, not gospel. Again, tune in to how you're feeling.

POWER METER

Power meters measure your workload in watts. Pedal softly and you'll be producing enough power to bring a reading light to a dim. Throw the hammer down and you can literally light up the house. Power meters provide instant feedback on how hard you're working. You can start pedaling and see that you're producing 150 watts without waiting for your heart rate to "catch up." They're also a nice reality check to use with heart rate training because with heart rate, you may be hitting 175 bpm, but maybe you're dehydrated or not feeling well, so you're not actually producing that much power, you're just suffering at a slower speed. While results from other monitoring methods may be up for interpretation, watts don't lie. You are either able to produce the prescribed amount of power or you aren't. If you aren't, that means you're too tired for that level of intensity and need an easier training day.

As with heart rate, training with power requires that you find your personal baseline numbers to work with. Most coaches like to use functional threshold power—simply the average wattage you can produce for a 1-hour time trial—as their anchor point. Since you're not likely to ever go out and be able to create an uninterrupted, all-out 1-hour time trial (TT) for yourself, power training experts like Hunter Allen recommend performing a 20-minute TT and multiplying the average wattage by 0.95, since your hour-long wattage would be about 5 percent lower.

When paired with a heart rate monitor, power meters allow you to experiment with cadence and gearing to find the sweet spot relative to your speed, wattage, and heart rate. Popular brands include SRM, CycleOps, Ergomo, and Polar. The only downside? The price. Power meters don't come cheap. The lowest-cost ones come in at about a grand. So it's a really serious investment, but also the most powerful training tool available for those who are really serious.

Training Efforts

Once you choose the tools you'll use to monitor your efforts, you need some efforts to monitor. The hallmark of training is working your body at varying intensities to accomplish specific fitness goals and become accustomed to riding at higher intensities. That means intervals—which are specific effort levels maintained for a certain amount of time. On page 149, you'll find a super simple mix-and-match training plan based on the following interval intensities.

MAX

To raise your max VO_2 (the maximum volume of oxygen your body can use), you need to push your efforts to the max. These intervals are to be done at full throttle, as hard as you can—Zone 5, or a 10 on the RPE scale. The good news: Because they're so hard, they're also very short, lasting only 20 seconds to 3 minutes.

THRESHOLD

If max VO_2 is your roof, then lactate threshold (LT)—the point at which you start working anaerobically—is your drop ceiling. To get fast, you want to raise your LT so you have more aerobic room before you bump into that overhang. There are lots of ways to train for raising your LT, including hill climbing and sustained efforts. These efforts are done at an RPE of 7 or 8, or Zone 4.

TEMPO

These efforts push you just above your comfort zone, so you're breathing faster and working harder than you would on a typical aerobic endurance ride. You're not working so hard, however, that you can't sustain it for a long period of time. The value of these efforts is underrated, in my opinion. Done regularly, they improve your body's ability to clear and use lactic acid, so they also help raise your LT. They're done at an RPE of 5 or 6, or Zone 3.

ENDURANCE

Long-Sunday-ride pace. You're working hard enough to feel like you're exercising, but you can carry on a conversation, cruise for hours, and enjoy the ride. These efforts build capillaries and endurance. Cruising rides are done at an RPE of 3 or 4, or Zone 2.

EASY

For hard intervals to work their magic, you need easy rides and rest periods to let your body heal, adapt, and get stronger and fitter.

Get in the Zone

ZONE 1: Light and relaxed breathing—barely above normal.

ZONE 2: Deep, steady, relaxed breathing. That's your aerobic, endurance-training zone. It's an RPE of 3 or 4.

ZONE 3: Slightly labored. This is a steady "tempo" pace, where you're working just a bit above your endurance comfort zone. It's where you'd be if you were riding with someone just slightly faster than you. It's an RPE of 5 or 6.

ZONE 4: Short, fast rhythmic breathing. This is your lactate threshold zone, right where you're hitting your sustainable upper limits. Also known as race pace, it's an RPE of 6 to 8.

ZONE 5: Hard, heavy breathing. This is your maximum VO_2 training zone, at the top of your effort, where your body is using as much oxygen as humanly possible, as hard as you can go. It's an RPE of 9 or 10.

TRAINING ZONE	% MHR	RPE
Zone 1 (recovery, easy day)	60–64	1–2
Zone 2 (aerobic endurance)	65–74	3–4
Zone 3 (high-level aerobic—"tempo")	75–84	5–6
Zone 4 (lactate threshold—race pace)	85–94	7–8
Zone 5 (maximum effort)	95–100	9–10

Your easy days and recovery periods between intervals should be ridiculously easy. Your only goal is to boost your circulation and promote repair and recovery. These rides hover within Zone 1, at 1 or 2 on the RPE scale.

Putting It All Together

No matter what monitoring tool you choose, the following chart will help you work in the proper training zone.

Mix-and-Match Training

You can find hundreds of training plans online, and everyone has their own training philosophy. But at the very heart of it all, training is nothing more than combining hard, medium, and easy days into every week. For example, a week could include 2 fairly hard days, 2 medium-effort days, 2 easy days, and 1 day with no riding. Don't ride 6 days a week? You can substitute cross-training of a similar intensity, maybe doing some hatha yoga on an easy day or CrossFit on a hard day. So long as you get in the intensity and the recovery you need, you will enjoy training gains.

As a bonus, adding intensity makes you far more likely to stick to your workout plans. Research shows that when women started exercising for fitness and weight loss, they enjoyed their workouts more and were less likely to throw in the towel when their weekly workouts included high-intensity sessions, compared to when they just exercised moderately day in and day out.

To that end, see the chart on the opposite page for a sample week with a variety of intervals for each intensity zone. Simply pick your intervals and go. How long you ride is really a matter of how much time you have. For hard interval days, you want to be sure you warm up for at least 10 to 15 minutes before launching into the efforts. Recovery or easy days should be kept to about an hour or so. Long days can be as long as you like, but generally 2 hours or so makes a nice long ride.

Interval Mania

By nature, intervals are short and hard. Do those twice a week (though you can pepper your long rides with harder efforts if you're feeling fresh). Longer, less intense tempo intervals are important as well, so don't overlook them even though there's not quite as much

PACE	ZONE	RPE	BREATHING	% MHR	% FIELD-TESTED POWER
Easy	1	1–2	Light and relaxed	60–64	30–40
Endurance	2	3–4	Deep and steady	65–74	50–70
Tempo	3	5–6	Slightly labored	75–84	75–85
Threshold	4	7–8	Short and rhythmic	85–94	85–95
Max	5	9–10	Rapid and heavy	95–100	100–130

DAY	MON	TUE	WED	THU	FRI	SAT	SUN
Effort	Easy/rest, easy to endurance	Hard	Medium, tempo to threshold	Medium, tempo to threshold	Easy/rest, easy to endurance	Medium to hard, long ride	Medium to hard, long ride
Zone	Zone 1–2	Zone 4–5	Zone 3–4	Zone 3–4	Zone 1–2	Zone 2–4	Zone 2–4
Notes	Monday is generally a great day to take off or do a little yoga as you dive back into the workweek after a good weekend of riding.	Short, sweet, and sweaty. I like to call it Turbo Tuesday. Blow off some stress, fire up your metabolism.	Nice solid ride that's not too hard or too easy, but just right for midweek.	Back-to-back medium days build muscular endurance and overall fitness.	TGIF. Do as you'd like.	Weekends are made for bike riding. Longer rides with a few hard efforts sprinkled in are perfect fitness builders. Group rides are great for this.	Repeat Saturday or take a nice Sunday cruise with a few hills thrown in for good measure.

variety involved. Remember to warm up at least 10 to 15 minutes before your hard efforts and cool down after. You'll see improvement in your performance in as little as 2 weeks.

HARD: ZONE 4 TO 5: THRESHOLD TO MAX VO$_2$

TRIPLE THREAT

Crank up your intensity until you're working very hard (a 9 on a 1-to-10 RPE scale). Hold that intensity for 3 minutes. Recover with easy spinning for 3 minutes. Repeat 3 times.

BENEFIT: Boosts max VO$_2$.

FLYING 30S

Sprint all-out for 30 seconds. Recover with an easy spin for 2^1/$_2$ minutes. Repeat for 12 sprints.

BENEFITS: Research shows that even seasoned cyclists can improve their max VO$_2$ by

3 percent and their 40-kilometer time trial speed by more than 4 percent in just 4 weeks by doing intervals of 30 seconds at supramaximal effort (that's science-speak for an all-out effort lasting less than 2 minutes).

FLYING 30S UPHILL

On a moderate incline, stand out of the saddle and charge up the hill as fast as possible for 30 seconds. Coast back to your starting point. Repeat, this time seated. Alternate between standing and sitting for six climbs. Recover for 10 minutes. Do another set.

BENEFITS: Raises fitness ceiling and develops mental toughness.

TABATAS

Sprint as hard as possible for 20 seconds. Coast for 10 seconds. Repeat 6 to 8 times.

BENEFITS: These intense efforts train your body to use more muscle and increases the intensity you can sustain over a 60-minute time trial, which corresponds to your lactate threshold.

MAX OUT

Go as hard as you can for 1 to 2 minutes. Spin easy for 1 minute. Repeat 4 to 6 times.

BENEFITS: Stronger top end and better ability to recover between hard efforts.

MINI TTS

Push steadily and as hard as you can sustain for 8 to 10 minutes. Recover for 5 minutes. Repeat 2 more times.

BENEFITS: Improves overall speed and endurance, even on easy rides.

UPHILL SPRINT 20S

Find a hill that takes 10 to 15 minutes to climb. Start climbing at your threshold. After 2 minutes, stand up and attack at just below all-out sprint intensity (9-plus on a 1-to-10 scale) for 20 pedal strokes. Sit and go right back to climbing at your threshold. Repeat every 1 to 2 minutes (depending on your fitness) all the way up the hill. Perform the drill 1 or 2 times.

BENEFITS: Not only raises your threshold, but also makes you a monster climber.

ROCKIN' ROLLERS

Find a short climb or series of climbs that take about 2 minutes to crest. Wind up before you hit the climb so you're at threshold as soon as the hill starts. Climb at threshold for 90 sec-

onds, then go as fast as you can for the final 30 seconds all the way to the top. Repeat 4 to 6 times.

BENEFITS: Improves fitness and power on varied terrain.

OVER 'N' UNDER

Increase your effort to threshold and hold it steady there for 5 minutes. Dial back your effort to just below threshold for 5 minutes. Repeat 3 or 4 times.

BENEFIT: Increases your tolerance for riding at your threshold.

40S

In a medium to large gear, push hard for 40 seconds, then recover for 20 seconds. Repeat 10 times. That's one set. Do up to four, resting for 5 minutes between sets.

BENEFIT: Muscular endurance as you build power and train your body to recover quickly between efforts for events that demand repeated surges.

MEDIUM: ZONE 3 TO 4: TEMPO TO THRESHOLD
TEMPO X 3

Increase your effort to where you're working at a hard, but sustainable, effort level (7 to 8 RPE). Hold that pace, without letting off, for 15 minutes. Spin easy for 3 minutes. Repeat 3 times. As you improve, lengthen the tempo time to 20 minutes.

BENEFITS: These are what some coaches call "fun fast" intervals—hard without making you cry for mercy. Improves your ability to clear lactate. Improves your sustainable "race pace."

STEADY AS SHE GOES

Increase your effort to a moderately hard pace where you are breathing hard, but your legs aren't burning (about 6 to 7 RPE). Hold for 30 to 40 minutes. Spin easy for 5 to 10 minutes. Repeat. Work up to one continuous steady-state effort of an hour.

BENEFIT: Makes you a monstrous fat burner.

BIG GEAR CHURNING

On a long, gradual hill or false flat (a stretch that looks flat, but actually has a low grade), climb at a moderate exercise level. Then after about 2 minutes, click into a harder gear and pedal at a lower cadence (about 70 rpm) while keeping your effort moderate (about 7 RPE) for 10 minutes. Click into an easier gear to pedal normally for 5 to 10 minutes. Repeat 1 or 2 more times.

BENEFITS: Improves muscular endurance and pedal force, and makes you more resistant to fatigue on climbs using your usual cadence.

Train Hard, Recover Harder

There's a saying in pro circles that the race is won in bed, which is to say all the training in the world will do you zero good if you don't rest. It makes complete sense. Training gains are based on a concept called super compensa-

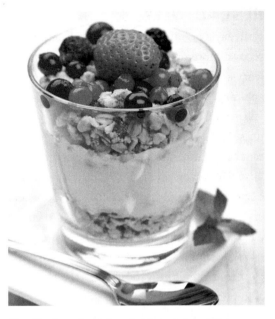

A healthy dose of protein and carbohydrates will help your muscles mend and recover quickly after a hard effort.

tion. You push yourself hard, break down your muscles, empty your fuel stores, and tax your central nervous system. You reach deep inside yourself, maybe even overreach to squeeze out every bit of speed and performance, leaving your body spent. If you follow that up with more reaching and digging, you'll find yourself in a hole.

Instead, you follow that overreaching with rest and recovery, so your body can repair and rebuild itself to be better and stronger than it was before. That way the next time you dig and reach, you're starting from a faster, fitter place. Then you rest and recover and keep progressing in a stepwise fashion. Here's what you need to know.

REST, ACTIVELY

Full days off are fine. But you'll generally recover more quickly if you move your body at least a little bit. Easy workouts—whether it's spinning, jogging, swimming, or yoga class—get your blood circulating to flush out waste products, bring in fresh nutrient-rich blood, and reduce inflammation, so you're ready for your next ride. When your training calls for a recovery day—generally after high-mileage weekends, hard interval sessions, or races—keep the pace embarrassingly slow. Keep yourself honest by just spinning to the coffee shop in your plain clothes or riding with your kids in the park.

Remember, too, to make active recovery part of every ride by dialing back your effort for the final 5 to 10 minutes of your ride. Easing up on the pedals enhances blood flow to help flush your legs of metabolic waste and fuel your depleted muscles. A study in the *Journal of Strength and Conditioning Research* found that when cyclists did a 15-minute cooldown spin at 30 percent of their max VO_2 after a hard effort, they were able to perform almost as well 24 hours later on an identical strenuous workout.

REFUEL THE RIGHT WAY

If you do a ride or race that leaves you depleted, you need to replenish yourself when you're done. The easiest way is with a little post-ride snack that delivers some carbs and protein. Chocolate milk is a crowd favorite because it's tasty and convenient, and it works. In a study of cyclists who rode until fully depleted, the pedalers who chugged chocolate milk afterward were able to hammer about 50 percent longer on their next ride before fatiguing than those who consumed a commercial carb-and-protein recovery drink. One essential note for women, however: Women need more protein for complete recovery than chocolate milk provides. Add a handful of almonds for the right ratio. Other good foods for recovery include smoothies with Greek yogurt and fruit, cereal and milk, and sandwiches.

Regarding timing, you may have heard that you have a 30-minute window after you're done for optimum recovery. That's true—but not always necessary. Yes, research shows that you have a 30-minute window immediately post exercise where your muscles are glycogen sponges and you can restock your stores most effectively by taking in carbs with a little protein (which speeds glycogen absorption and keeps your body from breaking down muscle tissue for energy). But this research has been done on fully depleted—on the verge of bonking—riders. That's not most of us most of the time. If you have eaten a meal or snack a couple of hours before a 2-hour ride, you still have fuel in storage. What's more, even if you ride longer and harder, research shows your glycogen stores will return to normal by the following day so long as you eat like a normal human being for the rest of the day.

The exception is if you're racing on back-to-back days, where after the first day you may be fully depleted and need to replenish for the second day ASAP, or if for some reason you don't eat regular meals. In that case, go ahead and chug that shake. Or better yet, do as I do and divide your meals. That way, I conquer my pre- and post-ride needs by eating half my morning or afternoon meal before I ride and half when I get home. "This strategy also prevents taking in more calories than you need—and stalling out any weight-loss efforts—by overdoing your recovery nutrition," says University of Pittsburgh–based sports nutritionist Leslie Bonci.

GET A MASSAGE

Many cyclists, myself included, swear by massage. Long hours in the saddle can leave muscles riddled with knots and adhesions that limit range of motion and, if left unchecked, lead to pain. By keeping those muscles smooth and "unstuck," a massage therapist can keep you rolling pain free.

Massage also speeds recovery. For one, it increases circulation—everywhere—even if you just get your legs rubbed down. In one telling study, Chicago researchers had 25 volunteers crank out enough leg presses to make their quads and hamstrings cry uncle. Then half the group got a massage while the others got zip. When the researchers measured everyone's circulation by testing blood flow in the upper arm, the leg pressers who got massage enjoyed improved overall blood flow for up to 72 hours post rubdown. The exercise-only group had hampered circulation for more than 48 hours.

Because circulation was boosted in the arm, far away from the legs, which did the work and/or received the massage, it suggests that massage triggers a systemic—full-body—response that encourages the blood vessels to open and improve blood flow. "That's important because, as we showed, exercise-induced muscle damage slows circulation," says study coauthor Shane A. Phillips, PhD, of the University of Illinois at Chicago.

The exercisers in the massage group were also far less sore. In fact, they had no lingering soreness 90 minutes post massage, while the exercise-only folks were still hobbling 24 hours later. "The increase in blood flow speeds recovery from muscle injury by providing more nutrition to the tissue and maybe also by improving the removal of waste products," says Phillips.

In another study on cyclists, those who got a massage on only one leg showed greater muscle regeneration in the treated leg. And researchers in Canada found that postexercise massage reduced inflammation and promoted the growth of new mitochondria—the parts of your cells that produce power.

Finally, numerous studies have shown that massage lowers levels of the stress hormone cortisol, which is released during hard efforts. Excess cortisol has been linked to overtraining syndrome, which is nothing more than a product of very poor recovery and can lead to a host of problems including irritability, weight gain, and muscle loss.

DIY Rub

No time or cash for a therapist's healing hands? Keep your muscles supple with a foam roller. A study recently published in *Medicine and Science in Sports and Exercise* reports that foam rolling reduces muscle soreness while improving range of motion and muscle activation (measured through a vertical jump test). Rest your leg muscles and glutes on the cylinder and roll slowly back and forth, pausing and pressing into the sorest spots for 30 to 45 seconds. (For more, see "The Science of Stretching" on pages 180–82.)

TAKE A COLD PLUNGE

Some studies suggest that a cold-water dunk after a hard ride helps speed recovery by reducing inflammation and that it helps athletes feel less fatigued and sore. A *Journal of Strength and Conditioning Research* study found that a group of cyclists who immersed their legs in cold water right after a hard effort performed even better on a second rigorous ride 24 hours later. Whether it leads to actual strength gains is up for debate. A recent review of 17 studies found that while it does reduce pain, cold-water immersion might not make muscles stronger. I've never been able to force myself to do the traditional ice-bath thing, where you soak in about 8 to 10 inches of 50° to 60°F water for 20 minutes. But if there's a stream or a cool pool that's convenient, I'll take a dip.

GIVE YOURSELF A SQUEEZE

Research suggests that compression tights can help reduce blood lactate levels and speed recovery. Studies show that athletes feel fresher and experience less muscle soreness after wearing them. For optimum effect, you may need to wear them during hard efforts, not just afterward. A good place to start is with compression socks. Your calves are known as your second heart because they help pump blood back up through the system to get oxygenated. Compression socks facilitate that process. If you notice a benefit, you can progress to full tights.

SLEEP TIGHT AND RIGHT

Sleep is essential for optimal recovery and performance. For one, too little makes you sick and slow. A tall body of research has found that folks who skimp on sleep (generally defined as fewer than 6 hours a night) are more prone to heart disease, diabetes, depression, weight gain, and, well, early death. A recent laboratory study revealed why. Researchers found that when they had volunteers sleep less than 6 hours a night for a week, key genes started switching on and off. Specifically, genes that govern the immune system, metabolism, stress response, and the sleep and wake cycle were suppressed, while those affecting inflammation were more active. Too little sleep = health havoc and poor recovery.

Proper sleep = improved performance. In two separate studies, when researchers had athletes (specifically, basketball players and swimmers) extend their sleep to a pro-level 10 hours a night (seriously, many pro athletes sleep nearly half the day) for about 6 weeks, they improved their sprint times, executed tricky moves faster, shot 3-pointers with greater accuracy, played harder, improved their efficiency, and just plain felt better.

None of this is surprising when you consider that the two most powerful stimulants of human growth hormone (HGH) are hard exercise and deep sleep, and that HGH is essential for muscle synthesis, fat metabolism, and other key elements of recovery and performance.

I did a sleep study at the Center for Sleep Medicine at New York-Presbyterian Hospital/ Weill Cornell Medical Center for a story a few years back. I didn't think I had sleep problems going in, but I learned so much, and I have never slept better since. Here's what the sleep experts there recommended for the soundest shuteye.

SKIP THE LATE-DAY STARBUCKS. Caffeine has a half-life of about 6 hours, so if you have a big Americano with 225 milligrams of caffeine at 3:00 p.m., by 9:00 p.m., you still have an espresso shot's worth flowing through your system. Ease up your coffee intake well before the end of the day.

CREATE A COOL CAVE. Your body temperature naturally drops at night, initiating your sleep cycle. If the room is too hot or cold, it's disruptive to falling and staying asleep because your body is struggling to stay in its comfortable sleep zone. What's the right temp? That's personal, say sleep experts. But most seem to zone

High-Tech Recovery

Many pros swear by electrical muscle stimulation (EMS) machines to speed their day-to-day recovery. These machines, like the portable Marc Pro, stimulate your muscles to contract, which pumps waste out and brings fresh blood in to facilitate muscle recovery and capillary development.

The technology has been used for years in rehab settings, but now athletes are hooking themselves up to simply recover faster and get stronger. A recent study published in the *Journal of Exercise Physiology* found that weight lifters who included muscle stimulation as part of their recovery saw greater strength gains and less fatigue than those who didn't. I was very skeptical—even a little skeeved out—the first time I stuck the Marc Pro electrodes on my heavy, post-race legs and watched my quads contract. But a half hour later, when the stairs from the basement seemed to have disappeared beneath me, I was sold. I took a unit with me to the Brasil Ride stage race (7 days of 40 to 90 miles of mountain bike racing) and used it every night. There's no question my legs stayed fresher. This freshness comes at a price, in this case $650. But if you get serious about training and racing, it's an investment that will keep you rolling with less downtime.

in on about the mid-60s. Then curl up under some covers and drift off.

KILL YOUR TELEVISION (AND IPAD . . . AND IPHONE). As darkness falls, your melatonin level rises, sending you into slumber. If you're lying

When to Pull the Plug

Pushing through a workout when you're still not recovered can put you in a hole. Here are six signs that warn you need to scrap your planned workout and do something else till you're raring to go.

1. Your heart rate is higher than normal when you wake up. *Take an easy or rest day.*

2. You can't stomach the idea of riding. *Do something else, like a walk or a mellow run or easy swim.*

3. Your heart rate on the bike is unusually high—or it's low plus you're irritable or don't feel well. *Decrease intensity and/or duration. (Lower heart rate can signal improved fitness. Keep a training log to become familiar with your body's normal responses.)*

4. You immediately feel horrendous on the bike and have a hard workout planned. *Spin easy or don't ride.*

5. You feel so-so on the bike and have a hard workout planned. *Do the first hard effort. If you still don't feel good, spin easy or call it a day.*

6. You didn't sleep well the previous night and don't feel rested. *Take an easy day.*

Source: Stephen Cheung, PhD

in bed staring at a giant screen, or even your iPhone, the light can suppress your melatonin and disrupt your sleep. Get it dark or at least very dim (maybe just a small reading light illuminating a good book) in your room 30 minutes before shuteye.

DIM THE NOISE. During my sleep study, the doctor was shocked at how often I woke up during the night. I thought it was normal. Turns out I just wake up to every little creak and squeak. I got earplugs the next day—life changing. Seriously. I sleep like the dead now. It's wonderful.

BE CONSISTENT. Your body is like a toddler. It likes routine. Give it regular bedtime and wakeup calls and it will throw fewer fits.

EASY ON THE BOOZE. That second (or third) pinot noir may make your eyelids droop, but alcohol-induced sleep is restless sleep. Too much alcohol before bed lengthens your non-REM sleep and shortens your REM sleep, which keeps you in more wakeful territory when you should be in deep slumber.

PUT THE MENTAL JUNK IN THE DRAWER. Your brain waves change as you cycle through the stages of sleep, going from the sleepy alpha waves in stage 1, the light-sleep theta waves of stage 2, the deep, slow delta waves of stage 3, and REM—rapid eye movement—sleep, where you start to dream. You cycle through these stages every 90 minutes until morning. Conversely, you have beta waves, which are your galloping workhorse, problem-solving brain waves. Lying in bed letting those horses run wild, especially at 3:00 a.m., is problematic because your brain can't get into those restful, restorative stages. The doctor who performed my study recommends that people with nighttime monkey brain keep a bedside worry journal. She tells them to write down everything that's preoccupying them in a list and assign a time to address them the next day. It helps those problem-solving beta waves calm down so you can sleep.

CHAPTER 15

Strengthen Your Human Frame

NOT MUCH IS MORE CONTROVERSIAL IN THE SPORT OF CYCLING than strength training. Some coaches strenuously discourage it, while others prescribe it as part of their plans. I for one believe that for most amateur cyclists especially, strength work pays off. Though research results have been a bit of a mixed bag on the subject, the most recent studies I've seen fall squarely in the benefit column.

One study in particular caught my attention because it was a scientific review that examined years of research on strength training and endurance performance. It concluded that performing sport-specific exercises, like squats and leg presses for cyclists, have many benefits. For example, workouts with heavy weight for 8 to 12 weeks in the off-season make your fast-twitch type II sprint fibers more fatigue resistant so they can hammer harder for longer, stiffen your tendons for greater stability in the saddle, and improve your neuromuscular efficiency—a fancy way of saying your brain can quickly recruit all the muscles you need to push your pedals. That all adds up to a fluid, efficient pedal stroke, improved power output, and higher threshold.

In another study, researchers had well-trained cyclists substitute explosive strength training for about a third of their endurance training. After just 4 weeks, the explosive trainers improved their max power and their time trial performance over those who strictly stuck to endurance work. They were also more efficient and were able to maintain higher short-term power (like that needed for sprinting) for 5 weeks longer than their endurance-only peers.

When I interviewed a colleague who has trained cyclists, including Olympians, for decades, he wasn't surprised. "I've incorporated heavy lifting in my cyclists' routines with great success for 25 years," says Douglas Lentz, director of fitness for Results Therapy and Fitness in Chambersburg, Pennsylvania. "As saddle time decreases in the off-season, we start to lift with the hips and legs, including heavy weight and plyometrics like box jumps." Once the riding season rolls around, all lower-body lifting stops, though core exercise continues.

Makes complete sense to me. In my experience, especially if you're a woman, strength training—done right—will nearly always make you stronger both on and off the bike. Plus it's good for your bones and can help prevent injury.

That bone thing is particularly important for us female cyclists. I haven't seen a great many studies on bone density in women cyclists in particular, but did see this: A study comparing male Masters cyclists (ages 53 to 71) riding about 200 miles per week with active peers less than half their age (ages 20 to 30) delivered some good news—and some bad news. The good news: The older cyclists were just as strong and able-bodied, scoring equally as well on lower-body lean-muscle and walking-speed tests as their younger, non-pedaling peers. The not-so-good news: Lower-body bone density—specifically, the femoral neck (the part of the thigh bone that sits between the ball that attaches to your pelvis and the long part of the bone), the femur's most vulnerable spot, was lower than in the active nonriders. That's not terribly surprising since cycling is a non-impact, non-weight-bearing sport. Although the study was on men, it doesn't take much of a leap to see how it's just as relevant, if not more so, to women, who start with lower bone density than men and are at higher risk for osteoporosis with age.

Our joints are also more vulnerable than men's. For one, our fluctuating hormones may make our tendons and ligaments more lax at certain times of our cycle (not much we can do about that). We also have wider hips, which makes us a bit knock-kneed and puts more stress on those joints. We tend to have less core strength, which is what provides the platform for pedaling stability. And we're generally smaller than men, so our joints and connective tissues are smaller and more vulnerable to injury. All that adds up to a recipe for knee pain, which is more common in women than men. Fortunately, it's nothing a little strength training can't remedy.

More Power to You

In general, if you're an avid cyclist who trains and maybe races, you're best off doing most of your heavy lifting in the off-season. Stick to core work when you're riding lots since you'll want to keep your legs fresh for rides and events. If you're more of a recreational rider, you can go ahead and lift all year long.

I'm also a fan of doing the least amount you can: I'm not doing biceps curls and bench presses and seven exercises for my legs when two will do. I also like moves that are highly functional, meaning that they hit many muscles in one shot and translate well to what I do on the bike. To that end, you'll find a mix-and-match approach to strength training in the workout sections that follow. There are three 3-move core routines, three 3-move leg routines, and three bonus plyometric moves (more on that in a bit).

Pick one workout or exercise from each section and do it 2 or 3 days a week. As mentioned earlier, you may choose to lay off the leg workouts during riding and racing season, but do core work year-round.

Core Matters

You need core strength to create a solid pedaling platform and prevent back pain. For cyclists, it's particularly important to strengthen what is known as the "inner unit" of the core—the deep muscles that attach to the lowest vertebra, lumbar 5, or L5, which include the transversus abdominis, the multifidis that run along your spine, the diaphragm above, and the pelvic floor below. The inner unit acts as an anchor, stabilizing your back, supporting your hips and shoulders, and helping to transfer force between your arms and legs in the cycling position.

When your core is weak, you not only slow down, but you also are at higher risk for hurting yourself. Research on competitive cyclists shows that when their core muscles fatigue, their pedaling mechanics break down, paving the way for poor performance and even injury as their knees flap from side to side instead of staying aligned.

These moves that follow strengthen your abs and obliques as well as key muscles in your middle and lower back to help reverse the cyclist's slump and better support your spine. Do one or two sets of each move, resting for 15 seconds between exercises. Aim for three sessions a week. If time permits, tack the routine onto the end of a ride. A study published in the *Journal of Strength and Conditioning Research* reported that cyclists who cooled down with a core workout had significantly better lactate clearance than those who did nothing.

Workout 1: Core

Plank with Alternating Knee Drops

Begin in the basic plank hold (in a pushup position with your forearms on the ground). Your elbows should be directly beneath your shoulders and your feet should be 8 to 10 inches apart. Slightly squeeze together your shoulder blades and keep your hips lifted so your body forms a straight diagonal line from your head to your heels. Slowly drop your left knee to the ground. Bring it back to the start position and drop the right knee. Continue alternating knees until you have touched each knee to the ground 15 times.

Power Bridge

Lying on your back, bend your knees and place your heels near your glutes. Your arms should be straight along your sides, with the palms down. In one smooth motion, squeeze your glutes, raise your hips off the floor, and push up from your heels to form a straight line from shoulders to knees, allowing your toes to come off the floor slightly. Hold for 2 seconds. Keeping your toes raised, lower yourself three-quarters of the way to complete 1 rep. Do 20 repetitions.

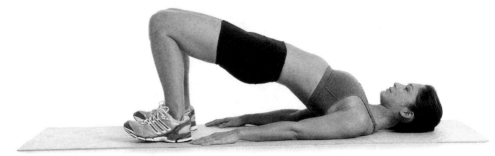

Scissors Kick

Lying on your back with your legs straight, place both hands palms down under your lower back. Pushing your elbows down into the floor and pulling your belly button toward your spine, raise your shoulders off the floor and look toward the ceiling. Raise your legs 4 inches off the ground and scissor them: left leg over right, then right over left. That's 1 rep. Work up to 30.

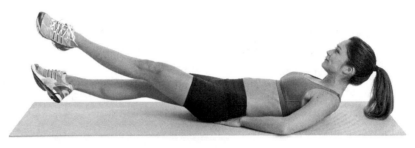

Workout 2: Core

Mountain Climbers

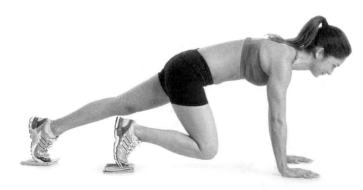

Start in a pushup position with a small towel under each foot (if you are on a carpeted floor, place a paper plate under each foot). Squeeze your shoulder blades together. Lengthen through the spine and pull your lower abs up toward the spine.

Without rocking or swaying the hips, slowly slide the right knee in toward the chest and slowly push it back out. Wait until the right leg is back in the start position before you pull in the left knee. Do 15 reps on each leg.

Sweeping Plank

Lie on your left side and raise your torso to assume a side plank position, with your left elbow under your shoulder and your forearm perpendicular to your torso for stability, and stack your right foot on top of your left. In one motion raise your right arm straight up toward the ceiling and lift your hips to create a straight line down your right side. Lower your arm to your side and your hips to a few inches off the floor. Do 10 to 15 reps, and then switch sides.

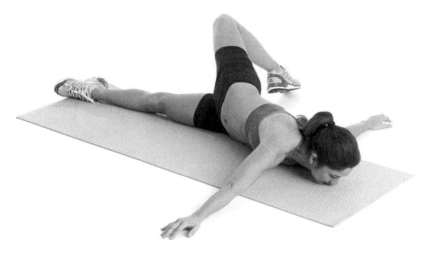

Scorpion

Lie facedown with your arms out to the sides. Lift your right leg and, twisting your torso, reach it across the back of your body toward your left hand. Return to the start position and switch sides. Do 10 to 15 total, alternating legs.

Workout 3: Core

Boat Pose

Sit, resting both hands lightly behind you, and lean back until your torso is at a 45-degree angle. Keeping your legs together, lift them off the floor as you extend your arms forward at shoulder height. Keep your abs tight, with your thighs and torso forming a 90-degree angle. Work up to holding for 60 seconds.

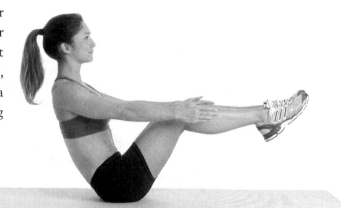

Swimming

Lie facedown with your forehead resting on the floor and your arms extended beyond your head, like Superman flying. Pull your navel to your spine and lift the left arm and right leg off the floor about 3 inches. Keeping your navel pulled in, lower your left arm and right leg and repeat the move to the opposite side. Alternate sides for a full set of 10 to 12 to each side.

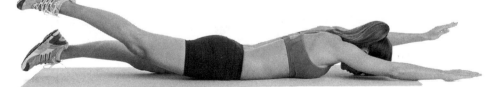

Side-Plank Crunch

Lie on the floor on your left side, legs extended, feet stacked. Prop yourself up on your left forearm so your elbow is directly beneath your shoulder and your forearm is perpendicular to your torso. Raise your hips off the floor so your body forms a straight diagonal line. Place your right hand behind your head, elbow pointing toward the ceiling. Using your obliques, two pairs of muscles at the sides of your abdomen, twist your torso and lower your bent right arm until it's parallel with the floor. Return to the start position. Complete a set of 12; switch sides.

She's Got Legs

Men can debate the merits of strength work off the bike all they want. For women, it works. We naturally have less lean muscle and we start losing it over time once we hit our 30s. You don't have to lift all year long if it makes your legs too tired and sore to ride and race as you like. But at the very least, carve out a 12- to 16-week period where you aren't riding or training on the bike as much—try winter if you live where it's cold, dark, and/or snowy—and dedicate some time to building strength. Even if you lay off the weights the rest of the year, you'll maintain a lot of those gains until you return to resistance training.

Workout 1: Legs

Squat

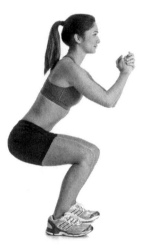

Stand with your feet hip-width apart, your abs tight. Clasp your hands. Bend your knees and lower body into a squat position as low as you can go, while maintaining a straight back and without wobbling. Push through the heels and squeeze your glutes to lift yourself back to the start position. For a more advanced exercise, hold a dumbbell in each hand. Repeat for a total of 15 squats.

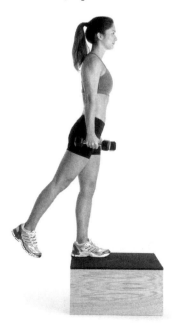

Planted Stepup

Hold a dumbbell in each hand and stand facing a bench or step about 12 inches high. Step onto the bench with your left leg. At the top of the move, contract your glutes and extend your right leg behind you. Keeping your left foot on the bench, bring your right leg back down, and lower your body until your right toe just touches the floor. Immediately repeat, completing a full set of 15 with one leg. Then switch sides.

Slide Lunge

Stand with your feet hip-distance apart. Place a paper plate or towel underneath your right foot. Shift your weight to your left leg and extend your arms straight out in front of you for balance. Bend your left knee and squat back 45 to 90 degrees while sliding the foot on the paper plate out to left as far as comfortably possible. Remember to keep your left knee over your toes as you lower yourself. Slowly pull the right leg back to the start position while straightening the left leg. Repeat for a full set of 15; then switch sides.

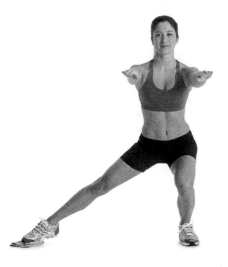

Workout 2: Legs

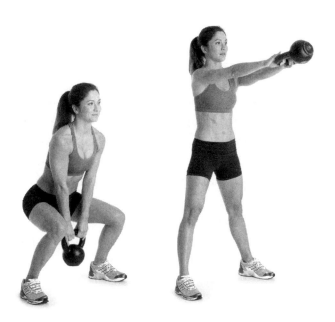

Kettlebell Swings

Stand with feet wide apart, holding a kettlebell with both hands, arms hanging down in front of you. Keeping your back straight, squat back, pressing your hips way back and swinging the kettlebell between your legs and behind your hips. Stand up, pressing your hips forward and swinging the weight up to chest level. Complete a full set of 15 reps.

No kettlebell? Substitute with a medicine ball or a dumbbell held by the ends.

Single-Leg Step Down

Holding dumbbells, stand on your right foot on a 6- to 12-inch-high step, allowing your left leg to hang in the air. Pull your navel toward your spine and, keeping your chest lifted and your back straight, slowly step down with your left foot and gently tap your left heel on the floor. Return to the start position, keeping your right heel firmly planted on the step. Do 15 reps on each leg.

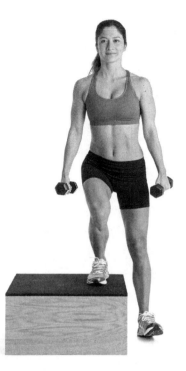

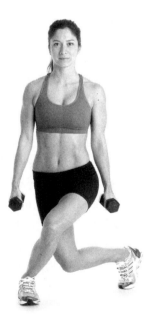

Curtsy

Stand with your feet hip-distance apart, holding dumbbells at your sides. Step back with your right leg to the 8 o'clock position behind you to the left. Bend both knees until the front knee is bent about 90 degrees (the knee should be in line with the ankle) and the back knee is close to the floor. Straighten legs and repeat for a full set of 15. Then switch sides.

Workout 3: Legs

Sumo Squat

Holding a dumbbell in each hand, hang your arms in front of you. Stand with your feet slightly wider than shoulder-width apart, toes pointing out to the sides. Squat a few inches, pressing your glutes back as you lift your arms out to the sides. Lift your heels and balance on the balls of your feet, deepening your squat until your thighs are nearly parallel to the floor. Pause, then lower your heels and rise back to the start position. Do 15.

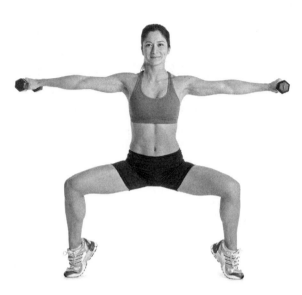

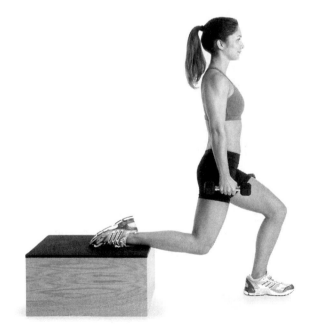

Dumbbell Bulgarian Squat

Stand holding dumbbells with your back facing a bench or sturdy chair (no higher than 18 inches). Extend a leg back and place the top of your foot on the seat. Bend your front leg until the thigh is as close as possible to parallel to the floor and forcefully press back to the start position. Repeat for a full set of 15. Switch legs.

Side Stepup

Stand to the left of a box or bench (either low or high). Step up to the side with the left leg, putting that foot on the box. Push with your left leg and bring your right foot up next to your left one. Step down to the start position. Complete a full set of 15, then switch legs. The cadence should be quick, but controlled.

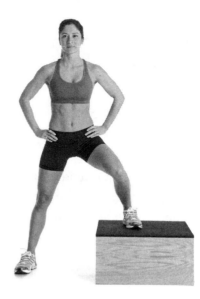

Go Ahead and Jump

Plyometrics, or jumping drills, condition your muscles to detonate on demand so you have the split-second force you need to crank up steep inclines, power over rolling terrain, and sprint to the finish line. And they work fast, too. Research shows that a twice-weekly plyometric routine can boost your power endurance (your muscles' ability to contract at near-maximum force) by 17 percent and increase your lactate threshold cycling power (the maximum power you can sustain for about an hour) by 3.5 percent in just 4 weeks. Bonus for women: Research also shows that jumping can increase bone density in the lower spine as well as the hips and femurs.

Add one jumping move from the choices below to your workout. Note: It's important that you have a decent base of strength before you start jumping. So if you're new to exercise, do 3 to 4 weeks of the leg and core work first, then add one jumping move to your routine.

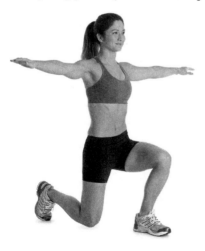

Scissor Jump

Stand with your left leg forward and your right leg extended behind you. Bend your left knee and dip your right knee toward the floor in a lunge. Hold your arms straight out in front of you or out to the sides. Swiftly jump up and switch legs. When your back knee touches the ground, jump again. Jump 10 to 20 times without resting.

Box Jumps

Stand facing a 12- to 18-inch-high box or step. Squat, then jump up, swinging your arms for momentum. Land firmly on the box with your knees soft to absorb the impact. Step down and repeat 10 to 15 times.

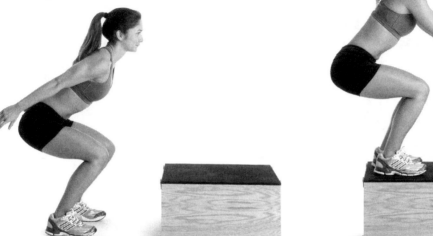

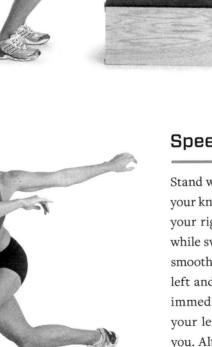

Speed Skater

Stand with your feet shoulder-width apart and your knees slightly bent. Shift your weight onto your right leg, bending it to about 45 degrees while sweeping your left leg behind you. In one smooth motion, sweep your left leg back to the left and jump from your right leg to your left, immediately bending into a half squat with your left leg as you sweep your right behind you. Alternate for a full set of 10 to 15 reps on each leg.

CHAPTER 16

Flexible Benefits

A FEW YEARS BACK I WAS TRAINING FOR LONG DISTANCE TRI-
athlons, racking up lots of miles and generally feeling great—until I wasn't. From
seemingly out of nowhere I developed a persistent ache in my right hip, which
didn't bother me quite as much on the bike as it did off of it. I stretched it. I rolled
it out on my foam roller. I tried working a tennis ball in there to break up adhesions.
No relief.

Fortunately, I was scheduled to take a media trip to Specialized's main office in
Morgan Hill, California. The trip included a meeting with Andy Pruitt, founder of the
Boulder Center for Sports Medicine in Colorado. He put me through a battery of flexibility tests and quickly identified the culprit: My vastus lateralis and vastus interme-
dius (prominent quad muscles) were wound so tightly they were pulling on my hip.
They loosened up enough when I rode that it didn't impede my performance, but
otherwise it was making me pretty uncomfortable. I stretched and rolled my quads
and have been pain free since.

And that's sort of the story with cycling and stretching. Lots of cyclists don't bother
because, eh, why bother? Cycling requires a very limited range of motion and there's
not a lot of compelling research that stretching will improve performance or prevent
injuries like pulls, strains, and sprains (which, let's face it, aren't very common on the

bike anyway). But then things start to hurt, like your low back and hips and knees and neck, and it becomes clear that there are definite benefits to flexibility.

Power Position

In fact, once you reach a certain level of training, improving flexibility might be the way to make your greatest gains, says Scott Holz, senior fit professor and global manager of Specialized's Bicycle Components University. Holz has worked with such Pro Tour riders as Fabian Cancellara and has seen the way pliant muscles help even the world's best cyclists find room to improve. "Flexibility is one of the biggest limiting factors for achieving your most powerful bike position," Holz says.

The upside of having supple muscles is huge: The more flexible you are, the more aero you can get—which helps you go faster with less effort. Regular stretching also quiets aches and strains that can limit your mileage, speeds the replenishment of muscle-glycogen stores, and helps counteract the effects of aging, which causes muscles to lose elasticity.

The key is to know what to do, and when. Holz recommends the following assessment, which is very thorough (and requires the help of a friend) to ID any potential trouble spots. And if you find any, he recommends getting to work right away—and staying at it. "Consistency is important," says Holz. "You're better off doing 10 to 15 minutes four days a week than an hour once a week." That's because gaining flexibility is a long-term process, he adds. "It takes 6 weeks to achieve a true length change in muscle or tendon structure," he says.

As for the question of when? Research shows that stretching before exertion can weaken muscles. Instead, take time for it post-ride (or later, after a hot shower), when your muscles are warm. Hold each for 20 to 30 seconds, unless otherwise indicated.

Iliotibial Band Stretch

The Test

Lie on a table or high bench and let half of your thighs extend off the edge. Dangle one foot and bend the other knee, pulling it toward your chest until your lower back touches the bench. Have a partner observe what happens.

If your dangling knee falls to the side rather than forming a straight line from the hip, your iliotibial (IT) band, which runs along the thigh to the calves, is tight. Repeat the test on your other leg.

Why It Matters

The IT band stabilizes the knee. If it's tight, it can rub against the knee and become inflamed, an overuse injury known as IT band friction syndrome.

The Fix: Leg Roll

Lie on your side with your thigh resting on a foam roller. Ease your leg along the cylinder, using your weight to apply pressure on the tissues. Roll up and down the band for 60 seconds, then repeat on the other leg. Spend extra time on tender areas. (For more, see "The Science of Stretching" on pages 180–82.)

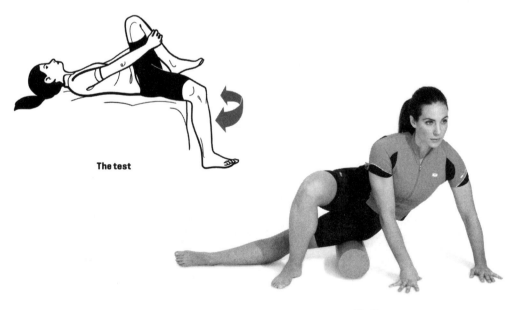

The test

The fix

Quadriceps Stretch

The Test

Lie on a table or high bench and let half of your thighs extend off the edge. Dangle one foot and bend the other knee, pulling it toward your chest until your lower back touches the bench. Have a partner observe what happens.

If the ankle on your extended leg sticks out beyond your knee, you have tight quads. The straighter the extended leg, the tighter the muscles.

Why It Matters

Your quads produce power, and a limited range of motion prevents some muscle fibers from firing, says cycling coach Carson Christen.

The Fix: Lying Quad Stretch

Lie facedown with your knees hip-width apart. Reach one arm back and grasp the opposite ankle. Slowly pull the heel in toward your butt. Keep your pelvis flat on the floor. Hold, then repeat on the other side.

Do It Anywhere: Stork

Stand with your left hand resting on a chair for support. Bend your right leg behind you. Grasp your foot with your right hand, keeping your back straight. Slowly pull your heel toward your butt until you feel tension in your quads. Keep your hips and knees aligned. Hold, release, and switch legs.

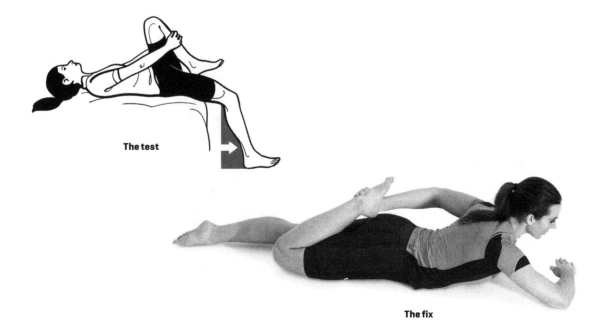

The test

The fix

Hip Flexors Stretch

The Test

Lie on a table or high bench and let half of your thighs extend off the edge. Dangle one foot and bend the other knee, pulling it toward your chest until your lower back touches the bench. Have a partner observe what happens.

If your extended thigh lifts so that the knee rises above your hip rather than remaining flat, your hip flexors aren't as flexible as they should be.

Why It Matters

The hip flexors pull the leg up and over the top of the pedal stroke; stretching prevents lower back pain when you amp up your intensity.

The Fix: Kneeling Lunge

From a lunge position, drop your back knee to the floor. Straighten your pelvis to align your pubic bone directly below your hipbones. Ease your hips down and forward, keeping your front knee directly over your ankle, and hold. Repeat on the other side.

Do It Anywhere: Step Lunge

Place the ball of your left foot on a step. Extend your right leg behind you, knee slightly bent. With your hands on your hips, keep your torso straight and lean into your left leg, pushing your hips forward. (Your left knee should not extend past your toes.) Hold, then repeat with the opposite leg.

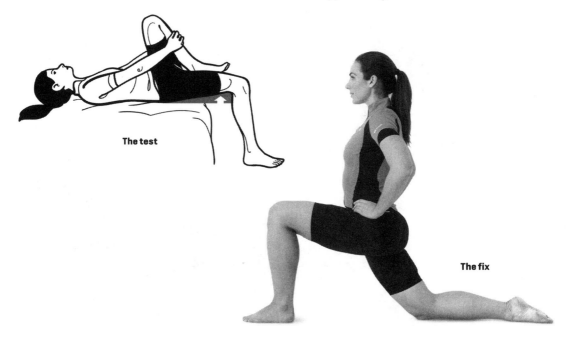

The test

The fix

Glutes Stretch

The Test

Lie flat on your back. Ask a partner to raise your leg as far as it can comfortably go, bending the knee. Estimate the angle your thigh forms to the floor: Less than 90 degrees indicates that you have tight glutes; 90 to 120 degrees is a typical limit. Test both legs.

Why It Matters

Tight glutes prevent you from achieving an aerodynamic position in the drops.

The Fix: Pigeon Pose

To work your glutes, kneel on one knee with the other leg bent at 90 degrees, its foot flat on the floor. Extend the knee on the floor straight toward the rear, so that your torso moves forward over your front leg, bending it to a 45-degree angle. Keeping your hips square, ease your pelvis toward the floor, lowering both legs to rest them on the floor, with the forward leg crossing in front of your torso. Next, tilt forward and lower your chest toward the floor. Hold, then repeat on the other side.

Do It Anywhere: Sitting Pigeon

Sitting in a chair, rest your right ankle on your left knee so your calf is parallel to the floor. Keeping your back straight, lean forward from your hips until you feel a stretch deep in your right glute muscle. Switch sides.

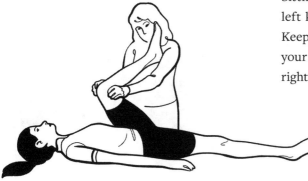

The test

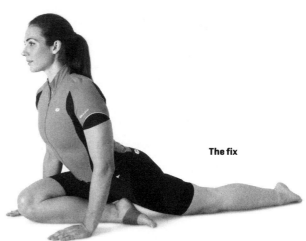

The fix

Hamstrings Stretch

The Test

Lie flat and have a partner raise one leg until your hamstring begins to tug. Estimate the angle formed with the floor: 55 degrees or less signals poor flexibility. Repeat with the other leg.

Why It Matters

Longer hamstrings let the pelvis tilt forward on the saddle, allowing for a more aero position. Plus, you'll get your glutes—the body's strongest muscles—more involved in pedaling.

The Fix: Standing Forward Fold

Stand with feet hip-width apart and slowly bend at the waist, tilting your pelvis forward and keeping your back straight. Pause for 10 to 15 seconds when you feel a slight stretch in the back of your legs, then deepen the pose until you feel the hamstrings relax.

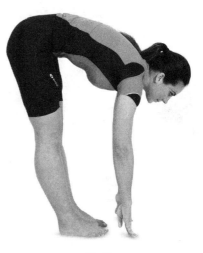

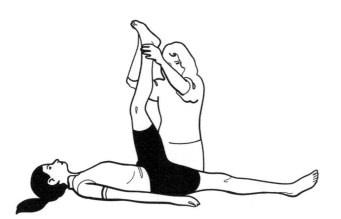

The test

The fix

Calves Stretch

The Test

Sit on a bench with your legs extended and your feet flat on the floor. Raise your toes while keeping your heels grounded. If you can't get your foot past 90 degrees, use the stretch at right.

Why It Matters

Tight calves and Achilles tendons force cyclists into an exaggerated, toe-down pedal stroke that transfers less power than a flatter foot. More flexible calves allow for a more powerful and efficient stroke—and also leave you less prone to cramping.

The Fix: Single-Heel Drop

Stand with the balls of your feet on a step. Lower one heel to stretch through the calf, ankle, and Achilles tendon. Hold for 10 seconds, then repeat a second time. Switch and stretch the other side.

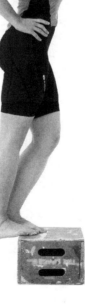

The test

The fix

The Science of Stretching

Every time you reach and hold, you change the properties inside the muscle. Within your muscles are receptors called spindles, which run parallel to the muscle fiber. As you stretch a muscle, the spindle records the change in the length of the muscle as well as the speed with which that length is changing and sends that info to your spinal cord. This trips the stretch reflex, which generates a contraction that is designed to protect the muscle from being stretched too far or fast. That's why stretching is best done slowly. As you lengthen the muscle to the point of feeling the stretch and then hold it for 20 to 30 seconds, the muscle spindle gradually gets used to the new length and eases back on its opposing contraction. Over time, the muscle and the surrounding connective tissues become more elastic.

Genetics, age, and even gender determine how flexible you are to start with. Research shows that women have a slightly greater range of motion than men in pretty much every joint. That said, we all get less flexible with age. Starting in your 30s, your muscles, tendons, and ligaments start to shorten and tighten, losing elasticity. If you sit a lot on (and maybe off) the job, that only worsens things, because your muscles aren't being taken through their range of motion, but instead are sitting (and tightening up) in a stationary position. It's also only fair to reiterate that cycling doesn't exactly stretch them out in any meaningful way, since you're sitting and draped over your handlebars. By stretching regularly you can improve—or at least maintain—the flexibility you have long term.

ROLL IT OUT

If you've ever gone to stretch and your muscles just feel stuck, it's because they are—literally! Exercise long and/or hard enough and eventually your muscles will develop adhesions, knots that make you stiff and sore. That's why foam rollers are all the rage—they're like a massage you give to yourself. They break the adhesions, stretch muscles, and give you instant relief (and the roller only costs a quarter of the price of a professional massage).

Follow these directions, rolling each body part over the foam roller 5 to 10 times. If a spot feels extra tender, try this: Start below the area, work your way up to it, and hold on it for a few seconds, then roll through it.

Calves

Sit on the floor with your legs extended straight out and your hands on the floor behind you supporting your weight. Place the roller under your knees. Slowly roll along the backs of your legs from your knees to your ankles and back up.

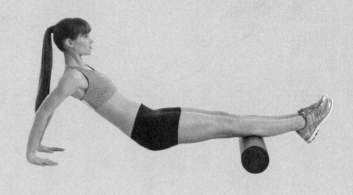

Hamstrings

Sit with the back of your right thigh on the roller; bend your left knee and put your hands on the floor behind you. Roll up and down from your knee to just under your right butt cheek. Switch legs.

Quads

Lie facedown on the floor with the roller under your hips supporting yourself with your hands. Lean on your right leg and roll up and down from your hip to your knee. Switch legs.

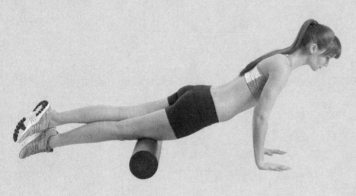

Back

Sit on the floor with the foam roller behind you. Lace your fingers behind your head and lean your upper back onto the roller. Tighten your abs and glutes and slowly move up and down the roller.

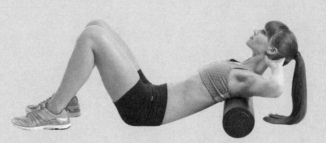

(continued)

The Science of Stretching *continued*

Outer Hip and Thigh

Lie on your side with the roller under your right hip. Bracing your abs and glutes for balance, slowly roll from your hip to your knee. Switch to the other side and repeat.

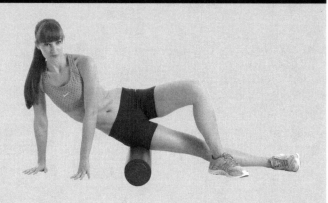

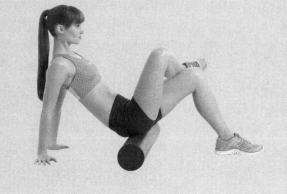

Butt

Sitting on the foam roller, cross your right leg over your left knee and lean toward the right hip, putting your weight on your hands for support. Slowly roll one butt cheek over the roller. Switch sides.

CHAPTER 17

Off to the Races

TALK TO ALMOST ANY RUNNER AND CHANCES ARE GOOD
they've done a 5K, 10K, and very likely a half- or full marathon—and if they haven't yet, chances are good that they plan to. By and large, people who run also race—even if it's generally against themselves or the clock. Ask most cyclists, especially women, if they race and you'll get a vigorous headshake.

There are many reasons for that. Bike racing is harder to get into. You need a license for one (though you can generally buy a one-day license at the venue). There are fewer races to be found. It helps to be part of a team. And, well, it looks intimidating. So it's understandable that so few riders actually ever race. But I think more should.

For one, racing makes you a better rider. You'll never push yourself as much on your own as you will in a race. So it sharpens your skills as well as boosts your fitness. It builds confidence off the bike as well as on. It gives you a goal to train for, which is highly motivating. Finally, for most of us who live fairly comfortable lives, it's demanding. There's also nothing else like it, which is kind of hard to explain to folks who don't ride, let alone race.

"Why do you do that to yourself?" is the question my mother and other well-intentioned people often ask during discussions that relate accounts of exerting yourself hard enough to taste bile in the back of your throat and suffering so greatly it feels as though your insides are being sent back and forth through a wringer.

"Because it's fun" doesn't seem to cut it with them as a reason. Though it most certainly is, especially when you cross the finish line in a thoroughly spent, grinning, grimacing heap of endorphin-saturated flesh. "Because it makes me feel fully and completely alive" is another reply that comes to mind. Because nowhere do I feel more utterly alive in the present moment than when I'm hammering down the pavement, drilling it off the line at a 'cross race, or floating, nearly hypoxic, over the roots and rocks aboard my mountain bike.

Race venues are also places to meet amazing people and make great friends. I know that sounds kind of funny, but once you start racing, it becomes like a giant family picnic on race day. You see all these familiar faces, and though you're competitors on the course, everyone chats up a storm (especially afterward) and enjoys the bond that you form in taking on a challenge together.

"There's a general feeling of camaraderie that exists alongside the competition, especially with women—maybe on some level we all sense the need to stand together," says Lara Goodman. "There are some women who don't approve and think that to fit in with, be equal to, or gain respect from men, you have to act like one, but to me that seems like accepting that there is something inherently wrong with being a female." And to that I say amen.

Bike Racing 101

So you're sold. Now you just need to find that first race. Fortunately, that's easy in the Internet age. Just click over to BikeReg.com and you'll find hundreds of races of every variety. You can search by race type and/or your location. You'll likely be surprised how many races there are just a short drive—or ride—from your doorstep. Here's a look at the various types of bike races and what you should know when you sign up.

ROAD RACES

If you've seen the Tour de France, you've seen a road race on the grandest scale. Of course right now women aren't allowed to race the Tour (but we're working on changing that). Women *are* able to compete in many other types of road races, however. And if you haven't raced, there are more to choose from than you'd imagine. Here's a snapshot.

GRAN FONDO

If you're brand new to racing, this is a great place to start. These are timed rides that technically are races, because they are timed and award prizes, but they are not conducted like races (you don't need a racing license, for example). Wildly popular in Europe for decades, the format has caught fire in the United States so fast that even casual riders and the century crowd are starting to embrace them.

This year, nearly every major North American city from San Diego to New York will host

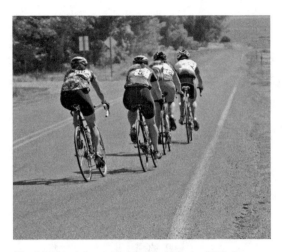

A healthy dose of protein and carbohydrates will help your muscles mend and recovery quickly after a hard effort.

one. American organizers have been careful to import the fondo's most appealing attributes: well-stocked aid stations, sumptuous post-event meals, and a chance to share the road with some big-name pros. Fondos are sometimes called by other names, such as *cyclosportif* or *l'étape*. The really good ones "have the kind of fanfare and entertainment that you see at the Tour de France," says Hunter Ziesing, who used to run mass cycling events for charity.

Expect a mass start in a downtown area and a route that stretches 100 miles or more along scenic and challenging terrain (many offer shorter, easier course options, too). Charity riders, take note: Because they're timed, fondos reward speed, so the pace can be brisk—and it picks up during timed climbs.

Take note, too, that many of these events are *big*, like thousands of people big. They also have all riders start at one time, which can be kind of chaotic if you aren't accustomed to it. A few tips to make it through the mayhem:

- **KNOW YOUR PLACE.** Most fondos start pros and licensed racers in front, with casual riders behind them. If you're unsure or intimidated, start toward the back. Ziesing also suggests joining a few group rides beforehand if you've never ridden en masse.

- **STAKE OUT TERRITORY.** Once you locate a spot, stand next to your bike to buy extra elbow room. A minute or two before the start, swing a leg over your saddle and prepare to ride: Make sure your helmet is buckled, your shoes are secure, and your bike is in the right gear to pedal as soon as the pack surges forward.

- **FIND YOUR FLOW.** If you're not starting at the front, don't try to gun it out of the gate. Stuck in a hard-charging pack? Maintain a comfortable speed and drift to the right. Then, without slamming on your brakes and causing a pileup, let speedier riders pass.

TIME TRIAL

Also known as the "race against the clock" or "the race of truth" (because there's no one out there to help you—it's all you and your strength), a time trial is a race where riders compete individually over the same course to see who can complete it in the shortest time.

The "Me" in "Team"

In general, road racing is very much a team sport. If you're going to join the fun, you should join a team or a club. Your local bike shop can help you find a few; in fact, they may even have their own team that you can race for. Teams are great for meeting other women you can get together with to train and practice techniques like drafting, sprinting, attacking (trying to break away from other riders), and group riding. Other tips:

BUY A LICENSE. Most events allow you to purchase single-day racing licenses, which is a good idea for trying it out your first time. However, if you're going to race more than once or twice a year, it makes economic sense to buy a license (and helps support the sport). You can register for one through USA Cycling (www.usacycling.org), the United States' official cycling organization.

When you sign up, you'll be asked to register for a racing category. Category 1 is reserved for elite riders. Category 4 is the beginner category for women. As you gain experience and get faster, you can work your way up the ranks. Races and events usually also divide racers by age, such as Juniors for those 18 and under and Masters and Seniors for racers in older age brackets, so everyone is racing against their peers.

KNOW THE RULES. Ignorance of the rules is not an excuse for breaking them. I've learned that one the hard way—more than once. The first was probably the worst. I showed up to my very first road race wearing a tank top—an official no-no. Race rules state that all participants' shoulders must be covered. Having only raced mountain bike events (where riders sometimes ride in unicorn costumes, or underwear), I had no clue. A very friendly race official pulled out his Swiss Army knife and we fashioned a makeshift jersey out of an event T-shirt. It was lovely and not at all as embarrassing as it sounds—not! The rules are online. It's a good idea to read them.

They're extremely low risk (if you crash, it's pretty much your own fault) and have a very low intimidation factor since you're basically out there on your own. Time trials can be of any length; 10 miles and 40 kilometers (about 25 miles) are common distances. Riders take the course one at a time with intervals of 1 to 2 minutes separating them. Drafting (riding directly behind another rider, should you catch her) is not allowed. Neither is any outside assistance. You're generally allowed to use special aero equipment, like aerobars, that are forbidden in regular road racing.

Most time trials are individual, but there are also two-person and team time trials, where two or more riders work together to score the fastest time against other pairs or teams.

CRITERIUM

Criteriums, or "crits," as they're commonly called, are probably the most prevalent type of amateur race in the United States. A crit is a short—usually less than 5 kilometers (3.1 miles)—race over a town or city loop that's been closed to traffic. You race for a certain number of laps or for a certain amount of time (e.g., 30 minutes and a final "bell" lap). Since these races are so short—30 to 90 minutes—the pace is at full throttle from start to finish. The winner is the one who crosses the finish line first without being "lapped" (passed by the lead riders). Often there are "primes" (pronounced PREEMS), which are prizes given to the winners of a predetermined number of laps, such as every third lap.

Because they feature mass starts, tight corners, and high speeds, crits are very exciting and, for beginners, pretty scary. Good bike handling is essential. If you're interested in racing criteriums, your best bet is to join your local cycling club. Many have "beginner" or training crits where you can learn the fundamentals of this type of racing along with people of similar levels of skill and ability.

OPEN ROAD

These are mass-start races on open roads. The courses may be big 50- to 70-mile loops, or smaller circuits of 10 to 20 miles that you repeat. Women's races often run about 50 miles, but pretty much anything goes.

Unlike crits, road races don't generally go out full gas from the gun, and the overall pace is a little slower because the race is longer. You'll find people working together in groups and riding pacelines. You'll also see a lot of racing tactics come into play. Riders will try to break away from the main group, and there's a lot of charging and chasing throughout the event. The first rider across the line wins. Open road races are somewhat less demanding technically than crits, but they still require good bike handling and awareness. Of all the racing types, road racing is the one that demands the most interaction among riders, and there's a great deal of etiquette (both explicit and understood) to learn. Joining a bike club will help teach you the ropes and make your road racing experience much more enjoyable.

STAGE RACES

Stage races are multiday—or on the very elite level, multiweek events. Large stage races, like the Tour of California, typically include all the elements of racing: hilly days, flat stages, time trials, and so forth. Unlike mountain bike stage races, which you can easily sign up for and compete in as an individual, you usually need to be on a team to take part in one on the road—another reason to join a bike club.

TRACK RACING

As mentioned earlier, velodrome or track racing is a very special discipline that takes place on steeply banked wooden or cement tracks. You use a bike equipped with only a fixed gear (one speed, no coasting) and no brakes. As you might imagine, track racing demands a great deal of skill, speed, and strategy. But it's also very fun. Many tracks offer introductory programs for riders of all ages and abilities. There are only about two dozen velodromes in the United States, so they aren't easy to come by. But if you ever have a chance, check one out.

MOUNTAIN BIKE RACES

Though mountain bike races all take place off-road, there are so many different types that each is nearly a separate sport in and of itself. For instance, I race cross-country, which includes some downhill segments. But I have never actually raced "downhill," which is a separate discipline using bikes built specifically to rage down mountainsides at high speeds. Whether or not you need a license depends on the type of race. There are many mountain bike races where no license is necessary. Just check the registration page to be sure. And as usual, if you do need one, you can buy a one-day license at the site. Here are the main selections you can choose among.

CROSS-COUNTRY

Cross-country (XC) mountain bike races are off-road races that are generally 10 to 30 miles in length and take about 90 minutes to 3 hours to complete. The course can be one big loop, but more often it's one smaller loop that's 5 to 10 miles long. How many times you go around the loop depends on your level of racing experience; beginners may do just 1 or 2 laps, while experts go around 5 or 6 times. Most XC courses aren't terribly technical, but they definitely may include some challenging sections with rocks, roots, logs, and/or steep descents.

Unlike road races, mountain bike races start

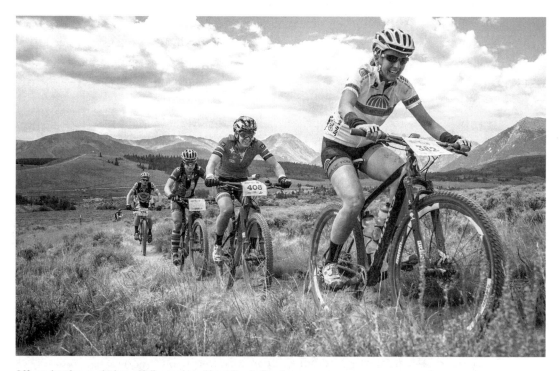

Off-road racing can be beautifully scenic and brutally challenging.

very fast because there's usually a "hole shot," a place where the course goes from a wide-open road to a skinnier trail in the woods and passing becomes impossible. The front of the pack will be gunning at full throttle to get there first. After the start, the pack generally thins out and you spend most of the race out there with a small group of riders. Some mountain bikers have teams, but it's much more of an individual sport than road racing is. Mountain bikers for the most part are not allowed outside assistance (though they can help each other), and they don't generally work together the same way road cyclists do, since, except on some open-road sections in long races, drafting isn't really a possibility.

SHORT TRACK

Like off-road criteriums, short track races tend to be very short, so they're good for spectators (it isn't unusual for them to be able to see much of the race while standing in one spot). These races often run by time. So instead of doing a certain number of laps, you race for 30 minutes plus a "bell" (final) lap. The winner is the rider who crosses the line first with the most laps completed. They're not as common as XC races.

MARATHON

Just like the running race of the same name, these events are *long*, some of them as long as 100 miles (which is a *very long* way to ride a mountain bike). Fifty-milers are also popular. These arduous events usually last for the better part of a day, with the winners typically coming in at 6 hours and the back of the pack trying to make it to the finish in under 12 hours.

STAGE RACES

These multiday events are increasingly popular among even casual mountain bike racers. Many are held in vacation destinations like British Columbia, South Africa, and the Rocky Mountains, so people save up their pennies (because they are *not* cheap) and make a vacation out of it. Some stage races have you travel from point A to point B over a specified number of days (generally 3 to 7). Others have a cloverleaf format, where you stay in one central location and race different loops starting there each day. These multiday races have a reputation as being the toughest competitions the sport has to offer.

24-HOUR AND ENDURANCE RACES

These races around the clock used to be wildly popular, but have faded a bit in recent years as other types of racing have taken over. Though some people do them solo, most often they are team competitions. Teams can consist of two, four, or sometimes five riders. For 24-hour races, team members take turns riding laps around a course over a 24-hour period (such as noon on Saturday until noon on Sunday). That means you ride through the night with lights on your helmet and bike. These races are often held at ski resorts or other camping-friendly venues and are famous for their very laid-back, festival atmospheres as racers camp out and cheer each other on.

More popular these days are endurance races, which are similar in spirit, but aren't 24 hours long. These events range in duration from 4 to 12 hours, so they're a good choice for riders who don't want to be racing through the night.

ENDURO

One of the fastest-growing segments of mountain bike racing today, enduro racing is like a big XC race where only certain downhill segments are timed and count toward the win. These are excellent for riders who are highly skilled, but not necessarily the fastest on climbs. It's a good idea to read the course description carefully when entering an enduro. Some are only moderately technical, while others can be extremely challenging and require full face helmets.

DOWNHILL

Downhill racing is a time trial–style event, where riders take their bikes on a ski lift to the top of a mountain and take turns seeing who can get down a designated trail in the fastest time. Races last for anywhere from less than a minute to about 6 minutes, depending on the course and the competition level. The courses are highly technical, including steep drop-offs and tight turns through rocks and trees. The bikes are much bigger and heavier, and riders wear full face helmets and light body armor that includes knee and shin pads, shoulder pads, and sometimes even spine protection.

CYCLOCROSS, ULTRACROSS, AND GRAVEL GRINDERS

These events, hybrids of road and mountain bike racing, are extremely popular and getting more so each season. Cyclocross and gravel races are also extremely beginner friendly. Here's what they're all about.

CYCLOCROSS

As mentioned in Chapter 11, 'cross was developed as an off-season training tool for European road racers, so 'cross races could be considered off-road races for roadies. Though the courses are unpaved, most competitors compete on 'cross bikes (see page 23), which resemble road bikes more than mountain bikes, though mountain bikes are allowed. Cyclocross is done on a short loop that racers compete around for 40 to 45 minutes plus a bell lap. Courses include man-made barriers like hurdles and stairs that force competitors to dismount and run with their bikes for short stretches to clear the obstacles before remounting. Races are held in the fall and early winter and mud, rain, and even snow are common. You generally need a license to race 'cross.

ULTRACROSS/GRAVEL

As mentioned on page 129, road-type races on unpaved roads are exploding in popularity, so much so that manufacturers are making special "gravel bikes." These races are typically pretty long—at least 40 or 50 miles—and quite challenging. Some ultracross races feature not only unpaved roads, but also sections of singletrack trail, which is both very fun and very challenging on your relatively skinny 'cross tires.

Race-Day Readiness

Warning: You will wake up on race day feeling like a butterfly bomb exploded in your belly. This feeling never really goes away. Think of it as potential energy and a sign that you care. It's not pleasant, but it's good to be nervous about something once in a while. Races make everyone nervous—even those folks who look calm and collected (don't believe it, it's just good poker face). Being well prepared can help calm those nerves. Here are a few tips that will help.

MAKE A LIST AND CHECK IT TWICE

Two days before a big race, I'll make a list of everything I need (see list that follows) and then start gathering my supplies, checking them off the list as I go. When possible, I like to be mostly packed early, well before the night preceding the race so I can just chill with my feet up rather than running around like a madwoman searching for my sunglasses. Do this regularly and it will become a habit and you'll never show up to the venue without your helmet or shoes, which happens more than you'd think. (A friend of mine once had to run to a store to buy a helmet for a race he'd traveled 90 minutes to get to.)

Also include a quick bike check. Check that the tires are inflated and the gears are shifting smoothly. Then leave the bike alone. Do not make any major adjustments, perform any sig-nificant maintenance, or put anything new on the bike. You want to race your bike just as you've been training on it.

RACE-DAY PACKING LIST

To be well prepared, bring:

- Helmet (can't race without one)
- Jersey and shorts (unless you're going to wear them there; then lay them out)
- Cycling shoes and socks
- Gloves
- Glasses
- Water bottles or hydration pack
- Food, water, sports drink—everything you plan on eating and drinking before, during, and after the event
- Tools, including at a minimum a spare tube, pump, and tire levers
- Wallet with money, ID, and license, if necessary (inevitably, a few people forget their licenses; I've done it, and it stinks)
- Paperwork, such as the accident waiver and anything else the race director may have sent you in advance (e.g., confirmation numbers, etc.)

SIGN IN, WARM UP

Aim to arrive at the venue 2 hours before start time if possible, 90 minutes at the latest. Sounds like a lot of time, but there's an awful lot to negotiate at race venues, including parking, signing in or registering, picking up your race packet, fastening your race numbers to

Crash Courses

I'd be remiss if I didn't talk about the risks of racing. Naturally, there's some risk involved in all sports, cycling included, whether or not you compete. But the level of risk does rise when you race. If you're going to race, you're going to go fast, often with many others nearby going fast, too. Your chances of crashing are certainly higher than when you're riding alone. Almost every mountain bike racer I know has crashed multiple times. It's simply part of the sport. Fortunately, most crashes are minor and usually result in nothing more than a few bruises and scrapes, though broken bones can happen, too. Road cycling has its share of wrecks, too, though I know plenty of women who race and have never wrecked.

It's up to you to assess your ability—how well you ride in close quarters and handle your bike—as well as your comfort level to find the type of competition that is right for you. Maybe you only time trial or choose races where you can line up in the back and stay out of heavy traffic. There's no wrong answer. Just be honest with yourself and as always, enjoy the ride.

your bike and/or jersey, using the portable toilets, and so on. There's nothing worse than feeling rushed, so leave yourself plenty of time.

Once you've fastened on your numbers and you're all set, go out and warm up, preferably with a lap or at least part of a lap on the course so you can see key parts, especially the start. The goal of your warmup is to burn off your prerace jitters, warm up your muscles, and fire up your fat-burning enzymes. It doesn't take long, just 15 minutes or so, including a few short hard efforts to get your legs going. The longer the race, the shorter your warmup can be, but don't skip this step entirely or you'll be forced to use the first 10 to 15 minutes of the race to get yourself in gear.

Mentally, form a race plan. What are your goals for the start? What are your mini goals throughout the race? Keep it simple, such as "start eating within 15 minutes" if you're in for a long day. Or, if you know your competition, you can plan who you will mark and try to stay with. Having little goals keeps your mind occupied and gives you concrete steps for success.

SETTLE IN TO THE RACE

My friend Rebecca is a perfect race pacer. She knows exactly how hard she can start and how much she can push herself into the red on any given day without blowing up before the end. Not everyone is so skilled at the art of pacing. Even well-seasoned competitors sometimes charge out too hard and blow up before the finish, or finish with energy to spare and feel like they missed out by not going hard enough. It takes time and practice, and also a little common sense, to get it right. If it's only 10 minutes into the race and you feel terrible, back off, breathe deep, and regain your composure. If you're feeling great, push it, but try to avoid burning too many matches too early. Making a hard push to muscle it up a particularly challenging climb is fine, but you can't stay at maximum intensity for too long and expect to finish strong. Your pace should feel hard, but not impossibly so.

What you do during the race depends on the type of race it is and its duration. When you're in a group, even in a race, riders will often take turns pulling at the front, then drifting back to take a break and draft with the pack. But there are no hard and fast rules here; road racing is all about tactics.

Sometimes teams will take the front and try to dominate. Sometimes they'll try to force other riders to the front so they can save their energy. You can discuss strategy with your teammates ahead of time. One of the most common techniques is the attack, in which small groups accelerate to try to break away from the main field; others usually then chase after them to reel them back in. Though some individuals attack on their lonesome for no apparent reason, most often, attacks are strategically planned to help a rider or group of riders get away from the pack so they have fewer competitors to contend with as they near the finish line.

Before you attack, consider what you hope to gain. Is the race winding down, making you think you can stay beyond the pack's reach until the end? Are you a stellar climber and feeling confident that you can beat everyone up a tough hill to gain time on your competitors? Are you trying to wear out the competition so a teammate can steal the lead down the

road? Don't waste energy attacking just because you feel like you should. Have a purpose in mind. The point of an attack is to get away. So unless you sense that you can get away, or that you can at least wear another team down without wearing yourself out, then it might not make sense.

Likewise, there will be plenty of times when you're on the other side of an attack and you have to decide if you should chase it down immediately or play a little wait-and-see. This is where team tactics come into play and you learn by trial and error. This is the fun, chess-match side of the sport that many road racers enjoy as much as if not more than the riding itself.

Most mountain bike races aren't quite as tactical, though you can find yourself in a pack in the larger, longer events, and then the same rules apply. In general, however, you will likely find yourself dueling with a few other racers throughout the event. As you do on the road, you'll want to attack when you feel like you've got the upper hand, such as on hard climbs or rocky, technical sections. With mountain bike racing in particular, you can be at a great advantage if you can break just far enough away that the competitor behind you can't see you and doesn't have you in her sites to chase. But don't waste too much energy when you are evenly matched. Instead, save yourself for a big push at the end.

Passing riders is often more difficult in mountain bike races than on the road, where you have a lot of open space. In fact, you'd never announce that you're passing in a road race, since you'd lose the element of surprise. But off road, where riders are skirting around rocks and roots and can't be expected to ride in a perfectly straight line, it's another story. Announce "On your left" or "On your right" to let riders know you'll be coming by and what side to expect you on.

No matter what happens or how the race plays out, hold your head high and be a good sport. Sometimes racers get caught up in the emotions of the day (usually mostly about their own performance or lack thereof) and start yelling at volunteers and generally misbehaving. Don't be that person. Even if it's not your day—heck, even if it's never your day—you can still show up and ride your best and finish with pride because you had the guts to line up to begin with.

LOOK BACK AND LEARN

Racing provides you with endless opportunities for growth and progress. After each race is over, let yourself settle down. Have a beer. BS with your friends. Then sit back and evaluate how the race went—right and wrong. Did you follow your race plan? Did you eat and drink enough? Did you sit in the peloton too long or not long enough?

If you decide you love racing and want to improve, consider hiring a coach. There are many online services that will provide you with an experienced coach who will assess your abilities, fitness level, and skills; build a structured training plan; and often dramatically improve your race results.

Or just keep it casual. I've known too many racers who get so serious that it stops being fun and they quit the sport they love because of the stress. That's bad. Think of it this way: Very few racers actually ever win. Most are there for the personal challenge, to have a good time, to become a better bicyclist, and to enjoy riding their bikes as fast as they can with a bunch of people just like them in places they've never been to. When you look at it that way, racing just gives more meaning to your everyday rides, and maybe to life itself.

CHAPTER 18

Conquer the Century

THERE'S NOTHING QUITE LIKE WATCHING YOUR ODOMETER click over into triple digits on your bike. Tell people you rode 100 miles and they'll generally reply wide-eyed, "I don't even like to drive that far!" That's the allure of the century ride—the holy grail of cycling achievement—you're achieving something most people would never dream of even attempting.

Daunting as it might sound to the uninitiated, hitting the 100-mile milestone on your bike is attainable—and even *enjoyable*—with proper preparation. The biggest roadblock for most women I've coached and consulted on the topic is time. There are only so many hours in the day, and most cyclists who have jobs and/or kids can reserve only so many for the bike. Obviously, the more you can get out, the better, but you can easily train for a century in just three rides a week.

Make the Training Rides Count

Each week, you need to fit in a long ride, a speed ride, and a steady ride. On other days, you can do some cross-training or, if you have time, one or two easy spins. Progressively make those rides a little longer and harder for 8 weeks and you'll be ready to conquer a century. Here's how they're done.

LONG RIDE

This is the meat of the training plan. It begins with 1½ to 2 hours on the bike—about 20 miles—and progresses from there. Do your long rides at a steady, but not taxing, pace, about 70 to 75 percent of your maximum heart rate. Most cyclists find that Saturday or Sunday works best for their long ride, but what day it is doesn't matter; just get it done. Note: If you're already comfortable with a ride that's longer than Week 1 (see the opposite page) prescribes, start from 2½ to 3 hours and follow the same guidance for mileage building, topping off at about 85 miles before the event.

STEADY RIDE

The bread and butter of the plan—steady or tempo rides should be done right at your threshold effort (as if you're riding with someone who's slightly faster than you). These rides should simulate your goal century pace and will train you to ride more briskly in comfort, so you can finish your century faster *and* fresher. Aim for two to four longer efforts (15 to 30 minutes in length) that increase your breathing and get your MHR up around 80 to 85 percent.

SPEED RIDE

This is the secret sauce of the plan. Distance riders often skip speedwork because they think they need volume, not intensity, to go long. As mentioned in Chapter 14, speedwork improves your endurance by raising your lactate threshold, the point at which your muscles literally scream, "Slow down!" When you raise this ceiling, you can ride faster and farther before your muscles slam on the brakes. Aim to do 4 to 6 very hard or maximum efforts on a challenging stretch of road like a hill or into a headwind to get these done.

Enjoy the Day

So pedaling is just a small part of what makes a successful century. You also need to pace yourself while riding in a large pack, stay fueled and hydrated, and of course be prepared for any weather, like wind and rain. Here are the essential steps to enjoying your big ride. Ideally, you should practice all of this in training so it will be second nature when it's go time.

DO A BIKE CHECK

About a week before your event, take your bike to a trusted mechanic for a tune-up. If you do your own maintenance, be sure to address these key things: Confirm that the bike is shifting and braking smoothly, and that the bolts securing the stem and headset are tight. Also pay attention to the places where the bike meets your body or the road: saddle, pedals and cleats, handlebars, and tires. Check for loose bolts, worn rubber, and peeling tape, and make whatever repairs are necessary.

FUEL YOURSELF

You could be out there for anywhere from 5 to 8 hours—a full day of saddle time. Some centuries have lunch stops, but most just have aid stations set up where you can refill your bottles

8-Week Century Training Plan

The days of the week are only suggestions. Do the rides when they fit into your schedule, reserving a day of rest, easy riding, or cross-training after each of them.

	MON	TUE	WED	THU	FRI	SAT	SUN
Week 1	Cross-train, rest, or an easy ride	Speed ride, 1 hr	Cross-train, rest, or an easy ride	Steady ride, 1 hr	Cross-train, rest, or an easy ride	Long ride, 1½–2 hrs, 20–25 miles	Cross-train, rest, or an easy ride
Week 2	Cross-train, rest, or an easy ride	Speed ride, 1 hr	Cross-train, rest, or an easy ride	Steady ride, 1¼ hrs	Cross-train, rest, or an easy ride	Long ride, 2–2½ hrs, 25–30 miles	Cross-train, rest, or an easy ride
Week 3	Cross-train, rest, or an easy ride	Speed ride, 1¼ hrs	Cross-train, rest, or an easy ride	Steady ride, 1½ hrs	Cross-train, rest, or an easy ride	Long ride, 2½–3 hrs, 35–45 miles	Cross-train, rest, or an easy ride
Week 4	Cross-train, rest, or an easy ride	Speed ride, 1¼ hrs	Cross-train, rest, or an easy ride	Steady ride, 1¾ hrs	Cross-train, rest, or an easy ride	Long ride, 3–3½ hrs, 45–55 miles	Cross-train, rest, or an easy ride
Week 5	Cross-train, rest, or an easy ride	Speed ride, 1¼ hrs	Cross-train, rest, or an easy ride	Steady ride, 2 hrs	Cross-train, rest, or an easy ride	Long ride, 3½–4 hrs, 55–60 miles	Cross-train, rest, or an easy ride
Week 6	Cross-train, rest, or an easy ride	Speed ride, 1½ hrs	Cross-train, rest, or an easy ride	Steady ride, 2¼ hrs	Cross-train, rest, or an easy ride	Long ride, 4–4½ hrs, 60–65 miles	Cross-train, rest, or an easy ride
Week 7	Cross-train, rest, or an easy ride	Speed ride, 1¼ hrs	Cross-train, rest, or an easy ride	Steady ride, 2 hrs	Cross-train, rest, or an easy ride	Long ride, 4½–5 hrs, 70–75 miles	Cross-train, rest, or an easy ride
Week 8	Cross-train, rest, or an easy ride	Speed ride, 1 hr	Cross-train, rest, or an easy ride	Steady ride, 1½ hrs	Cross-train, rest, or an easy ride	CENTURY!	Cross-train, rest, or an easy ride

Emergency Last-Minute Century Training

Your plan was to be triple-digit fit by September. Now that 100-miler you registered for light-years ago is a calendar flip away, and you've barely cracked 40. It happens. Fortunately, cycling is more forgiving on the body than, say, running. So while I would never suggest that anyone crash train for a marathon, if you're generally fit and have been riding a few times a week, you can get away with going big by cramming your training a bit. Here's how.

SHOOT FOR 65. Coaches advise that you should be able to do a 75-mile ride before your century. But you can squeak by with 65. If you take it easy, you can increase your weekly long ride by a safe 10 to 15 percent for 4 weeks: week 1: 45 miles; week 2: 51 miles; week 3: 57 miles; week 4: 65 miles.

1 STEADY, 1 SPEED, 1 SPIN. Ride 3 or 4 days a week between now and the event: ride long 1 day and at a fast pace another, with 1 or 2 easy-spin days between. Speedwork improves endurance because your body learns to recover faster, and it helps you tackle headwinds and hills. Try this: Warm up for 20 minutes, ride fast for 20, cool down for 20. Inch up the mileage on your midweek rides by a mile or two as you progress toward the event.

TAKE YOUR TAPER. Don't cram in miles the week before the ride. Keep your rides short so you can be rested and ready.

KEEP IT CASUAL. Avoid injuries by starting out slowly and spinning for the first 50 to 60 miles. Use the rest stops to stretch and fuel often, but limit each pit stop to 10 minutes.

and grab a banana, some PB&J, or some cookies and go on your way. Everyone has different preferences and tolerances for what they can eat when they ride, but fueling is a must. Aim for about 200 calories an hour in whatever form works best for you. Again, practice during training and avoid eating anything new and different on the actual ride itself. Most rides will tell you what foods they will have at the aid stations, so you can prepare accordingly.

Also, you don't need to gorge yourself the night before like you're preparing for famine. Just have a normal dinner and a good breakfast and remember to keep your tank topped off as you ride.

BRING TWO BOTTLES

You'll likely see some riders wearing hydration packs. But for a fully supported century, they're really not necessary. Instead, bring two water bottles filled with your favorite hydration drink. Plain water is okay, but at least half of your bottles should contain electrolytes to replace what you are sweating out. If it's very hot, both bottles should contain electrolytes.

You can buy low-sugar, low-calorie electrolyte drinks like those from Osmo Nutrition (which makes drinks just for women), Skratch Labs, and Nuun. These companies also make little sleeves and/or tablets of mix that you can easily carry with you for refills. Plan to drink about a bottle an hour. And contrary to what you've heard, your level of thirst is a good guide.

PRACTICE RIDING IN A GROUP

The bigger the better. You'll be less nervous and far safer than if your first ride in a pack is on event day. Ideally, you'll be riding with a few friends whom you're comfortable turning wheels with. If not, you'll soon find a similarly paced bunch you can ride with at least for some of the day. These rides generally attract hundreds—sometimes thousands—of cyclists. So you don't need to ride alone unless you really want to (and even then you often can't avoid company, so embrace it; it's easier to get to the finish fresher when you can sit in and catch a draft for a while).

SAVE THE PARTY

Everyone is all excited the night before a big ride, and it's easy to get swept up in the energy and maybe have one more than you mean to. Instead, prehydrate, eat a good-sized meal, put your legs up, rest, and go to bed early. Celebrate after the ride.

PACK IT ALL—AND THEN SOME

Rain is a drag. Riding soaking wet from miles 65 to 90 because you didn't bother to bring your jacket is worse. If you think you'll need it, bring it. It's always better to be looking at it than looking for it. Also, pack a little cash and a credit card in a zipper-lock bag, just in case.

ARRIVE EARLY

Leave time to sign in, change, and hit the restroom.

START EASY

Even if you plan to finish fast, it will be a long day, so begin easy. Give yourself a few miles to warm up and work your way through the crowd before turning up the juice.

CHANGE POSITION

Consciously change your position a few times an hour. Switching from the drops to the hoods to the top bars will prevent any one spot from getting too sore or fatigued.

MAKE SPEEDY STOPS

Don't spend more than 10 minutes at rest stations. It's much harder to ride that last 20 miles if you've been sitting around stiffening up for a half hour beforehand. Go steady, and keep going. You'll finish faster and fresher.

PART VI

EAT TO RIDE, RIDE TO EAT

Women have gotten the short end of the stick when it comes to medical research. There are myriad reasons, but largely it's because it's more convenient and less risky to study men. Men don't have pesky menstrual cycles, which involve hormone-level variations that can muddy the waters when it's time to analyze and interpret data. They also can't get pregnant, so there's no risk that testing would inadvertently cause harm during those early weeks of development before a woman may even know she's pregnant.

The downside of this is that, though we know that our genes are expressed differently than men's, hormones and body size and body composition affect how we respond to medications, and we actually have different symptoms and signs of heart disease—and die from it more often—than men in all of those areas.

While women remain a bit of a medical mystery and are vastly understudied, it's getting better. But there's a lot of catch-up work to be done. What does any of this have to do with cycling nutrition? Quite a bit, actually. Because guess what? When it comes to sports nutrition, women burn different macronutrients—carbohydrates, protein, and fats—at different times of the month. They also have different hydration needs and different recovery needs than men. We know this because some tireless scientists like Stacy Sims, PhD, a Stanford-based exercise physiologist and cutting-edge nutrition researcher who has consulted for pro teams, including Team RadioShack, have dedicated their life's work to studying these issues—and coming up with solutions.

"Women are not small men" is Sims's motto, one that she has used to promote a line of sports nutrition products tailor-made for women. She has faced her share of skeptics and critics, with many people asking, "Is women's specific nutrition really necessary?" Considering what we know about how very different the sexes are physically, metabolically, hormonally, and chemically, I'm going to go out on a limb and say, no, it's not necessary. Women have been competing fairly successfully without it for decades. Is it a good idea and could it help your performance? You bet.

To that end, the next four chapters delve into the fundamentals of fueling and how to make your riding and eating work better together. What exactly are women's sport-specific needs and how can you best meet them? You'll find answers to those questions in the chapter that follows. Of course, you'll also find the basics that both sexes need to know to ride and recover strong.

Because hydration is both extremely important and extremely misunderstood, we dedicate a full chapter to just how much—and what kind of—fluids you need. You'll want to check that one out if you ride, race, and/or train long hours, especially in the heat. Much of what we've been told about hydration simply isn't true. Women are more likely than men to succumb to hyponatremia, the potentially fatal condition of having a dangerously low blood sodium level from drinking too much fluid. So it's important that we get it right.

Finally, many women (and men) turn to cycling to help them shed some pounds as well as to have fun and get fit. The sport can definitely aid in weight loss, but again, there are an awful lot of myths and misconceptions that can and do get in the way of successfully meeting your goals. Contrary to what you've been told (and told and told), weight loss is not simply a calories-in versus calories-out equation. The quality of those calories is what ultimately determines your success with the scale.

You'll find concrete eating and riding advice to get you started and keep you rolling toward your best on-the-bike performance and your healthiest, happiest weight.

CHAPTER 19

Fuel for Life and the Ride of Your Life

ON THE FACE OF IT, FUELING TO RIDE IS A SIMPLE THING. YOU eat food. Your body turns it into energy. You use that energy to turn your cranks. Simple, right? Yeah. Right. The accepted principles of sports nutrition, an ever-evolving, often hotly contested science, have been in greater flux and more debated over than ever in recent years.

The result has been nearly fanatical followings for certain eating styles, like paleo, gluten-free, and vegan, while even dietitians and other experts struggle to make sense of the disparate science and resultant food factionalism. Amidst all the noise, however, there are two things most objective experts agree on: No diet should be taken to extremes. And there's no one diet that works for everybody. You have to do some trial and error to figure out what works best for you.

Case in point: myself. When I first started training and racing, I was a carb-heavy vegetarian. It worked fairly well. But I had trouble keeping my weight stable and too often found myself bonking. I was running on nothing but starchy carbs, which I was also overeating when I didn't need to be eating, because, well, it can be tricky to not overeat starchy carbs. Once I started training for ultra endurance events like Ironman and mountain bike stage racing, I took a good hard look at my diet and started reading up on how to manipulate my fuel to be a better fat burner.

I focused on fruits and vegetables for the bulk of my carbohydrates and ate plenty of lean protein, as well as lots and lots of fats in the forms of nuts, olives, oils, avocados, and so on. I saved the starchy carbs for right before a race or hard ride. I pretty quickly shed nearly 10 pounds, never bonked again, and frankly never felt better. Again, that may not be the answer for everyone. But it was the answer for me (and a few others who I and some fellow coaches have worked with).

You Ride How You Eat

Though there is much personal leeway, there *are* some fundamentals to fueling that pretty much any cyclist can benefit from following. There are also a few fundamentals that are specific to women. Here's what you need to know.

A CALORIE IS NOT A CALORIE

For far too long we were sold a bad bill of goods that told us that at the end of the day, what mattered most, especially when it came to weight loss, was calories, particularly how many you took in versus how many you expended. Take in 3,500 more than you burn, they said, and you'll put on a pound, whether the calories came from beets or banana cream pie. That is simply not true.

"Foods close to their natural state, such as fresh vegetables, whole grains, and lean, whole cuts of meat, require action—energy—from your body. You need to work to chew them and to digest them. They create a thermic response, which means you burn more calories just processing them. Your body gives up nothing in the way of work when you eat a cream pie," says Leslie Bonci, director of sports nutrition at the University of Pittsburgh Medical Center.

She and other experts partly blame the preponderance of "lazy calories" for the current obesity epidemic. "Our food is so heavily processed, it's practically predigested," she says. "That fast-food burger has gone through so much pulverization, you barely have to chew. We're losing the ability to burn calories as we naturally would during the eating and digestive process." Not to mention that many of these lazy-calorie foods are also calorie dense, so there's more to store.

Then there are the macronutrients—fats, protein, and carbohydrates—which all play specific roles in your body and are processed differently. Sports nutritionist Cynthia Sass pulls out the car analogy when addressing those. "They're as different as gasoline, motor oil, and brake fluid in terms of the roles they play in keeping your body operating optimally," she says. Many of her clients, she notes, might eat the perfect number of calories, but they have cut their fat intake too much. So the jobs that fat does, such as repairing cell membranes and optimizing hormones, go undone, and the surplus carbs are stored as fat. Sass says that by correcting her clients' balance among carbs, protein, and fats without changing their calorie intake, she has helped them lose weight, improve their immune systems, gain muscle, and boost energy.

In general, you want to have a representative of each macronutrient group at every meal. How much of each depends on how much and what type of riding you do as well as what you find works best for you. Sass recommends about 50 percent carbs (fill half your plate with vegetables, fruits, and some whole grains), 30 percent fats (olive oil, avocado, and so on), and 20 percent protein (lean meats, fish, eggs, and poultry). If you want to skew your carbohydrate intake lower—say, closer to 40 percent carbs, 30 percent fat, and 30 percent protein—then cut back your carbs at all your meals except the ones before your rides or training, so you have plenty of fuel on board to make those rides and workouts count—and enjoy them, too!

CARBOHYDRATES COME IN MANY FORMS

At some point, "starch" became synonymous with "carbohydrate." While pasta and bagels are carbohydrates, and you do need carbs for fuel, they're often not the best sources, especially if you're trying to lose weight or stay lean. Starchy carbs are easy to overeat, and any surplus goes to your fat stores. "Your brain operates on sugar, and when you eat bagels or

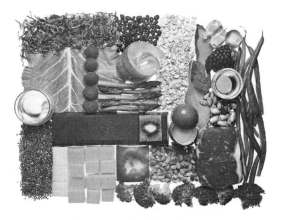

Whenever possible choose food that is easily recognizable as something that has come from the earth.

potatoes, your body turns them into sugar and delivers them to your cells quickly, which makes your brain happy and leaves you wanting more," explains legendary endurance sports coach Joe Friel, who used to be a carb loader like everyone else back in the day, but has since changed his tune to the point that he coauthored the *Paleo Diet for Athletes.*

Fruits and vegetables, in contrast, are rich in carbs, but often lower in calories and also digest more slowly. You're less likely to plow through so many berries and carrots that you end up with more fuel than you need. As a bonus, plant foods are loaded with vitamins, minerals, and immunity-boosting phytonutrients that make you healthier and stronger, so you can ride better and burn more calories.

The bottom line for everybody, frankly, is that you should choose carbs wisely. Eat starchy, refined quick-digesting carbs only during, right before, and after training rides or races, when it's important to have food that can be quickly digested and converted into fuel. Otherwise, get your carbs from fruits, vegetables, and whole grains.

How much is enough? If you're eating considerably more than Sass's recommended 50 to 55 percent, especially from starchy sources, then you risk changing your metabolism, says Friel. "When I see someone who has started eating lots of starch," he says, "they not only have gained fat, they've also changed their metabolism from fat-burning to sugar-burning." It doesn't happen over one plate of pasta, but the body is adaptable. "Over the course of a few of months," Friel says, "it will switch over to burn whatever you're feeding it most."

When possible, pair your carbs with some protein. Lean meats, nut butters, fish, and eggs slow digestion, so you feel full sooner, get energy from your meals more steadily, and stay full longer. The amino acids in protein also help repair, build, and maintain muscle tissue.

Where the Carbs Are

Fruits and vegetables are more substantial sources of carbohydrates than most people realize.

Raisins, seedless (¼ cup), 32 grams

Brussels sprouts, cooked (½ cup), 7 grams

Peas, cooked (1 cup), 25 grams

Strawberries (1 cup), 11 grams

Spinach, cooked (1 cup), 7 grams

Succotash, cooked (1 cup), 47 grams

Carrots, cooked (½ cup), 8 grams

Orange (1 medium), 14 grams

Collard greens, cooked (1 cup), 12 grams

Corn, sweet, cooked (1 ounce), 7 grams

Cantaloupe (1 cup), 15 grams

Squash, winter, acorn, cooked (1 cup), 30 grams

Sweet potato, baked, with skin (1 large), 44 grams

Artichoke, cooked (1 medium), 13 grams

Watermelon (1 cup), 11 grams

Green bell pepper (1 cup), 10 grams

Broccoli, raw (1 cup), 4 grams

Peach (1 large), 17 grams

Banana (1 medium), 30 grams

For comparison's sake, here are carb counts for common pastas and grains.

Spaghetti (1 cup), 40 grams

Spaghetti, whole wheat (1 cup), 37 grams

Tagliatelle (1 cup), 44 grams

Wheat bread (1 slice), 12 grams

Rye bread (1 slice), 15 grams

Mixed-grain bread (1 large slice), 5 grams

French bread (5 inches), 18 grams

Pita, white (6-inch), 33 grams

Long-grain white rice (1 cup), 45 grams

Short-grain white rice (1 cup), 37 grams

POWER UP WITH PROTEIN

Protein has been a diet darling for a few decades now. Cyclists need to pay special attention to keep their intake at the higher end of the recommended dosage, particularly if they're also trying to lose weight.

When researchers put 39 active men and women on a diet for 3 weeks, they all lost about 7 pounds. But those given twice the recommended amount of protein (1.6 grams per kilogram of weight—108 grams for a 150-pound adult—rather than the recommended 0.8 gram per kilogram) dropped most of their lost weight—70 percent—in the form of fat, while those sticking to the Recommended Dietary Allowance (RDA) dropped more than half in the form of fat-free mass, like muscle.

When you cut back your food intake, your body goes "catabolic" and starts breaking down protein faster than it makes it new, explains Donald K. Layman, PhD, a professor of nutrition at the University of Illinois. "You can reduce—maybe reverse—this effect by eating extra protein throughout the day." Layman recommends 30 grams at all three meals. For reference, one can of tuna has 42 grams, 2 eggs deliver 12 grams, and 3 ounces of beef has 21 grams. As a bonus: Extra protein helps your body make infection-fighting white blood cells, which may boost your immunity to protect you from getting sick when you're training hard.

Even if you're at your happy weight, you still need plenty of protein. Without enough, your body borrows from muscle to meet its needs, which are high for cyclists. As a woman, you also start with less precious lean muscle mass than your male peers, so you want to hang on to every powerful ounce.

Though everyone talks carbs and fat when it comes to fueling your rides, protein also plays an important role when you're in the saddle. Because protein slows digestion and lowers a food's rating on the glycemic index, it prevents high-energy carbs from sending your blood sugar soaring, then crashing. That's especially valuable during long days in the saddle, when steadily released energy keeps you from bonking. During fuel shortages, your body sends protein to the liver, where it gets turned into backup carbs.

The power of protein doesn't stop there. Its amino acids act like recovery agents that refresh your body for the next go-round: After a muscle-ravaging ride, protein rebuilds tissues and prepares them for more. To optimize its muscle-mending powers, eat 15 to 25 grams of protein within an hour of finishing a ride. Aim for the highest-quality proteins possible, meaning those that offer the most muscle-building amino acids. Eggs and dairy products (like milk) are high on that list because they're considered "complete," meaning that they contain enough of all the essential amino acids needed to rebuild cells. Milk is particularly high in branched-chain amino acids, including leucine, which has been found to trigger muscle recovery.

Except for certain grains, such as quinoa, most plant proteins are "incomplete," or lacking a few key amino acids. To build and repair tissues, those proteins need to be paired in the right combination with others. If you're a vegetarian, traditional food pairings like beans and rice deliver overall protein quality. But don't worry excessively about pairing them in the same meal. So long as you eat them all in the same day, you'll be fine.

Proteins are also absorbed at different rates (similar to fast- and slow-release carbs). Whey, a milk protein, is digested quickly—which is why it's preferred in recovery beverages. But another milk protein, casein, is slowly digested, so it's ideal for minimizing blood-sugar spikes

THE FOOD	PROTEIN IN GRAMS
Steak (4 ounces)	34 grams
Chicken breast (4 ounces)	26 grams
Tuna/fish (4 ounces)	26 grams
Pork (4 ounces)	26 grams
Salmon (3 ounces)	19 grams
Shrimp (3 ounces)	18 grams
Greek yogurt (6 ounces)	18 grams
Whitefish (3 ounces)	16 grams
Yogurt, low-fat plain (1 cup)	13 grams
Eggs (2)	12 grams
Tofu (4 ounces)	11 grams
Lentils (1/2 cup)	9 grams
Cheese (1 ounce or 1 slice)	7 grams
Peanut butter (2 tablespoons)	8 grams
Pasta (1 cup)	7 grams
Nuts (1 ounce)	7 grams
Mixed vegetables (2/3 cup)	2 grams

throughout the day. Soy, a plant-based protein source containing antioxidants, is as digestible as milk proteins.

Here's a look at some high-quality protein sources that add up.

BEFRIEND FAT

Remember when avocados and nuts were "bad" for you and bagels were a health food? Yeah. That. The tide against foods we used to think were bad—some really bad—has turned and is swelling daily. Most recently, research in the *Annals of Internal Medicine* reported that people who ate higher-fat diets (even saturated fat, which is no longer the diet demon we once believed)—focusing on nuts and fish, but also including butter, cheese, and red meat—along with less starchy carbs not only lost more weight than low-fat eaters, but also maintained more muscle and reduced their risk for heart disease.

It's no coincidence that Americans got heavier as fat consumption went down. For years, the government preached low-fat, carb-heavy diets. "This wasn't only misguided; it was flat-out wrong," Friel says. This is *especially* important for endurance athletes like cyclists, who burn fat, and lots of it, for fuel. As a woman, it's especially, especially important because women are better fat burners than men. And the more conditioned you are, the better fat burner you become. You need ample amounts of fat, which, contrary to widely held belief, won't make you fat. In fact, starchy foods turn to stored fat far more quickly.

What's more, evidence is stacking up that

unsaturated fats are essential for firing up your fat-burning metabolism. In a study of 101 men and women, Harvard researchers put half the group on a low-fat diet and half on a diet that included about 20 percent of calories from monounsaturated fatty acids (MUFAs). After 18 months, the MUFA-eating group had dropped 11 pounds; its low-fat-eating peers had shed only 6. Fat is also slower to digest than carbs, so it helps you stay hunger-free longer.

Fat will also help you ride longer so you can burn more calories, says Friel. Research shows that athletes who get about 50 percent of their diet from fat produce better average times to exhaustion in exercise tests than those eating typical low-fat, high-carb diets.

Add fat, especially the metabolism-revving unsaturated types, to every meal. Sass recommends getting about 20 percent of your calories from MUFAs, or about 55 grams per day at 2,500 calories, which is what most cyclists eat as training ramps up. "Because most athletes don't have time to count fat grams, the simpler message is: Include small portions of good fats, like almonds, avocado, and olive oil, with all meals and snacks," she says. Try nuts and seeds, olive-based tapenades, and even the occasional chunk of dark chocolate. Some healthy portions to shoot for:

- **NUTS AND SEEDS:** Everything from pecans to pine nuts, almond butter to tahini. A serving size is 2 tablespoons.
- **OLIVES:** Black, green, mixed, or blended in a spreadable tapenade. A serving is 10 large olives or 2 tablespoons of spread.

- **OILS:** Canola, flaxseed, peanut, safflower, walnut, sunflower, sesame, or olive. Cook with them, drizzle them, eat them in pesto. One serving is 1 tablespoon.
- **AVOCADO:** As guacamole, or just slice and serve. One-quarter cup equals one serving.
- **DARK CHOCOLATE:** Go for $\frac{1}{4}$ cup of dark or semisweet, which is about 2 ounces.

FUEL YOUR FEMININE PHYSIOLOGY

It's an exciting time in sports nutrition thanks to scientists, researchers, and sports nutritionists who are finally taking our unique physiology into account when considering how athletes need to fuel themselves for optimum performance.

A woman was the driving force behind this change, of course, and that woman was sports nutrition and performance researcher Stacy Sims. Sims, an elite-level athlete herself as well as a research specialist in how hormones affect thermoregulation, macronutrient usage, hydration, and recovery, recognized early on that sex differences extend far beyond ponytails and sports bras.

To boil it down to basics, women have two hormone phases each month: high and low. During the low (follicular) hormone phase, we are physiologically similar to men in our carbohydrate metabolism and recovery. When our hormone levels rise during the other half of the month (the luteal phase), however, it becomes a different story.

Fuel the Ride

When it comes to on-the-bike performance, your daily nutrition is important. But if you're going to be racing and/or going out for long rides, what you eat before and during can make or break your outing.

PRERIDE SNACK FOR HARD DAYS (30 MINUTES PRERIDE)

Top off with 100 to 200 calories of carbs. Pick from among such choices as:

1 banana drizzled with 1 teaspoon honey

A fig bar

½ of a PB&J

ENDURANCE RIDES (RIDES OF 90 MINUTES OR LONGER)

Aim for about 120 to 200 calories of carbs per hour (along with electrolytes like sodium and potassium), such as:

Lärabar

Energy chews

Energy bar

Banana

Cooked, salted fingerling potatoes

The high estrogen level makes us spare glycogen and increases the amount of fat we use for fuel—not exactly what you're looking for when racing or doing threshold intervals. High progesterone delays our sweat response and turns up our core temperature, increases our sodium loss, and increases muscle breakdown (while also hindering our ability to synthesize muscle because we can't access amino acids as well as men). The one-two punch of high estrogen and progesterone shifts fluids into the cells (hello, bloat), decreases our blood plasma volume by about 8 percent, and makes us more predisposed to central nervous system fatigue (fatigue that is from chemical changes in the brain and neuromuscular system rather than the muscles themselves). All of this means we're quicker to tire, our heat tolerance decreases, and exercise feels harder so we don't have the mojo to really go.

To counteract these hormonal effects, Sims created a special hydration system (more on that in Chapter 20). But you can also help yourself by fine-tuning your nutrition to give your body more of what it needs during certain times of the month. Specifically, before you train or race, be sure to take in foods and fluids with branched-chain amino acids (BCAAs), specifically leucine, isoleucine, and valine, such as whey protein powder (a smoothie can work well), nuts, and cottage cheese. Also be sure to have ample amounts of sodium (see "Salt of the Earth," on the opposite page), which helps offset any reduced plasma volume and increased sodium loss.

On the bike, you're looking for sodium and potassium to keep that fluid loss and balance in check. Also be sure to take in a blend of sugars like glucose and sucrose, since depending on where you are in your cycle, your body might be having a harder time accessing those glycogen stores.

Finally, when you're done with a hard training session or race, make sure to replace your depleted energy stores with some carbs along with a healthy hit of protein, particularly of the whey variety. "It shuts down the breakdown effects progesterone has on exercise and increases the amount of circulating amino acids to promote muscle synthesis," says Sims. Chocolate milk is easy to find and tastes good but, as mentioned earlier, is a little off the mark for women, since we need more protein for recovery. Add some nuts or go with a protein smoothie or drink.

Your other nutrient needs should be covered if you generally eat a healthy, well-rounded diet. However, if you're premenopausal, you might also consider taking an iron supplement (check with your doctor about this first, though). In a meta-analysis of studies on iron supplementation and female exercise performance, Australian researchers found that it may improve your cycling performance on nearly every level, including how hard you can ride when you're going at full throttle and your exercise efficiency so you can put out more watts at a lower heart rate.

The effect was most pronounced in women who were iron deficient and athletes in training. But low iron is common in menstruating women, especially active women, because hard training can cause iron loss and interfere with its absorption. It's worth getting screened, especially if you feel fatigued or if you're not riding as well as you should be, says study author Sant-Rayn Pasricha, PhD. If you train and race, it could be worth getting screened even if you feel "normal," says Pasricha, because you can be low in iron and not know it. "Female athletes ought to consider iron-status screening because the benefits of supplementation to those who are iron deficient or at risk for iron deficiency are so clear," he says. Women ages 19 to 50 need at least 18 milligrams a day.

SALT OF THE EARTH

Sodium has been vilified in recent years, but as an active cyclist, you need more than your fair share. Sodium's primary job is to maintain the balance of fluid inside and outside your cells, but it also plays a role in muscle and nerve function, especially during strenuous exercise. You can't make it on your own, so it has to come from your diet. While it's easy to get plenty of the mineral from foods, it can be tricky to dial in that delicate balance between how much you eat at the dinner table and how much you take in on the bike. Here's what you need to know. (More on sodium and hydration during exercise in "Drink According to Thirst," page 217.)

PERSONALIZE YOUR INTAKE. Though the Centers for Disease Control and Prevention recommends a daily maximum of 2,300 milligrams of sodium, the average American consumes one and a half times that. But recent research suggests that it actually may be more dangerous to

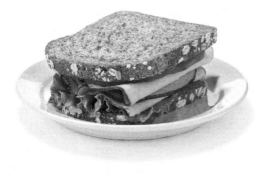

Sodium comes in many forms. If you're loading up before a big event, choose one that provides other important nutrients as well. A turkey sandwich can be a good choice.

blacklist the saltshaker than to shake it freely. A study in the *American Journal of Hypertension* found that people who consume between 2,645 and 4,945 milligrams of sodium a day have a lower mortality rate, as well as fewer cardiovascular events like heart attack or stroke, than those who stay within the recommended amount. Wait, what? "We know that some people are salt sensitive and that their blood pressure rises more easily when they consume salt," says Andrew Getzin, MD, clinical director of sports medicine and athletic performance at Cayuga Medical Center in Ithaca, New York. But it isn't true for everyone. "And if you're not getting enough salt, your body doesn't retain as much fluid, which can put you at risk for dehydration and low blood pressure," he adds. That's especially important if you're a salty sweater—i.e., you have a white film or crystals on your skin and clothes after you ride.

If you're planning to ride for many hours in the heat, make sure there's some sodium in your preride meal. A turkey sandwich, for example, contains about 1,500 milligrams. On the bike, a good rule of thumb is to consume between 500 and 700 milligrams per hour, which is about how much you can absorb within that time. Start with that amount and see how you tolerate it. If you feel sluggish or dizzy or experience muscle cramps, you may need to increase it. If you develop stomach issues such as diarrhea, you may be taking in too much; salt draws water into your gut and can lead to the runs. After you get off the bike, plan to eat a salty snack such as pretzels or toast with peanut butter. You'll replenish the sodium you lost through sweat and better retain fluids as you rehydrate.

SALT 'N' PEP. Not all energy products that contain salt are created equal. Read labels and experiment with different sources and quantities of sodium during and after your rides to find the ones that work best for you.

And Now, for Something Completely Different

Special diets are so common they're really not all that "special" anymore. Lots of athletes experiment with radical changes to see if they will yield radical results. Honestly, they rarely do. If you've been kicking around the idea of radically changing the way you eat but are wondering how it will affect your energy when you ride, here's some food for thought. David Zabriskie rode the 2011 Tour de France on a vegan diet. And the entire Garmin-Transitions team went gluten-free while training for the 2010 Tour de France. The key is to find a fueling plan that includes a healthy balance of nutrients, carbohydrates, protein, fats, and fluids—even if it doesn't feature piles of pre-ride pasta. With any diet, "the right foods can mean the difference between finishing first and bonking," says Esther Blum, author of *Cavewomen Don't Get Fat*.

All five of the following popular eating approaches can provide the health and performance benefits you need as a cyclist—as long as you're willing to follow (and possibly bend) some rules and make a few tough sacrifices. Here's what you need to know.

VEGAN

This plant-based diet nixes all animal products, including meat and dairy—even honey, whey, and gelatin. Research shows that filling up on fruits, vegetables, whole grains, legumes, nuts, and seeds can fend off chronic disease, lower blood pressure, and increase longevity. And there's evidence that diets based on these foods, which are typically high in antioxidants, can reduce injury and speed recovery, says Virginia Messina, author of *Vegan for Life*. But you miss out on key nutrients like protein, iron, and vitamin B_{12}, which are critical for athletes. The B vitamins, for example, help repair cells and convert protein and carbs to energy, especially during hard workouts. "Vitamin B_{12} comes from animal foods, and getting enough can be tough," says Michelle Babb, a nutritionist in Seattle.

FUEL UP: The best vegan sources of B_{12} include fortified breakfast cereals and soy products, nutritional yeast, and dietary supplements. Protect lean muscle mass with protein sources like tofu, almonds, black beans, and oatmeal. Preserve your iron stores by pairing iron-rich foods with vitamin C for better absorption: a bean burrito and salsa, steel-cut oats and strawberries, and spinach salad with citrus.

ENERGY SOURCE	MILLIGRAMS OF SODIUM / SERVING SIZE
GU Peanut Butter Energy Gel	65 mg/1.1-ounce packet
Honey Stinger Energy Chew	80 mg/1.8-ounce bag
Nesquik Low-Fat Chocolate Milk	160 mg/14-ounce bottle
Gatorade Thirst Quencher	160 mg/12-ounce bottle
Clif Bar, Banana Nut Bread	190 mg/2.4-ounce bar
PowerBar PowerGel	200 mg/1.44-ounce packet
SaltStick Caps	215 mg/capsule
Mini pretzels	250 mg/20 pretzels
V8 Original Vegetable Juice	650 mg/8-ounce can
Beef jerky	670 mg/1 ounce

PALEO

Fans of this throwback plan eat only foods that were available before the invention of agriculture. These include grass-fed meats, pastured poultry and eggs, fruits, vegetables, fish, nuts, and seeds. The idea is that by eating like your Stone Age ancestors you can shrug off modern-day disease, not to mention lose weight, improve sleep, get better skin, and gain more energy. Starting the day with meat and nuts for breakfast does raise levels of feel-good hormones like dopamine and serotonin, says Blum. "You'll feel energized, focused, and ready to ride." But take note: The diet is short on the complex carbs you might rely on for energy on the bike, says Babb. Also, coffee is discouraged—that means no midride espresso.

FUEL UP: Fill your plate with wild salmon, wild meat (such as bison), free-range eggs, greens, coconut, and sweet potatoes. For sustained energy, you'll also need to eat plenty of complex carbs such as grains, dairy, and beans.

PALEO POWER SWAPS

For a boost of on-bike energy, substitute these recipes for packaged fuel.

Power Gel

2 tablesoons raw organic honey

2 tablesoons raw almond butter, apple butter, or ¹/₂ banana

1 teaspoon lemon juice

Combine in blender until smooth and creamy. Transfer to a fuel belt bottle or EZ Squeezees pouch ($6.99 for a three-pack) and carry.

Sports Drink

1 cup coconut water

¹/₂ cup pomegranate juice

¹/₂ cup water

¹/₈ teaspoon organic sea salt

1,000 mg carnitine tartrate (found in vitamin and health food stores)

Combine ingredients and shake well.

Recipes created by Esther Blum, author of Cavewomen Don't Get Fat

RAW

Put your stove on Craigslist. Nothing in this diet can be heated above 118°F. Proponents claim that heat destroys foods' natural enzymes and nutrients that promote good digestion and optimal health, says Anne Guzman, a registered holistic nutritionist and sports nutrition consultant in Toronto. Raw foodists boast of having boundless energy, glowing skin, and mental clarity—as well as needing minimal sleep. Some stick to a vegan approach (see page 213 for how to make up for missing animal-based nutrients); others allow raw fish and meat, and raw (unpasteurized) dairy. Since nothing is cooked or processed, you'll avoid the nutritional void of certain prepackaged foods. Devotees rely on preparations that add variety to the diet, including juicing, fermentation, and dehydration. Whether or not the benefits are real, there's nothing inherently wrong with going raw—as long as you're vigilant about preventing foodborne illness. Wash and store your ingredients carefully.

FUEL UP: Prepare to eat a lot. Raw food is not only naturally low in calories but also has more water than cooked foods, so you'll have to eat more to get enough calories, carbohydrates, and protein, says Messina. Fill up on fruits and veggies (spaghetti squash and raw kelp noodles can replace pasta), nuts and seeds, sprouted beans and grains, fresh juices, dates and other dried fruits, plus cold-pressed extra-virgin olive oil and virgin coconut oil.

GLUTEN-FREE

Forgoing gluten, a protein found in wheat and related grains, provides relief for people with celiac disease, an illness in which the protein triggers an autoimmune response that affects digestion and overall health. But plenty of people who are not gluten sensitive have embraced the diet because of claims that it improves well-being and energy. Avoiding the protein isn't easy, however, especially for athletes. In addition to being an ingredient in such ride-fueling staples as breads and pastas, it's found in many energy bars and in other surprising places, like salad dressings and soups. The good news? Steering clear of gluten encourages you to pass on processed and packaged foods, which are often high in sugar and calories and low on nutrition, says Guzman.

FUEL UP: Switch to carb sources like bananas, sweet potatoes, almond flour, brown rice, polenta, and pastas made from rice and quinoa. Plenty of packaged energy snacks are now gluten-free, including KIND bars and Skout Organic Trailbars.

MACROBIOTIC

This low-fat, high-fiber approach to nutrition is more than an eating plan, it's part of a lifestyle meant to balance mind and body. What you eat: roughly 50 percent whole grains, 30 percent local in-season vegetables, and 10 percent beans and seaweed (such as dried nori and kelp). Fermented foods like miso, tempeh, and sauerkraut are also encouraged. You can cheat a little (use that remaining 10 percent): Meat, fish, dairy, and other normally forbidden foods are allowed occasionally, but artificial sweeteners, chemical additives, heavy spices, and caffeine are not. "A plant-based diet that relies on whole foods means more nutrients, less inflammation, and better recovery," says Guzman. That's a big plus for athletes. And fiber and fermented foods promote good gut bacteria for better nutrient absorption and a strong immune system.

FUEL UP: Good macrobiotic options include millet, oats, brown rice, quinoa, seaweed, fermented soybeans, and sauerkraut. But when half of your diet consists of high-fiber foods, digestion on the bike can be an issue, so cheat as needed for rides and recovery.

CHAPTER 20

Drink Up!

I LEARNED THE IMPORTANCE OF PROPER HYDRATION THE
hard way—more than once. The first time was in Philadelphia. I was at a mountain
bike race that started at high noon in May. And it was unseasonably hot—like, pushing 100°F hot. We were racing three laps, which I had figured would take $1\frac{1}{2}$ to 2
hours, so two bottles would do the trick. Well, on any other pleasant May day it might
have. But two laps in, I was out of water, getting tunnel vision, and suffering a case of
the chills—never good when it's actually 96°F out.

I started screeching at spectators. "I'm out of water! Anyone have water!?" Before
long, someone took mercy on me and gave me a spare bottle. I recovered and went on
to win the race.

The second hydration debacle didn't have such a happy ending. I was at another
mountain bike race and it was Africa hot, because it was in South Africa. It was day
2 of an 8-day stage race I was doing with my teammate Cheryl. We were looking at
a 6- to 7-hour day of racing in the hot sun. At the time, I was also using "liquid
nutrition," meaning I was drinking high-calorie energy drinks to get in more calories without having to try to eat and digest a lot of solid food. This had worked fairly
well during my training in Pennsylvania, where, because of the time of year, the
temps had been in the 40s. It was downright disastrous that day.

I had four bottles' worth of fluid on me—70 ounces in my hydration pack and a
bottle on my bike. Each bottle was packed with 250 calories. Less than 2 hours into
the race, I'd already drained nearly three bottles as I tried to stay cool and hydrated
in the oppressive South African heat. You do the math. That's nearly 800 calories in

about 2 hours. I'll spare you the details of the day, but it created a Molotov cocktail in my gut and I spent the rest of the race beating back nausea, dashing into the bushes, and desperately trying to get to the finish line so I could recover.

I learned a lot of lessons that day. First and foremost is that you can get some nutrients from your sports drinks, but the primary purpose of those bottles on your bike is to hydrate you. And there's an awful lot of confusion and misinformation about the topic. While hydration is very important, as the examples above illustrate, you can overdo it on the drinking. We've been so conditioned by sports drink companies to hydrate, hydrate, hydrate that a few people have actually drunk themselves to death by developing hyponatremia, a potentially fatal condition in which you have dangerously little sodium in your blood. Women, by the way, appear to be more prone to hyponatremia than men are, so it's important that we practice smart, healthy hydration.

Drink According to Thirst

Here's the deal. For years, cyclists have been told to drink enough while on the bike that they weigh the same after the ride as they did beforehand. The truth is, you can shed 2 to 3 pounds an hour while riding hard. But the body can't replace all of the fluid it loses, and not every ounce of weight is lost as sweat anyway. So aim to drink 50 to 75 percent of the amount of sweat you lose during a long ride, which generally adds up to 6 to 8 ounces

(two or three gulps) every 15 to 20 minutes, or about a large cycling bottle an hour, depending on your hourly sweat rate. How do you know your sweat rate? Simple, says Monique Ryan, RD, author of *Sports Nutrition for Endurance Athletes*, who once coached a heavy-sweating triathlete who routinely lost 40 ounces of fluid an hour. To determine how much you sweat out, simply weigh yourself before and after a short ride. "An hour ride is a good indicator of what you're losing through sweat alone," Ryan says.

If you're planning a hard ride or race in very hot weather, prehydrating is a good idea, as well. Hydrating before pedaling helps you avoid drying out on the road. For best absorption, sip 12 to 16 ounces of fluid 4 hours before hopping on your bike; 2 hours before, sip another 12 ounces. While riding, drink enough to match the intensity of the exercise, the heat of the day, and your body's needs. It goes without saying that the hotter it is, the higher your fluid needs are, so you might end up draining twice as much per hour on a 90°F day than you would when it's in the 60s or 70s.

FILL UP ON MORE THAN JUST FLUIDS

You sweat out more than just water. That fluid pouring out of your pores also contains electrolytes like sodium, calcium, magnesium, and potassium, which are essential for maintaining fluid balance and creating all the electrical impulses you need to live, from the most basic cell functions to neuromuscular interactions. Electrolytes are everything in exercise. And you lose a lot of them when you sweat, especially sodium.

Your sodium needs are about as personal as the type of pedals you prefer. "During exercise it comes down to how much you lose through sweat," says Pamela Hinton, PhD, associate professor of nutritional sciences at the University of Missouri. "Some people perspire more than others, and some have higher concentrations of salt in their sweat." Although you can figure out how much fluid you lose through sweat by weighing yourself before and after a ride, there's no simple way to calculate exactly how much salt you shed. Again, if you notice a white film or crystals on your skin or clothes after a ride, you're likely a salty sweater and may need more sodium during exercise than someone who sweats out less salt.

Air temperature has the greatest impact on how much you sweat, so if it's hot, you might need to up your sodium intake. In addition to perspiring more on warmer days, you lose more salt per unit of sweat. "As sweat travels from your glands to your skin, the body reabsorbs some of the salt," says Evan Johnson, PhD, an exercise physiologist in the Department of Health, Human Performance, and Recreation at the University of Arkansas. But as your sweat rate goes into overdrive on a hot day, there's less time for the body to grab on to the salt, and you end up with more of it in your sweat.

One study, published in the journal *Medicine and Science in Sports and Exercise*, found that athletes who downed a drink containing about 3,800 milligrams of sodium before running to

exhaustion in 90°F heat reported lower perceived exertion compared to when they preloaded with a low-sodium drink. Salt attracts fluid, so the more salt that's in your body, the higher your blood volume. "A higher blood volume decreases the amount of work your heart has to do," says Johnson, "because it doesn't have to beat as fast to move the same amount of blood throughout your body." As a result, exercise feels easier.

Your hydration status also influences how much sodium resides in your bloodstream. As mentioned earlier, endurance athletes can actually consume too much water and develop a fatal but rare condition called hyponatremia. "You essentially dilute the concentration of sodium in your blood," Hinton says. When the level dips too low, it affects your muscles' ability to contract, including the most important muscle—your heart. Hyponatremia is more common in newer athletes and those who ride at slower paces. If you're riding hard, it's difficult to overhydrate, Johnson says. "At a lower intensity, you can drink more easily and you don't sweat as much, so you don't lose as much of the excess fluid." The easiest way to avoid hyponatremia is to simply drink according to your thirst and no more. Also, choose an electrolyte drink that contains sodium over plain water.

The only way to find what drinks work for you is by testing them. "Some products may not taste good to you, while others may sit in your stomach in a bad way," says Douglas Casa, PhD, the director of athletic training education at the University of Connecticut at Storrs. If you're the type of salty sweater who finds white streaks on your jersey after a ride, you may need a drink with more sodium. For extreme salt sweaters, Casa suggests adding ¼ teaspoon of salt to 16 ounces of sports drink (that's 600 milligrams of sodium). If you find that a sports drink upsets your stomach, try diluting it with water. "Just never start a big event with a new product in your bottle," says Casa. "That's a recipe for disaster."

Whether or not you need other calories in the form of carbohydrates or protein in your bottles is a matter of contentious debate. If you're going to be riding for more than an hour or so, you will need to take in some calories to maintain your blood glucose and stave off fatigue. Most of that should be in the form of food. But a little bit of carbohydrate in the form of sugar in your sports drink can contribute to your fueling as well as help pull more fluid into your intestines and increase your blood glucose availability.

And protein? Protein muscled its way onto the sports drink scene after early studies showed that carb-protein blends seemed to shoot into the bloodstream and enhance endurance cycling performance better than carb-only beverages did.

Recent research on 10 trained cyclists performing an 80-kilometer trial showed that riders drinking carb-only beverages did just as well as those drinking carb-protein beverages, and both groups did better than those consuming flavored water. However, the International Society of Sports Nutrition recently reported that taking in BCAAs—branched-chain amino acids—during vigorous aerobic exercise can decrease muscle damage and depletion. "If you're on a long ride where you're also eating, you'll be taking in protein already," says Ryan, "so it's likely not necessary to also have it in your drink."

Finally, a word on caffeine (there'll be plenty more on it in Chapter 22, too). Caffeine has long been demonized as a diuretic. Conventional wisdom says it should lead to dehydration and heat stress, especially when you consider that it also raises your heart rate and increases your metabolism. Neither is true. In fact it may improve your carb burning.

A review of ongoing research recently revealed that caffeinated drinks don't make you pee that much more than equal amounts of beverages without the buzz. The stimulant also doesn't worsen the effects of summertime heat. In fact, caffeine makes you feel better. Numerous studies have shown that it lowers the rate of perceived exertion while improving strength, endurance, and mental performance. Even better, researchers from the University of Birmingham, in England, found that riders who drank a caffeinated sports beverage burned the drink's carbs 26 percent faster than those who consumed a caffeine-free sports drink, likely because caffeine speeds glucose absorption in the intestine.

Of course you *can* overdo caffeine, and nobody rides well when they feel jittery. But you also don't have to worry about the effects of having a midride espresso and can feel free to grab that Red Bull at the 7-Eleven if your energy levels are flagging and you've still got many miles to go.

For Women Only

As mentioned in the last chapter, women have unique fueling needs because our oscillating hormone levels have profound effects on our metabolism, especially during exercise. To recap, when our estrogen level is high during the luteal phase of our cycle, we tend to spare glycogen and burn more fat. A high progesterone level (also during the luteal phase) hinders our sweat response, raises our core temperature, increases our sodium loss, and hampers our access to amino acids, making it tough to synthesize muscle and causing more muscle breakdown. Worse, when it comes to hydration, our fluids shift from our bloodstream to inside our cells, so our blood plasma volume drops significantly.

Bad. Bad. Bad. That's why Stanford exercise nutrition expert Stacy Sims developed a special line of sports drinks made just for women. Note that this discussion isn't an advertisement for her product line, but the science is interesting and good to know. I also had the privilege of being one of her guinea pigs as she was developing the drinks. And, well, the proof was in the pee sticks.

See, Sims had a houseful of women athletes, primarily cyclists and triathletes, come to a training camp where we used the products before, during, and after strenuous workouts.

We stopped to pee on urinalysis strips along the way so we could see firsthand how our physiology was being affected by the drinks.

Upon arrival, we all went for a long, hilly ride up and down and around the east peak of Mount Tamalpais, near San Francisco. Then we returned to the house, cooked up some dinner, and sat around for a fireside chat about the menstrual cycle, with Sims schooling us on how our bodies respond to our ever-changing hormone levels.

The next day we downed her PreLoad Hydration product (which tastes a bit like a virgin margarita) as we kitted up in the morning, then filled our bottles with her Active Hydration for Women, stuffed some food and pee sticks in our pockets, and headed out for a hard training ride. PreLoad contains BCAAs that work with sodium to pump up our total body water content (for a little hyperhydration) as well as increase the amount of circulating amino acids to dampen the muscle breakdown effects of progesterone, speed up recovery, and keep stress hormones and central nervous system fatigue at bay. It also contains sodium bicarbonate and sodium citrate to help buffer lactate, so you can go harder without the hurt. The Active Hydration drink serves up more sodium for hydration and a bit of glucose and sucrose to counteract the glycogen-sparing effects of estrogen and give us some quick energy. And we needed it—all of it.

The day's task was a 40-mile ride that included four 12-minute threshold efforts up Route 1 from Muir Beach. After each effort, we were to roll back down the hill and duck behind a roadside construction pile to pee on our sticks and see how we were doing. Specifically, we were looking for our urine's specific gravity (were we staying hydrated?), pH (buffering), protein (were we becoming catabolic, eating into our own muscles?), and ketones (were we taking in enough food, or was our liver having to produce ketone bodies to fuel us because we weren't?).

Up the hill. Down the hill. Ducked and peed. Analyzed. What did I learn? Well, that I do a pretty good job of hydrating and a less-good job at eating, and I tend to lose protein, perhaps because of chronically high progesterone. Generally speaking, the test was successful in that I

Gonna Make You Sweat

Sweating and hydration go hand in hand. After all, hydration is nothing more than pouring back in a bit of what you're dripping out. Sweat works like central AC for your body. On hot days or as you're grinding up a hill, glands under the skin produce sweat and send it to the surface, where it evaporates. Each drop that turns into vapor pulls heat away from your body, and you feel cooler. The hotter you get, the more you sweat.

On days when there's a lot of moisture in the air, sweat can't evaporate as quickly, making it harder for your body to cool off. This is why heat-related problems like cramps, exhaustion, and heatstroke are more common in humid environments than in dry ones. Your sweat can also tell you important facts about your diet, fitness, and exercise metabolism. Here's how to decode yours.

IF YOURS STINKS

Your diet may be to blame. Caffeine stimulates sweat glands under your arms and in your scalp and groin that secrete a fatty, odiferous sweat. And if you eat a very-low-carb diet, your body breaks down protein and fats, creating acetone, which is excreted through sweat and has a distinctive ammonia smell.

IF YOURS POURS

You're hydrated and working hard. Seasoned riders may not sweat more than cyclists who aren't as fit, but they're able to work harder and produce more sweat. In hot conditions, however, fitter athletes have greater sweating capacity, according to research published in the *American Journal of Physiology.*

IF YOURS STAINS

You may be losing a lot of salt. Less-fit riders who aren't used to riding in heat shed more sodium than their fitter, heat-acclimatized counterparts. Choose a drink with 400 to 600 milligrams of sodium per serving.

IF YOURS STOPS

"You're not adequately replacing your fluid loss," says Appalachian State University sweat researcher Caroline Smith, PhD. You don't need to replace every drop but you do need to drink enough so your body's cooling system can work. This is a sign of heat exhaustion, when your core temperature can rise quickly, which can potentially lead to heatstroke.

Feed Your Thirst

On the bike, hydration is important, but off of it, your first priority should be staying on top of your daily hydration, which woefully few of us do, says Monique Ryan. Research on gym-goers found that nearly half began their workouts in a dehydrated state. "Many people don't consume enough fluids during the day," Ryan says. "If you hydrate properly on a regular basis, you won't need to worry as much about getting dehydrated during a typical moderate ride." The old eight-glasses-a-day dictum is a good guidepost.

Not a big water drinker? You can top off your tank with foods that are high in water, says Tara Gidus, an Orlando, Florida–based, sports dietitian. As an added bonus, their nutrients can replace the electrolytes you lose through sweat, replenish spent energy stores, and reduce inflammation. Reach for these waterlogged foods to take a bite out of your thirst.

MELONS

Made up of 90 percent water, melon is an ideal recovery food. "It replaces glycogen stores quickly," says David Grotto, author of *The Best Things You Can Eat.*

BERRIES

These gems contain up to 92 percent water and are rich in anthocyanins, which give them their deep hues and reduce postworkout inflammation and joint pain.

SOUP

It contains sodium, the most important electrolyte to replace. Choose brothy varieties or ones with vegetables, which offer nutrients to round out the electrolyte mix.

GRAINS

As they cook, grains such as quinoa, rice, and oatmeal soak up water, which your body absorbs as it digests them. Oatmeal's soluble fiber also sucks up cholesterol.

BELL PEPPERS

At 92 percent water, these are among the most hydrating of all vegetables. They're also packed with vitamins C (one red bell pepper has 253 percent of your Daily Value) and A.

LETTUCE

Iceberg leads the pack at 96 percent water, but other varieties, such as romaine, are more nutritious and nearly as aqueous.

CUCUMBER

A cuke is as water rich as lettuce, and its peel contains silica, which promotes elasticity in joints, skin, and fingernails.

CELERY

At 95 percent water, it's *low in calories* and *high in fiber*, both of which can aid in calorie management, as well.

was able to ride negative splits (I got farther up the hill with each repeat) and I recovered quickly between efforts.

We rolled home, downed some Acute Recovery, which is formulated to give you a big hit of protein (slow and fast release) as well as some glucose to shut down post–intense exercise muscle breakdown, counteract any catabolic effects of progesterone, and speed muscle synthesis and recovery and glycogen replacement. Sims has found that women have a shorter window for recovery than men, and we can restock our stores and mend our muscles best if we get what we need within 90 minutes of a hard ride, as opposed to the 3 to 6 hours that men have.

The next day, we went out for more testing. Only this time, we had our PreLoad in the morning, then another half-strength bottle of PreLoad before doing eight 1-minute full-throttle efforts up Mount Tam from Stinson Beach, punctuated by 2 minutes of recovery. The goal: more buffering, more available amino acids, less eating into our muscle stores as we throttled ourselves during day 2 of training camp.

We peed on our sticks at the bottom of the hill, then again up at the top to see what happened. This time, I made it a point to eat half of a bar about an hour into the ride, as well as sipping away on my bottles. It worked. Sims analyzed my stick. My protein level hadn't changed, I was not ketonic, and I was respectably hydrated. I also felt great, which in the end is what really matters.

Of course, all this begs the question of whether you need these special drinks during the lower-hormone phases of your cycle. The answer is probably not, but it won't hurt. Since we can't really pinpoint when our hormones start to rise (we know when they drop because we start bleeding) and we don't know how long our high-hormone phase lasts, it's simple enough to just follow one fueling protocol so we're sure we have what we need when we need it. Again, this isn't a paid advertisement for Sims' Osmo Nutrition, but it's good information to have so we women know what to look for in our foods and beverages for optimal performance.

CHAPTER 21

Pedal Off the Pounds

I'M A FIRM BELIEVER THAT WEIGHT LOSS SHOULD BE THE by-product of living an active, healthy life. The goal is to fully enjoy your sport—in this case, cycling—to its fullest rather than having weight loss itself as the end goal. Sure, a bike can be a vehicle for weight loss. But I always want people to get on a bike because they love it and enjoy the ride first and foremost.

That said, it is hard to argue with the fact that for some people, a little weight loss (sometimes a lot of it) could exponentially increase their enjoyment of the sport. After all, each pound you carry has potential, be it to put raw power into your pedals so you can outsprint the masses to the line or ascend the likes of Mont Ventoux, or to weigh you down so you're slower on the bike or maybe shorten your life by packing on too many pounds of fat. Of course, you can go too far in losing weight, too. Shave off too many pounds and you risk losing some of your crank-churning power. That's why, of all the measurements that avid cyclists track, from heart rate to mileage to speed, perhaps none outrank the one on the bathroom scale in importance.

Most coaches, in fact, devote a good deal of time to helping cyclists achieve a weight goal alongside their other riding goals. "I spend a lot of time helping riders achieve their ideal weight because the rewards are so great," says Hunter Allen, founder of Peaks Coaching Group and coauthor of *Training and Racing with a Power Meter*. "Every extra pound you carry above that weight makes you 15 to 20 seconds slower for each mile of a climb."

Off the bike, the rewards are just as substantial. The Centers for Disease Control and Prevention reports that if you're overweight, losing just 5 to 10 percent of your total body weight can lower your blood pressure, improve cholesterol levels, and protect against diabetes and cancer. Even if you never compete, slimming down will help you enjoy riding more because your heart won't have to work as hard. Maybe you'll even drop some of those leaner-than-thou types on the group ride. You get the idea.

It's only fair to acknowledge that some people lose weight more easily than others. I've seen some women drop significant weight through a series of little steps like ditching added sugars and adding some intervals to their riding. I've seen others struggle until they make more major changes. What is the same in the success stories, however, is consistency. Most often, those who bring structure to their riding plan as well as their eating do best.

Nancy Beeman, a longtime cyclist, learned that firsthand. Her desk job and subsequent retirement to the Midwest, where winters are long and unforgiving, left her with more than 30 unwanted pounds. She wasn't losing weight by just riding around when the weather was nice, so she bought a training book and started following a plan. Then she tackled her eating. "I didn't know how to start a diet, and more importantly didn't have the confidence that I could stick to one," she says. So she downloaded MyNetDiary on her iPhone to help her count calories as she learned to modify her diet and establish new eating habits (more on that in a bit). "It was fun—like piecing together a puzzle. I had to select the foods that would fuel me, as well as stay within the limit I had set for myself."

She also made plans for getting through the long Midwest winters. "I joined a spin class once a week and made a commitment to get on the trainer at least 3 to 4 hours a week," she says. She also "reimagined" herself as she wanted to be and made it a priority to become that person. It worked. "That first 15 pounds came off in the first 3 months and I was so excited I set another goal. This time I only went for another 5. When I lost that too, I went in for the kill—the final 10 pounds. It took me about 8 to 9 months, but I finally did it. I lost all 30 pounds and two pant sizes!" Because she had done it so deliberately and systematically, Nancy also knew it would be sustainable.

The Sweet Spot

Note that this is about being strong, not skinny. Fat plays a key role in immune system function—if you don't have enough, your energy will flag and you'll get sick. Become so lean that you start to burn muscle, and your power will plummet. The idea is to find a sweet spot where you can ride strong, yet be healthy, too.

Where is that sweet spot? It depends. I spent many years fielding that question from clients and readers. "What should I weigh?" "What should my body composition be?" "How much weight should I lose if I want to climb better?" So I devoted a few weeks to consulting experts and the research and coming up with some solid equations to answer those questions. In the end, I found that the answers depend on numerous factors, including your current weight, height, and body frame. Below, you will find three ways to calculate a target ideal weight you can live, ride, and even race with for life. Focus on the one that best fits your goals, or try all three. Then, check out the training and nutrition advice that will help you achieve your ideal cycling weight—and stay there for good.

OPTION 1: SHED EXCESS POUNDS

If you fit one or more of the descriptions below, use the accompanying steps to estimate an ideal target weight for your height and body frame.

—You ride a few times a week, primarily for recreation.

—You used to ride all the time, and maybe even raced, but work, family, and other responsibilities have forced you to scale back.

—You know you've got some weight to lose before you can think about improving your performance on the bike.

Your current weight: _____

Your height: _____

To find your baseline healthy weight, use the following formula:

100 pounds for the first 5 feet of height plus 5 pounds for each additional inch

For example, if you're 5 feet 6 inches, your ideal weight is 130 pounds (100 + 30).

Baseline target weight: _____

NOW, FACTOR IN YOUR FRAME SIZE

Just as mountain bikes come in small, medium, and large, so do our skeletal frames. That's why there's a range of medically recommended weights for any given height. A standard measurement of frame size is your wrist circumference in relation to your height. Use a tape measure to measure your wrist in inches at its widest point and then locate your frame size in this chart.

Match your wrist size to your height.

If your frame size is:

SMALL: Subtract 10 percent from your baseline target weight: _____

MEDIUM: Keep your baseline target weight: _____

LARGE: Add 10 percent to your baseline target weight: _____

HEIGHT	WRIST	FRAME
< 5'2"	< 5.5"	Small
	5.5" to 5.75"	Medium
	> 5.75"	Large
5'2" to 5'5"	< 6"	Small
	6" to 6.25"	Medium
	> 6.25"	Large
> 5'5"	< 6.25"	Small
	6.25" to 6.5"	Medium
	> 6.5"	Large

This number is your adjusted target weight. Standard body-weight formulas are based on averages, which means that results for some people may be slightly skewed. If the number you calculate is equal to or greater than your current weight, or if it's too low to be attainable, try Option 2, which focuses on your body composition.

OPTION 2: GET LEANER AND FASTER

If you fit one or more of the descriptions below, use the following steps to estimate a weight and body composition to help you maximize performance.

—You ride 4 or more days a week, including hard-charging training rides.

—You want to be competitive in a Gran Fondo, do a hard century, or race occasionally.

—You want to maximize your body composition and gain more power.

Determining your body composition gives you a breakdown of the percentages of your weight that are fat and lean pedal-pushing muscle. You'll get the most accurate reading from a special body composition scale (which you can purchase for home use, but most fitness centers have one). To get the most precise reading, make sure the one you use takes your fitness level into account, and follow the directions carefully. Your hydration level and menstrual cycle will affect the reading. Like your weight, the figure will fluctuate, so aver-

age your numbers from readings taken over a couple of weeks. Avoid online calculators; they don't provide accurate readings for active people.

Next, compare your reading to the percentages in the chart below, which are listed according to fitness levels.

Your current body fat: _____ percent

Essential fat: 10 to 12 percent

Athletes: 13 to 20 percent

Fitness: 21 to 24 percent

Acceptable: 25 to 31 percent

Healthy body fat ranges from 18 to 30 percent for women (who naturally have more fat than men). Athletes in top form may fall below these numbers. If your body fat percentage is higher, decide on a goal number within the healthy range. But be realistic; don't just target the lowest possible percentage. "Having a bit more body fat is better for your immune system and for consistency on the bike," Allen says.

Your body fat goal: _____ percent

Next, use these formulas to come up with a goal weight based on body composition.

Step 1

Figure out how many pounds of body fat you have.

Your current weight x your body fat percentage

= _____ pounds

(Example: 200 x 0.28 = 56 pounds)

Step 2

Next, figure out your lean body mass.

Your current weigh - pounds of body fat = _____ pounds

(Example: 200 - 56 = 144 pounds)

Step 3

Now, subtract your goal body fat percentage from 1.00.

(Example: 1.00 - 0.20 = 0.80)

Your answer: _____

Step 4

Divide your lean body mass from Step 2 by your answer in Step 3.

(Example: 144 pounds ÷ 0.80 = 180 pounds)

Your answer: _____ pounds

This is your target ideal weight based on your desired body composition.

OPTION 3: GET COMPETITIVE

If you fit one or more of the descriptions below, use the following guidelines to figure out how your weight compares with the riders at cycling's highest levels.

—You are a competitive racer who trains 10 to 15 hours a week.

—You're already lean, but you aspire to achieve a racing weight comparable to that of the fastest racers.

—Your body fat is at the low end of the healthy range (or lower).

Caution: This weight may not be realistic or even healthy for you to maintain over the long term. For many cyclists, these numbers may be aggressively low. Unless you get really serious about racing, you might want to set your sights a little higher.

As mentioned in the climbing section, cycling coach Joe Friel, creator of the Training Bible series of books, has calculated that top women riders come in at 1.9 to 2.2 pounds per inch. That means a 5-foot-5 woman would tip the scales between 123 and 143. Elite climbing specialists are often even lighter. Extra weight exacts far less of a penalty on flat ground as it does when you head toward the heavens on 10 percent grades. (This ratio isn't the same as your power-to-weight ratio, which is considered the gold standard for determining your most competitive cycling weight. But it's close, and it doesn't require an expensive power meter to figure out.)

There are exceptions, says Friel. Even a cursory glance at the others in your cycling club will tell you that fast, successful riders come in all sizes. Some riders—even in the top ranks—are simply built bigger, but that doesn't make them slower. If you tend to be muscular, it can be unrealistic, if not downright counterproductive, to try to achieve an unnaturally low weight.

Use the ranges described above to see how close your goal or current weight is to a weight that would best serve your ability to compete (assuming you have the corresponding fitness). If your goal or current weight is less than your competitive weight, go back to "Option 2: Get Leaner and Faster" to make sure your body fat is within a healthy range. If it's not, hit the gym to put on lean muscle tissue. And be sure you're properly fueling during and especially after your rides to avoid becoming catabolic and eating into your precious muscle stores. Be especially sure to meet your daily protein requirements by including some in every meal and snack.

Ride It Off

Now that you know how much you want to weigh, it's time to plot how to get there. The following 2-week plan from coach Hunter Allen will jump-start your weight loss by training your body to become a fat-burning machine. "It combines intense efforts with on-bike fueling strategies to teach your body to burn fat more effectively," he says. "It's not about drilling it every day. It's about becoming a strong, well-rounded rider and an excellent fat burner." You'll get noticeable results fast.

HOW IT WORKS

The program assumes you hop on your bike (or a stationary bike at the gym) 4 or more days a week. If you've been riding less than that, take the easy days as full rest and begin with the fewest number of intervals indicated on a given day.

Keep your calorie intake in check by limiting snacks on easy and rest days. On days that include hills, intervals, and/or other hard work right after your warmup, have a preride snack.

For endurance rides (days 6, 7, 13, and 14), when you'll pedal at a lower intensity, roll out the door on an empty stomach, ideally in the morning before breakfast or a few hours after a meal later in the day. But take plenty of food with you. You can fuel up after the 90-minute mark, before you drain your glycogen stores and bonk. "The idea is to train your body to become an efficient fat burner while still properly fueling your ride," Allen says. At first, it may be difficult to wait this long to start eating. Remember to ride at an easy to moderate effort. You should be able to carry on a conversation easily. If you're really flagging, have a bite or two at the 1-hour mark and extend that time on subsequent rides.

YOUR QUICK START PLAN

DAY 1 Lengthen your planned ride by 30 minutes and add one to three 10-minute intervals at an effort close to what you could maintain in a 60-minute time trial, or a rate of perceived exertion (RPE) of 5 on a scale of 1 to 10. Pedal lightly for 5 minutes between each interval.

DAY 2 Include two to five 3-minute intervals in your planned ride, maintaining the hardest steady effort you can. Pedal lightly for 3 minutes between each interval.

DAY 3 Lengthen your planned ride by adding 45 minutes, structured as one 8- to 10-second sprint every 2 minutes at 80 percent of your all-out effort (RPE 8), maintaining a moderate to somewhat strong effort in between, or RPE 3 to 4.

Rate of Perceived Exertion (RPE)

0	Very easy
1–2	Easy
3	Moderate
4	Somewhat strong
5	Strong
6–7	Very strong
8	Extremely strong
9–10	All-out

DAY 4 Include five to ten 1-minute intervals in your planned ride. Do these aggressively (RPE 7 to 8) and attack so that you're fading (but still pushing) in the final 15 seconds. Pedal lightly for 2 minutes between each interval.

DAY 5 Spin easy for an hour or take a rest day.

DAY 6 Endurance ride. Aim for 2 hours at an easy to moderate effort (RPE 2 to 3). If you haven't done a ride of this length recently, extend your longest recent ride by one-third.

DAY 7 Endurance ride. Aim for 3 hours at an easy to moderate effort (RPE 2 to 3), or extend your longest recent ride by one-third.

DAY 8 Spin easy for an hour or take a rest day.

DAY 9 Include two to four 10-minute intervals in your regular ride at an effort close to what you could maintain in a 60-minute time trial (RPE 5). Push yourself hard during the last

2 minutes. Pedal lightly to recover for 5 minutes between each interval.

DAY 10 Include five to ten 15-second all-out sprints (RPE 10) in your regular ride. Pedal lightly to recover for 4 minutes between each interval. Alternate between small- and big-ring sprints.

DAY 11 Include the following anaerobic intervals in a regular ride: three 2-minute intervals at RPE 7 with 2 minutes of easy pedaling between them. Ride 5 minutes easy. Then do three 1-minute intervals at RPE 8 with 1 minute of recovery in between. Ride 5 minutes easy and finish with three 30-second intervals, going all out, with 1 minute of easy pedaling in between.

DAY 12 Lengthen your regular ride by 45 minutes and pedal that final stretch at nearly your time trial pace or upper-tempo pace (RPE 4).

DAY 13 Endurance ride. Aim for 2.5 to 3 hours at an easy to moderate effort level (RPE 2 to 3), or extend your longest recent ride by one-third.

DAY 14 Long endurance ride. Plan to pedal for 3 to 4 hours at an easy to moderate effort (RPE 2 to 3), or extend your longest recent ride by one-third.

Fuel Your Way Lean

Of course, the riding part is only half the equation. What you eat has an equal if not larger impact on what you weigh. Moderately active women (those who ride or do some activity for 30 to 60 minutes on most days of a week) need between 1,800 and 2,200 calories a day to maintain their weight, slightly less if they're looking to lose. Active women (those who are generally active for more than an hour a day) need 2,200 to 2,400 to maintain and slightly less to lose.

I never recommend that someone become a slave to calorie counting, because eating should be enjoyable and eventually intuitive. But if you have trouble maintaining a healthy weight, it is a good idea to get a feeling for what those calorie counts look like in real life. And now you can, thanks to the Go Faster Eating Plan on page 232 that was formulated by Anne Guzman, a sports nutrition consultant for Peaks Coaching Group. This plan provides 2,000 to 2,500 calories day, including 500-calorie breakfasts, lunches, and dinners and energizing 250-calorie snacks. Choose from the options on pages 233 to 237 to design your own daily meals (or use the weeklong calendar as a starting point) .

The beauty of this plan is that it's easy to adjust. If you're riding less or looking to lose a little weight, you can easily lower the calorie count by eliminating a snack or shaving some of the portion sizes (e.g., going from $1\frac{1}{2}$ cups of rice to 1 cup). When you're super active and training hard, just mix and match and follow along to your heart's content. Note: This plan assumes your endurance riding days will be Saturdays and Sundays. If they're not, swap the Saturday and Sunday meals for other days.

The Unhealthy Pursuit of Thin

I'd be remiss to write about finding your ideal cycling weight without addressing the perils of obsessing about weight—eating disorders. As someone who suffered through one during her college years, I know the risk is real. I also know far too many cyclists (and runners and other athletes), male and female, who have fought through or continue to battle eating disorders or disordered eating (skirting the edges of a full blown disorder).

It's true that cycling is a power-to-weight sport, so losing some excess weight if you indeed have some excess weight can help you ride, especially climb, faster. But it's very important to not get fixated on the numbers on the scale as the end all, be all of performance. It's not. Great cyclists come in all shapes and sizes. And for some, getting too light is a detriment to performance, because they are no longer as powerful. I think women in particular tend to forget that side of the power-to-weight equation.

So go ahead and run your numbers and see what you get. But then concentrate on the strength exercises in Chapter 15 and the intervals in Chapter 14 rather than worrying excessively about your food intake. High intensity work is a healthy way to get strong (boosting your power) while winnowing away some excess fat, so you get the best of both worlds without going down any unhealthy roads.

Go Faster Eating Plan

MEAL	MON	TUES	WED	THU	FRI	SAT/ Endurance ride	SUN/ Endurance ride
Preride + On Bike	Refer to the Ride-Specific Fueling Guidelines for preride and on-bike nutrition choices tailored to easy and hard days.						
Breakfast	Banana-Berry Smoothie	Coconut Quinoa Yogurt Bowl	Nutty Oatmeal Bowl	Fruity Quinoa Bowl	Maple Berry Kamut	Eggs and Whole-Grain Toast	Nutty Oatmeal Bowl
Snack	Crackers and Hummus	Yogurt and Berries	Crackers and Hummus	Yogurt and Berries	Crackers and Hummus	Banana and Chocolate Milk (30–60 minutes post-ride)	Dressed Potato (30–60 minutes post-ride)
Lunch	Chicken Primavera Rice Bowl	Grilled Chicken sandwich, veggies, and hummus	Smoked Salmon Bowl	Savory Sandwich Wrap	Chicken Primavera Rice Bowl	Maple Berry Waffles	Grilled Chicken sandwich, veggies, and hummus
Snack	Fruit and Nuts	Crudités and Hummus	Turkey Wrap	Fruit and Nuts	Crudités and Hummus	Crackers and Hummus	Fruit and Nuts
Dinner	Mediterranean Bulgur	Spicy Thai Curry	Grilled Turkey Burger with Oven-Baked Fries and steamed spinach	Hibachi Stir-Fry	Chicken Fajitas	Zesty Spaghetti and Meatballs	Oven-Roasted Salmon and Oven-Baked Fries (sweet potato) with steamed vegetables

Recipes

Breakfasts

Banana-Berry Smoothie

1 whole banana

1 cup organic unsweetened rice milk

2 cups strawberries, fresh or frozen

1 cup fat-free Greek yogurt

½ cup dry oats

2 tablespoons fresh ground flaxseed

Blend ingredients until smooth.

Makes 1 serving

Coconut Quinoa Yogurt Bowl

1 cup cooked quinoa

1 banana, sliced

½ cup fat-free Greek yogurt

¼ cup shredded coconut, raw and unsweetened

1 cup berries, fresh or frozen

Mix the quinoa, banana, and yogurt together. Sprinkle with coconut and top with the berries.

Makes 1 serving

Nutty Oatmeal Bowl

1 cup cooked oatmeal

1½ cups berries, fresh or frozen

1 banana, chopped

1 tablespoon almond butter

½ cup fat-free Greek yogurt

Mix the ingredients together.

Makes 1 serving

Fruity Quinoa Bowl

1 cup cooked quinoa

1½ cups berries, fresh or frozen

½ cup fat-free Greek yogurt

1 banana

1 tablespoon tahini

Mix the ingredients together.

Makes 1 serving

Maple Berry Kamut

1 cup cooked Kamut

1 cup berries, fresh or frozen

½ cup fat-free Greek yogurt

1 tablespoon 100 percent maple syrup

2 tablespoons fresh ground flaxseed

Mix the ingredients together.

Makes 1 serving

Eggs and Whole-Grain Toast

2 slices whole-grain bread, toasted

2 eggs, boiled or poached

Serve the eggs on top of the toast or on the side.

Makes 1 serving

(continued)

Recipes *continued*

Lunches

Chicken Primavera Rice Bowl

1½ cups long-grain brown rice, cooked

1 cup broccoli, steamed

1 cup diced carrots, steamed

4 ounces grilled or roasted chicken breast, sliced

Toss ingredients together. Season to taste with salt, ground black pepper, and herbs.

Makes 1 serving

Grilled Chicken on Whole-Grain Bread

2 slices whole-grain bread

Mustard to taste

4 ounces grilled chicken breast or tofu, sliced

1 cup fresh raw spinach

SERVE WITH:

1 cup carrots or other fresh vegetable

2 tablespoons hummus

Spread the bread with mustard and layer the chicken or tofu and spinach between the slices.

Makes 1 sandwich

Smoked Salmon Bowl

1 cup cooked long-grain brown rice or quinoa

2 cups fresh or frozen mixed vegetables, steamed

1 tablespoon pesto

4 ounces smoked salmon

Toss ingredients together. Season to taste with salt, ground black pepper, and herbs.

Makes 1 serving

Savory Sandwich Wrap

1 large whole-wheat wrap

2 tablespoons hummus

Mustard to taste

2 slices roasted turkey or ⅓ can tuna or 2 ounces chicken

½ avocado

4 slices fresh tomato

1 cup romaine or fresh spinach

Spread the wrap with hummus and mustard. Layer the rest of the ingredients on the spreads and wrap up.

Makes 1 wrap

Maple Berry Waffles

2 Kashi Waffles 7 Grain

1 cup fat-free Greek yogurt

1 tablespoon 100 percent maple syrup

1 cup berries or other fruit

Top the waffles with yogurt, maple syrup, and berries.

Makes 1 serving

Dinners

Mediterranean Bulgur

1 cup cooked bulgur

1½ cups cooked lentils or chickpeas

½ cup feta cheese

1 tomato, chopped

⅓ cup chopped red onion

½ cup kalamata or black olives

1 red bell pepper, chopped

1 stalk celery, chopped

2 cloves garlic, chopped

¼ cup fresh lemon or lime juice

2 teaspoons chopped fresh mint

¼ cup chopped fresh parsley

2 teaspoons dried dill

1 teaspoon sea salt

Ground black pepper to taste

1 tablespoon olive oil (optional)

Let the bulgur and lentils or chickpeas come to room temperature. Toss all ingredients in a large mixing bowl.

Makes 2 servings

Grilled Turkey Burger

4 ounces lean ground turkey

1 egg

Salt, ground black pepper, and spices to taste

Mix all the ingredients in a medium bowl, then grill to desired doneness.

Serve on a whole-grain bun with lettuce, tomato, pickles, and mustard and ketchup to taste.

Makes 1 serving

Spicy Thai Curry

16 ounces cubed chicken breast, tofu, or shrimp

2 tablespoons olive oil, divided

3 cloves garlic, chopped

3 teaspoons chopped fresh ginger

3 tablespoons soy or tamari sauce

2 large red bell peppers, thinly sliced

3 scallions, chopped

16 ounces fresh baby spinach

½ cup low-fat coconut milk

4 teaspoons green curry paste (or to taste)

4½ cups cooked brown rice

⅓ cup fresh basil

½ cup chopped unsalted peanuts

½ teaspoon crushed red pepper flakes

1 lime, quartered

Cook the chicken in a tablespoon of the olive oil over medium heat until just done. Remove it from the pan. Add the remaining oil and sauté the garlic and ginger on medium heat. When the oil is absorbed, add the soy sauce, then add the bell peppers. Cook for 2 minutes, then add the scallions and spinach. Cook for 2 more minutes. Add the coconut milk and green curry paste and stir until well combined.

Serve the chicken over the rice, seasoned with the basil, peanuts, crushed red pepper, and a squeeze of lime.

Makes 4 servings

(continued)

Recipes *continued*

Hibachi Stir-Fry

4 ounces chicken, fish, beef, or tofu

1 cup chopped zucchini or other vegetable

½ bell pepper, chopped

½ cup chopped onion

1 clove garlic, chopped

1 tablespoon olive oil

Soy or tamari sauce to taste

1½ cups cooked long-grain brown rice

Toss meat or tofu, vegetables, and garlic together in a medium pan and sauté the mixture in the olive oil over medium heat until the meat or tofu is cooked through. Sprinkle with tamari and serve over the rice.

Makes 1 serving

Chicken Fajitas

4 ounces chicken breast, sliced

¼ onion, chopped

1 bell pepper, sliced

1 tablespoon olive oil

4 small corn tortillas or 2 small whole-wheat wraps

½ cup fat-free Greek yogurt

2 tablespoons salsa

2 tablespoons guacamole

Sauté the chicken, onion, and pepper in the olive oil over medium heat until the meat and vegetables are cooked. Wrap the mixture in the tortillas. Garnish with the yogurt, salsa, and guacamole.

Makes 1 serving

Zesty Spaghetti and Meatballs

4 (1-ounce) premade meatballs made from extra-lean beef, turkey, chicken, or bison

1 cup pasta sauce, jarred or homemade

1½ cups cooked spaghetti (or other pasta, preferably whole wheat)

Heat the meatballs and sauce, then toss with the pasta.

Makes 1 serving

Oven-Roasted Salmon

1 (5-ounce) salmon fillet (or other fish)

1 tablespoon butter

Salt, ground black pepper, and other seasonings to taste

Preheat the oven to 350°F. Place the fish on a foil-lined baking sheet. Top it with the butter and seasonings. Bake for 15 minutes, or until desired doneness.

Makes 1 serving

Oven-Baked Fries

1 potato (baking or sweet), cut into wedges

1 tablespoon olive oil

Salt, ground black pepper, and herbs to taste

Preheat the oven to 400°F. Place the potato wedges on a foil-lined baking sheet, sprinkle them with the olive oil, and season with salt, pepper, and herbs to taste. Bake for 20 to 30 minutes, or until potatoes are fork-tender.

Makes 2 servings

Snacks

Crackers and Hummus

12 rice or whole-grain crackers

4 tablespoons hummus

Yogurt and Berries

1 cup fat-free Greek yogurt

2 cups fresh or frozen mixed berries

Banana and Chocolate Milk

8 ounces 1% chocolate milk, no added sugar

1 banana

Dressed Potato

1 large baked potato

½ cup fat-free Greek yogurt with chopped chives

Salt and ground black pepper to taste

Fruit and Nuts

1 apple

1 orange

15 almonds

Crudités and Hummus

2½ cups sliced raw vegetables (carrots, celery, broccoli, bell pepper, cauliflower, etc.)

4 tablespoons hummus

Turkey Wrap

2 small corn or 1 regular-size whole-wheat wrap

1 cup fresh spinach or romaine lettuce

1 tomato, sliced

2 slices turkey

2 tablespoons hummus

RIDE-SPECIFIC FUELING TIPS

In addition to your regular meals, you need to fuel your body while you're riding. Follow these guidelines for type of ride you're doing today.

Preride snack for hard days (30 minutes preride): 1 banana drizzled with 1 teaspoon honey.

Endurance rides (90 minutes or longer): Aim for a total of 70 grams of carbohydrate per hour (280 calories) in the form of a 5 to 8 percent electrolyte sports drink and food. *Examples:* Eload Endurance Formula Drink (1 serving = 110 calories) + 1 banana + 2 Fig Newtons squares OR Secret Drink Mix (1 serving = 80 calories) + 1 5-oz. cooked potato + ¼ cup raisins (or 2 dates).

Easy days: Drink a low-calorie electrolyte beverage, such as nuun or Elete Hydration, on the bike.

CHAPTER 22

Performance Enhancers (What Works— And What Doesn't)

TALKING ABOUT "PERFORMANCE ENHANCERS" IN CYCLING IS risky business. It's no secret the sport has a long, rather sordid history with illicit and illegal performance enhancers of all types. So we're not going to talk about any of that because, honestly, there are plenty of ways you can boost your on-bike performance without breaking the law.

As mentioned in the previous chapters, training and achieving a healthy weight and strong muscles are undoubtedly your primary performance enhancers. A nutritious diet both on and off the bike also can propel you forward in your goal to get faster. You got the fundamentals in Chapter 21. Now let's talk about some add-ons. Lots of riders reach for supplements and special foods and/or drinks to help put more endurance in their legs and power in their pedals. Here's a look at what works and what you can safely skip.

Probiotics

Probiotics have grown in popularity since the likes of Dr. Oz have touted them on daytime television. Since then, the science on these good-for-your-gut bacteria has flourished and the verdict is that what's going on in your gut can mean the difference between not just general healthiness and sickliness, but also a good day on the bike and a bad one. After all, your digestive system is where you process all those nutrients that fuel your ride. When it's out of whack, your riding will suffer.

It all comes down to microbe management. Your gastrointestinal tract is home to trillions of bacteria. Some are beneficial and keep you healthy; others are the kind that can make you sick. As long as there's a balance between the good and bad, your system will function normally, says Shekhar Challa, MD, author of *Probiotics for Dummies*. But when that equilibrium is thrown off—thanks to anything from taking antibiotics (they kill all bacteria) to stress, age, even exercise—you start feeling lousy. You can restore a healthy balance using probiotics, or beneficial bacteria, which are found naturally in your body and in fermented foods like yogurt, kefir, and sauerkraut. Here's how probiotics can improve your health—and your ride.

SETTLE YOUR STOMACH

Heartburn, cramps, nausea, and gas are common among cyclists, especially before, during, and after a race or event. By improving your digestive function, probiotics can help reduce those complaints. Introduce them to your diet slowly to allow your stomach time to adjust to the new cultures, says Jo Ann Hattner, author of *Gut Insight*. "And start taking them at least 2 weeks before an event to prevent surprises, like gas and bloating," she says. Hattner also suggests consulting a physician before you start using probiotics.

FIGHT OFF COLDS

Upping your training time can make you more vulnerable during cold and flu season. All that pedaling gets blood flowing to your heart and limbs, but diverts it from your gut, which is where 90 percent of your immune system resides. Probiotics work by crowding out the bad bacteria to form a protective barrier inside the intestine, and a study in the *British Journal of Sports Medicine* concluded that they enhance immune function in endurance athletes.

WHITTLE YOUR WAIST

Researchers at the Washington University School of Medicine in St. Louis reported that people who are overweight have fewer good bacteria in their digestive systems than those who maintain a normal weight. And researchers in Japan found that taking a daily probiotic supplement may help you shed fat around your belly.

POWER YOUR PERFORMANCE

Probiotics help the body make B vitamins, says Challa, which improve endurance and help process muscle-mending protein. What's more, they promote absorption of vitamins and minerals, improving your body's ability to recover from hard rides.

Your A, B, Cs—And Other Vitamins and Minerals

The issue of vitamins and minerals used to be a no-brainer. Of course they were good for you. They're vitamins and minerals! And it's true that they most definitely are good for you— when they come in the form of food. What's become less clear in recent years is how beneficial it is to pop them—especially megadoses of them—in pill form.

Yet many of us still do. In fact, 40 percent of Americans start their day by swallowing at least one vitamin-and-mineral supplement. When you move to the ranks of elite athletes, that percentage soars past 90. Though you're likely not a pro racer, chances are you do, too. Research shows that active people believe more in the power of vitamin pills than the sedentary set. But as Spider-Man says, "With great power comes great responsibility." And responsible vitamin use is something too few of us practice.

"I see a lot of athletes overloading on supplements," says sports nutritionist Leslie Bonci of the University of Pittsburgh Medical Center. "It's often not even intentional. It's just part of their lifestyle." Think about it. Say you wake up and pop a "high performance" supplement designed for active people. You've just ingested up to 300 percent of most essential vitamins and minerals. Pour yourself a bowl of cold cereal and you've just consumed another 25 to 100 percent of the Daily Value

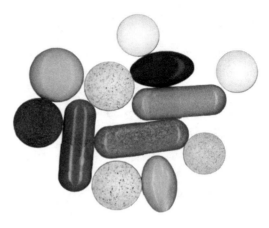

A little supplementation goes a long way. Too much will give you pricey pee at best and may be detrimental to your health at worst.

(the amount the FDA recommends you take in each day)—or twice that, because most active people eat more. Add a PowerBar, replete with 100 percent of C, E, and B vitamins and another one-third of minerals like iron and zinc, before your nightly ride and, voilà, you've met the daily nutrient requirements five or six times over.

A, B, C OD

Even cyclists who know they're taking a truckload of vitamins are rarely concerned. "It's a common misconception that because you're more active, you need significantly more vitamins and minerals," says Bonci. "That's not necessarily true." Yes, studies suggest very active people may require slightly higher levels of a few vitamins. But the reality is that because you ride more, you eat more, and by eating more, you get more nutrients, says Bonci.

THE NUTRIENT	THE RECOMMENDED AMOUNT	WHY YOU NEED IT
Vitamin A	5,000 IU	Healthy skin and eyes
Vitamin C	60 milligrams	Stokes immune system; maintains healthy cartilage, connective tissue, and bones
Vitamin D	400 IU	Helps your body absorb calcium for strong bones and teeth
Vitamin E	30 IU	Neutralizes tissue-damaging free radicals
Vitamin B_1 (thiamine)	1.5 milligrams	Helps transform carbohydrates into energy
Vitamin B_2 (riboflavin)	1.7 milligrams	Helps produce energy in your cells
Vitamin B_3 (niacin)	20 milligrams	Helps your body use fatty acids and sugars; necessary for production of hormones
Vitamin B_6	2 milligrams	Helps break down amino acids; helps produce antibodies that fight infection
Vitamin B_{12}	6 micrograms	Protects lining of nerve cells; helps synthesize red and white blood cells
Folic acid	400 micrograms	Essential for making DNA for new cells; helps reduce harmful homocysteine levels
Calcium	1,000 milligrams	Builds bones and teeth; fights high blood pressure
Iron	18 milligrams	Part of hemoglobin, which carries oxygen to cells
Potassium	3,500 milligrams	Helps maintain healthy blood pressure
Sodium	2,400 milligrams (recommended limit for most people)	Essential for normal body function and muscle contraction
Magnesium	400 milligrams	Needed for healthy nerves and muscles
Copper	2 milligrams	Needed for healthy connective tissue in heart and blood vessels
Zinc	15 milligrams	Assists with wound healing and immunity

For the most part, a heavy supplement habit results in little more than pricy pee. But overdoing it in the long term can have consequences beyond your bank account. Some vitamins, such as A, D, and E, are said to be "fat soluble" because in the intestines they have to be absorbed by fat in your food to be used by the body. Excess fat-soluble vitamins are stored in your body fat and liver. Having too much in storage can be toxic. A recent study has shown that those taking more than the recommended Daily Value (5,000 IU) of vitamin A from both dietary and supplemental sources had 10 percent lower bone mineral density and twice the risk of hip fracture as those taking the recommended amounts—a serious concern for cyclists, especially women cyclists who are at a higher risk for osteoporosis by virtue of their sex. Even the health benefits of long-heralded vitamin E have been called into question in recent research that suggests too much of this antioxidant may actually decrease longevity.

Even vitamins and minerals your body doesn't stockpile can be harmful in high doses. Megadoses—amounts that are more than 10 times the Daily Value—of the B vitamins niacin and B_6 can actually impair performance. Micronutrients also work together in the body, so taking too much of one, such as zinc, can inhibit the absorption of another, like copper.

ONE "KITCHEN SINK" SOURCE

The best advice says that if you want to supplement, choose one "kitchen sink" supplement that provides up to 100 percent of all the vitamins and minerals from A to Z. Since the sports foods you eat are also fortified, avoid megadoses of anything, says Bonci. Then, just eat a diet rich in whole foods. Even the effectiveness of calcium supplements is being called into question. But if you're a cyclist with a family history of osteoporosis and don't drink milk, fortified beverages, or dairy foods, you should probably take an additional calcium supplement.

Here's a quick rundown of commonly supplemented essential micronutrients, what they do, and how much you need.

SPORTS-SPECIFIC SUPPLEMENTS

You can walk into any GNC and come out with an armful of potions and pills and powders promising to make you lean, strong, and fast. But the sports supplement business is very much one of "buyer beware." There's rarely any gold-standard-level research behind the benefit claims. There's no real government regulation or oversight. Even word of mouth doesn't generally get you very far because the same supplement one person swears by will leave another rider shrugging it off as a waste of money.

That said, there are a handful of supplements that seem to stand up fairly well to scientific scrutiny and others that have simply stood the test of time and continue to be used by cyclists and coaches. Here are a few that may be worth looking into. Just remember that no pill or potion can take the place of hard training, good nutrition, and a healthy lifestyle. They're just icing on the cake.

Natural Alternatives to "Vitamin I"

Some cyclists (and many other recreational athletes) take so much ibuprofen before and after—and maybe during—hard efforts that it's become jokingly known as "vitamin I." The idea, of course, is to head off inflammation and the soreness that comes with it before it happens. But before you pop another Advil, research now shows that using ibuprofen in this way may hurt your performance, recovery, and even your health long term.

In one study published in *Medicine and Science in Sports and Exercise*, researchers found that when distance runners took 600 milligrams of ibuprofen before an event, they actually ended up with more tissue-damaging oxidative stress afterward than those who took nothing. Another study on cyclists found that ibuprofen can damage the gut during exercise and lead to a leaky small intestine—not good. Finally, animal research has shown that vitamin I can actually hamper your muscles ability to recover after exercise.

THE TAKE-HOME: Save the ibuprofen for when you're actually injured. If you want to head off muscle soreness from a particularly hard session, turn to natural anti-inflammatories such as tea or cherry juice instead.

Black and green tea have natural antioxidative properties that have been shown to decrease muscle damage and speed recovery. In one study, cyclists taking black tea extract had less soreness following an intense interval workout after taking black tea extract. In another study at the University of Vermont, students who were given 12 ounces of tart cherry juice before and after strenuous exercises suffered only a 4 percent reduction in muscle strength the next day compared with a 22 percent loss found in subjects given a placebo.

BETA-ALANINE

Beta-alanine is an amino acid that is found in chicken, beef, pork, and fish. It is also naturally produced by the body and is readily used by your fast-twitch muscles to fuel sprinting. It's created a few waves in the cycling world because it's actually been researched. In one study of 25 cyclists, those taking the supplement improved their scores in a cycling performance test by 13 percent after just 4 weeks. Another later study found that riders taking 6 grams a day for 4 weeks improved their time to exhaustion in a cycling time trial by more than 12 percent, while those taking a placebo improved by just 1.6 percent on the same test.

Sports nutrition advisor Stacy Sims is a longtime advocate. "It improves muscle fiber firing rate and recovery," she says. The recommended dosage is between 3.2 and 6.4 grams a day. Beta-alanine is available as a standalone supplement, or you can find it bundled with other ingredients in sports supplements like OptygenHP (see following page).

OPTYGENHP

OptygenHP contains a number of active ingredients, including the mineral chromium, which helps stabilize blood sugar for more even energy production, beta-alanine (see above), and rhodiola, which was made legendary by Tibetan Sherpas, who reportedly took it to improve their endurance and ability to use oxygen when climbing in thin air. Rhodiola is an adaptogen, which means it helps your body adapt to stresses by lowering your level of the stress hormone cortisol. Research is mixed on how effective it actually is. Some studies show significant benefits, while others show none.

Those who use OptygenHP (and, full disclosure, I do, as do many racers I know) do so because they feel like it makes hard efforts easier and that they can train and race better with less recovery time. It is a "load and sustain" supplement, which means you need to take it for at least a week to see effects.

SPORTLEGS

This is a favorite of many a charity rider I know, because unlike other sports supplements, you can take this one when you need it (like on the MS 150) and it works right away. The special ingredients here are the lactate forms of calcium and magnesium. Your body produces lactate for extra fuel when you're exercising at high intensities. Problem is, lactate production creates an acidic environment, which eventually leads to the burning sensation in your legs that slows you down. SportLegs preloads your muscles with lactate, so you can ride longer in that tough zone before you have to produce more on your own.

The supplement itself has not been studied in athletes, but the individual ingredients have,

and with success. It's also been around for more than a decade and is still selling strong, which in itself is generally a positive indication that a product works. It won't turn you into a mountain-mashing machine, of course. Rather, people who use it generally say it makes them feel like they're having a good day on the bike. On long rides and multiday rides and races, riders often carry some pills with them so they can reload every 2 to 3 hours.

The Espresso Express

Caffeine may be the most widely used stimulant drug in the world, especially among cyclists. From roadies who sip espressos to downhillers who pound energy drinks before a race, the allure of a preride pick-me-up transcends cycling's cultural differences. The jolt is very real. Caffeine is an endurance performance booster, says Sims. "It increases your power output and time to exhaustion, and lowers your perceived exertion." In other words, you'll pedal longer and more powerfully, and feel less tired.

HOW IT WORKS

During endurance efforts, caffeine helps the body utilize fat as fuel, so you don't burn through your carbohydrate stores as quickly, says Sims. But a preride cappuccino could improve your town-line sprint as well. "Caffeine increases the calcium content of muscle, which enhances the strength of the muscle contraction," she says—good news for riders looking to hammer big gears. Also, many studies attest to

How Big Is Your Buzz

DRINK	MG CAFFEINE
Starbucks coffee, 16 ounces	330 milligrams
Vivarin, 1 tablet	200 milligrams
Double espresso	150 milligrams
Latte, 16 ounces	150 milligrams
Red Bull, 8.46 ounces	80 milligrams
Clif Black Cherry Shot Bloks (3)	50 milligrams
GU Espresso Love gel, 1 packet	40 milligrams
Stash green tea (steeped 3 min), 8 ounces	36 milligrams
Coco-Cola, 12 ounces	30 milligrams

the substance's ability to improve reasoning and memory in sleep-deprived people, which could be useful for ultra endurance cyclists.

KNOW YOUR DOSE

Whether you take caffeine from foods, drinks, or supplements, the International Society of Sports Nutrition has concluded that 1.36 to 2.72 milligrams per pound of body weight is most effective. (See how your favorite caffeine source stacks up in the chart above.) For the best results, take 40 to 50 percent of the desired amount 1 hour before a big event; consume the rest throughout your ride.

As with any drug, you can develop a tolerance. Most of my riders limit their daily consumption so they'll feel more of a boost when taking it before major training sessions and races.

LISTEN TO YOUR BODY

Caffeine affects everyone differently. If you're not accustomed to it, don't start slamming espressos. Ease into it, experimenting with small doses. Some people get fluttery heartbeats and get too amped to focus even with relatively low doses. Even those who are hard-core coffee drinkers (including yours truly) can overdo it without knowing it. Case in point: I was doing a 4-hour endurance mountain bike race last summer and had unknowingly bought some energy chews that were caffeinated. So pretty much everything I ate for the entire race was delivering an espresso shot's worth of caffeine. A little over 3 hours in, I felt like hell. My stomach was cramping. My energy was shutting down. It was pretty awful. So, use caffeine with care. It's strong medicine.

PART VII

FOR WOMEN ONLY

Back when I played high school and college sports, there wasn't much advice available for women athletes in terms of how to handle our unique needs and concerns. We were just happy that we finally had equal playing time. There was no way we could expect any real advice on playing through PMS and periods. In fact, I'm not sure there was much information to be had, anyway. It was still very much an "Oh, it's in your head" era for women's issues. So we played and dealt with it as best we could.

Later, when I'd become a cyclist, the story was still pretty much the same. Not much concrete advice was out there beyond the usual "Take ibuprofen if you have cramps" and "Find a tampon that doesn't leak." It was worse when I got pregnant. There wasn't just a dearth of information, there was bad information. My midwives, who I thought were otherwise fairly well informed, were still cautioning women against getting their heart rate above 140 beats per minute—a recommendation that American College of Obstetrics and Gynecology made in the 1980s and then unceremoniously tossed in the mid-1990s because there was no scientific grounding for it. Though they never told me I couldn't ride, I know it made them apprehensive that I did.

A major reason for the paltry advice was because research on sports was being done by men, and on men. Nobody knew how the menstrual cycle or menopause affected sports performance because nobody had studied it. Women also were not competing and participating in endurance sports in the numbers that they are today. So information was sorely lacking. Fortunately, all that has started to change.

Fast-forward to today, when I have friends and fellow racers who are approaching or going through menopause and are mystified by (and because of) the sheer lack of information on how to tackle the challenges of staying active during this major metabolic change.

Thanks to the presence of more women in sport, there now is more interest in these issues. Thanks to more women working in sports science, there are more researchers who have a vested interest in these topics. We now know in great detail how the menstrual cycle affects our physiology, and how that in turn affects our sports performance. We have far better guidelines for exercising through pregnancy and managing menopause.

You'll find the most up-to-date information on all issues female, including how to avoid being at the mercy of your menstrual cycle, what to eat to turn down the heat on hot flashes, how to avoid saddle sores and urinary tract infections even when you're logging maximum saddle time, how to safely and comfortably pedal through pregnancy, and a whole lot more.

I'm going to go out on a limb and say that I bet you will find much of the information eye-opening, if not life altering. I sure did. During the researching and writing of this section of the book, I discovered feminine hygiene options I didn't even know existed (good-bye forever, tampons, can't say it's been fun) and discovered that now that I'm a little older, I can power myself far better with protein and fat than I ever could with a ton of carbs. And I've never felt better. I hope you read it and will say the same.

CHAPTER 23

Menstrual Cycle Facts, Myths, and Management

"UGH. GOOD THING IT'S NOT A HARD DAY TODAY. I JUST GOT MY period this morning. I feel sluggish, sleepy, and gross," said my friend Erica as I rolled over the grass into her backyard before a long ride out toward Hawk Mountain last summer.

And the banter began. "I hear you, sister," I replied. "My worst day is the day before, which of course was the Neshaminy race last week. It makes my thermoregulation and digestive system go a little haywire, which didn't help matters since it was so hot and tough to eat to begin with."

Erica's husband, Mike, walked by us, smirking. I didn't let him get away unscathed. "Dude, it's true! If men menstruated they'd never stop talking and strategizing about it. 'Oh, we were going to have Andy attack today, but he's premenstrual and had wicked cramps, so we figured Paul would be our best bet.' You wouldn't be all hush-hush and nearly ashamed to admit it. You'd be crowing about it. Making crude jokes about it. Bragging about what you did despite it. In this day and age, it's still kind of crazy that something so widespread, so natural, and so frequent is talked about so little."

Mike gave me that patient look he gives me when I'm up on my soapbox waving my arms, daring him to knock me off, and calmly replied, "I agree with you 100 percent."

I believed him. But I still wasn't sure that, as a man, he completely got it. Women have a long history of being shamed into being quiet about their menstrual periods. I remember my male classmates joking that a woman could never be president because "she'd bomb the world every 30 days." I mean it's even called "the curse." When the world views something as a negative, as a form of weakness, the last thing you want to do is bring it up and use it as an excuse in any way, shape, or form.

One day, sitting at my desk, thinking of column ideas, it dawned on me that in all the years I'd done my *Bicycling* blog and column, I had not once mentioned the menstrual cycle, let alone my own, despite the fact that I am indeed a woman and that I've thought about it, planned around it, and bemoaned its timing on and off throughout my entire athletic life. So I talked about it—and now I'm going to talk about it some more. Because if we women don't talk about it, it won't get the attention it deserves.

Facts and Feelings

We all have been active, if not competed, while dealing with the effects of our menstrual cycle. How we feel about those effects not only varies from woman to woman, but also from month to month for each woman. So it's hard to draw conclusions about how your monthly cycle affects your cycling.

Some studies have been done on the subject, but these types of studies are hard to do, and they're rarely conclusive. Most recently, for instance, there was a roundup of rowers where researchers monitored heart rate, oxygen consumption, blood lactate level, glycogen and fat oxidation, and power output throughout an hour-long endurance test conducted during different phases of their menstrual cycle. Some women were on the Pill. Some weren't. It didn't matter. No matter what their cycle phase, all the variables remained consistent.

That's good news. Women have set records, won races and games, and earned medals in every phase of their cycle. This study confirms that our bodies are generally cooperative (even if we feel lousy), though it's impossible to take into account all the variables, psychological and otherwise, that are affected by hormone fluctuations and impact performance.

It's also maybe not such good news. Most studies examine women who are already athletic, so they've learned to manage their periods. There are women out there who are made so miserable by the migraines, cramps, and nausea they experience that they never get that far. Undoubtedly, many women would and could perform even better than they do if there were more open discussions about managing some of the challenges of menstruation in the sporting life, and if experts didn't take a broad brush and say, "Don't worry, you're fine."

Fortunately, the tide is turning. As women have flooded the playing fields (and the research labs) over the past 40 years, more bright minds have begun examining these issues among all women. I've sung the praises of Stacy Sims an awful lot in these pages because she was the first person I ever heard utter "menstrual cycle" in a presentation at a cycling coaching conference. I couldn't believe my ears, and I have been in regular contact with her since.

So here's what we know (this was explained in greater detail in Chapters 19 and 20, so we'll recap quickly). Women have greater glycogen needs during the luteal (premenstrual) phase of their cycle because the body is in glycogen-sparing mode. We also need to pay special attention to hydration because our core temperature is higher, our plasma volume is lower, and it's harder to cool ourselves because our sweat response is delayed.

You might also feel moody and bloated (yay!) à la PMS during this phase. But that's no excuse to skip your ride. In fact, you'll likely feel far better if you saddle up and go for a spin. Exercise releases endorphins, those pain-relieving proteins in your brain that also improve your mood. In other words, you'll feel happier and less crampy if you get yourself in motion. Boosting your circulation may also decrease some of the fluid retention that gives you that bloated feeling and ease the gastrointestinal distress that sometimes accompanies all the hormone fluctuation. As discussed in Chapters 19 and 20, taking good care of your nutrition and hydration needs, particularly during this phase, can also ease symptoms and make efforts easier.

Then there's that other part of your cycle—menstruation in the low-hormone phase. Ironically, your physiology most resembles a man's during your period and the days that follow. That's because your levels of progesterone and estrogen are at their lowest, explains Sims. Guess what? You'll feel stronger like a man, too. Even

better, you're likely to feel less pain and recover faster, according to her research. "Your body isn't gearing up for the possibility of carrying a fertilized egg and being pregnant," says Sims. "That takes a lot of energy." Once you're clear of the possibility of pregnancy, the body goes into a more chill mode, explains Sims, and all those energy systems are at your disposal to use for exertion.

If you take birth control pills, you're pretty much always in the high-hormone phase, since they raise your estrogen level, even during the sugar pill week. NuvaRing may be a better choice for cyclists since it releases lower levels of hormones, says Sims. "The higher levels of progestin [with vaginal rings] can still impact muscle integrity and recovery, but overall the hormonal effects are not as pronounced." What's interesting about the effects of contraceptive hormones is that for years, athletes have used the Pill and the ring to manipulate their cycles when they don't want to have their period during a big event (I know I was tempted to do so for an Ironman competition). But realizing that it's actually during that time that I may be the strongest has made me realize that it could actually be counterproductive to do so.

So yes, the bottom line is that your cycle, especially the PMS part, can affect your performance. Fifty percent of polled athletes in a 2014 *ESPN the Magazine* survey reported that menstrual cramps affected their game at some point. But remember, too, that a woman can win a world championship during any phase of her cycle, and that you can optimize your performance by understanding and working with your cycle, so there's no reason to let it hold you back.

Missing Punctuation

For many years, most of the research on active women and menstruation focused not on the effects of menstruation on exercise, but how exercise affects menstruation—specifically, the way it sometimes stops it from happening. Amenorrhea, the absence of menstruation, can occur when women exercise to an extreme, though it appears to have less to do with the amount of exercise than it does energy intake and body weight.

High amounts of exercise (think pro-level marathoners or Ironman triathletes) performed by those of very low body weight—typically less than is recommended for their height—can put their body in a state of emergency that causes it to shut down any functions that aren't essential for survival, like reproduction. Some women seem more vulnerable to this than others. I have put in 17- to 20-hour training weeks without ever once missing a dot, while friends have occasionally been affected under heavy training loads, despite not being excessively thin.

Though it could be tempting to regard it as a blessing in disguise (hey, no more periods!), the consequences go beyond interrupted reproduction. The underlying cause of amenorrhea is hormone disruption, particularly a lowering of estrogen, which not only fuels fertility but also protects our bones and cardiovascular health. So though it's unlikely that you'll be pushing yourself to the point of pausing your periods, if you do, it's important to get them back. In general, that means eating larger quantities of a healthy diet to give your body the fuel and fat stores it needs.

GOING WITH THE FLOW

I've had my period during more big events than I can count. Probably the biggest was Ironman Louisville in Kentucky. I had been rigorously training for the better part of a year. Then, as the event neared, I got bloated and moody and started having GI issues. Layer that with how cranky you also get during a tapering-off week before a major race and, well, it wasn't pretty.

So I was oddly relieved when my period started the day before the race, because all the PMS stuff was out of the way and all I had to deal with was the bleeding. To be perfectly blunt, I wasn't going to really worry about it. I'd be swimming in the Ohio River, biking for 112 miles around Kentucky horse country, and running 26.2 miles around Louisville, all in a very dark skin suit with a padded chamois. At the time, I used tampons. So I would just put one in at the beginning of the day and not worry about it. Note: This is *not* something I'd typically do, because tampons generally should be changed at least every 8 hours, but in this one case, I made an exception. (I do not use super-absorbent tampons, and whether leaving a regular tampon in for longer is dangerous is still debated). I wanted to win that day, and there was no way I was going to stop to change tampons. That's what laundry detergent is for.

I know other women who have light flows who don't bother with anything and just take the wash-up-later approach. In the end, there's no right answer on how to best ride out your flow, but here are a few suggestions you might want to consider.

THINK TWICE ABOUT PADS. Pads are the worst choice for cycling. For one, they're very difficult to adhere to a chamois, many of which are channeled and therefore don't have a flat, smooth surface to securely attach the pad to. Even if it does stick, you can bet it's going to move and bunch up as you sweat and sit and stand and move around on the saddle, which sets you up for rubbing and chafing and, honestly, the mess you were trying to avoid in the first place. So while a pad is probably okay for an easy spinning day, you may want to consider another option (including the laundry one) for harder efforts. You'll also want to be prepared to change the pad if you're riding longer. From a hygiene standpoint, menstrual blood and sweat can make pads brew up a perfect storm of bacteria, setting you up for infection.

TUCK THE TAMPON STRING. Tampons are a popular choice among women cyclists because they're convenient and generally minimize mess. One bit of advice I learned the hard way: Tuck that string in a bit. I've actually had rope burns on my sensitive tissues, which is as comfortable as it sounds. And if you're on an extended outing, carry a spare so you can put in a fresh one after a few hours. Leaving a tampon in all day can cause toxic shock syndrome (TSS), a potentially lethal bacterial infection. To keep matters in perspective, TSS is extremely rare and was more common in the 1980s when women were using extremely absorbent tampons (no longer on the market), which increased the likelihood of bacteria collecting and causing staph infection. But it's still wise to change tampons regularly and to use those with less absorbency (i.e., regular rather than super) when you can just to be as safe as possible.

CONSIDER THE CUP. Before writing this chapter, I had never tried "the cup," which is shorthand for the DivaCup or Softcup. But so many active women were gushing about them that I was compelled to run out and buy a box so I could give a firsthand account. And I can say unequivocally, I'm sold. They are, as they sound, medical-grade silicone cups that collect rather than absorb your flow. They reportedly hold at least three times as much fluid as a super tampon, are less prone to leaking than a tampon, and can be worn for 12 hours. They're also convenient. You just remove, rinse, reinsert, and go. Yes, it's a little messy, but you're going to wash your hands anyway, right? You don't have to carry a spare, dispose of some pretty gross garbage, or worry about a bacterial infection. They're also way better for the environment.

I found them to be remarkably easy to use and to leak far, far less than any tampon I have ever tried. Any woman who has used NuvaRing as birth control will get it positioned correctly immediately. Others might have to practice to get the cup in the right place. But if you follow the instructions on inserting it, the device really does slip right into place without much trouble. I use the Softcup, but more brands are coming on the market all the time, so the odds are good that if you don't care for one style, you'll be able to find one that works for you.

CHAPTER 24

Riding for Two: Pregnancy

WHETHER OR NOT YOU RIDE WHEN YOU'RE PREGNANT IS YOUR personal choice. I rode all the way up to delivery, though I changed my routes and certainly didn't do any extreme mountain biking. I never felt unbalanced or unsafe and really didn't think twice about it. Nor did my doctor once I assured her I wasn't doing anything stupid. A few of my other friends rode all the way through theirs, as well. Others stopped riding as soon as they started to show. Some stuck to the stationary bike as soon as they got the plus sign on the test stick.

Even the typically conservative American College of Obstetricians and Gynecologists (ACOG) doesn't single out cycling as a "don't" during pregnancy. (They do single out horseback riding, gymnastics, downhill snow skiing, ice hockey, soccer, vigorous racquet sports, scuba diving, and basketball, in case you were curious.)

Mary Jane Minkin, MD, clinical professor of obstetrics, gynecology, and reproductive services at the Yale School of Medicine, a very active woman I have worked with many times, says it best: "Common sense should rule. If you're a good rider who has been riding for years and is comfortable on the bike, keep riding," she says, adding that you should pay attention to how you feel once you get out of the first trimester or so. "Some women feel out of balance as their center of gravity changes. You don't want to be on a bike if you feel off-balance. That's common sense. It's the same advice I give skiers. You don't want to be falling. So use your head."

Navigating Pregnancy

That's always good advice, of course, but sometimes it's hard to do, especially when you're wading into the often-unpredictable waters of pregnancy. You will be bombarded with advice whether you want it or not. You will second- and third-guess your every move. Total strangers will criticize you if they don't like what you're doing. So here's a guide on how to be safe and smart when you're riding for two. It is obviously not a substitute for medical advice. Every pregnancy is different, even for the same woman. Riding may not be safe during some high-risk pregnancies, so always consult and work with your doctor.

KEEP ACTIVE

First and foremost, exercise is good for you. The American College of Sports Medicine and ACOG recommend 30 minutes or more of moderate exercise a day on most, if not all, days. Regular physical activity provides all the same benefits to you when you're pregnant that it does when you're not—it strengthens your heart, helps you maintain a healthy weight (even as you gain during pregnancy), improves mood, and lessens the chance of developing gestational diabetes, a type that is caused by pregnancy and can affect your baby's health as well as your own.

The general advice on how much exercise to do depends on what you were doing before you got pregnant. For an Ironman-level triathlete, a 2-hour bike ride is just something you do before breakfast. For someone just starting out, it could be your longest ride. You want to stay well within your comfort zone, and don't go trying to break any records or push your limits. Doctors no longer set heart rate limits for pregnant women (years ago, they put the ceiling at 140), but instead recommend that you keep your efforts moderate (i.e., you can still talk while you ride).

TAKE IT TRIMESTER BY TRIMESTER

Again, every pregnancy is different and you'll feel different throughout each pregnancy. In general, though, the first trimester is when there's a sea of change in hormones; your body is working overtime to establish the pregnancy and create the placenta, and you're most likely to be plagued by morning sickness, fatigue, and a general "Wow I just don't feel like myself" feeling. Or you may feel pretty much fine. Ride accordingly. I remember feeling pretty normal, but out of breath more easily— and a lot hungrier when I was done. Like Minkin says, just use your head.

Usually that early malaise lifts as you go into the second trimester and get your energy back. This could be when you feel best on the bike. It might also be when you start to get bigger and your center of gravity changes, so stay in tune with how you feel—likewise, of course, going into the third trimester. I carried low and actually felt more stable in the saddle. But by 8 months in, some friends have felt so unwieldy even trying to get on their bikes that they racked them until the baby was born. Do what feels right for you.

GIVE YOURSELF MORE TIME— AND SPACE

It goes without saying that you're going to be a little slower as your belly grows and there's less room for deep breathing. There's a little person growing inside of you, taking up some of that energy you'd be using for pedaling. Your usual loops will start to take longer, so plan accordingly, and shorten them if need be.

Also, you're going to be bigger and heavier physically, which impacts your bike handling. You're going to need more time to slow down and to stop. You might find it trickier to corner. I, and many of the women I rode, worked, and trained with, decided to stay away from big group rides and heavily trafficked roads at some point during our pregnancies. It just felt safer to do that. And that's exactly what you want to feel when you literally have a baby on board. Bike paths and rail trails, which tend to be wider, smoother, and flatter than most roads, can be your best friends during those final months.

FINESSE YOUR FIT

As your bump gets bigger, you might have a harder time bending over the bars and need to adjust your bike fit to stay comfortable in the saddle. Raising your handlebars can help by putting you in a more upright position. You'll be sitting more heavily on the saddle, too, so you may want to use a wider saddle, like those on comfort bikes, which are designed to support your seat when you're sitting up more.

Likewise, you will probably need to adjust your riding clothing by investing in a few larger-sized items to accommodate your expanding girth.

PACK FLUIDS AND FOOD

Don't underestimate your energy needs. I'll never forget one mostly flat 20-mile ride with two of my friends, another of whom was also pregnant, on a route I'd done a million times before. I had eaten a good breakfast and didn't think twice about heading out with them for a lunchtime spin. With about 5 miles yet to go, I hit the wall. Out of nowhere, I just got vapory and began to bonk. Of course none of us was carrying any food. I had $2 in my pocket. I kept telling myself that if I could just make it back to the edge of town, I could stop at the pizza shop (and I don't even like its pizza) and buy whatever I could get for $2. I got a breadstick and it got me home.

It's even more important to stay well hydrated when you're pregnant. You need more water so your body can perform pregnancy-related functions as well as all the usual ones. Plus it's easier to overheat when you're pregnant because your metabolic rate is higher and your body isn't able to rid itself of heat as easily. Carry twice as much fluid as you normally would and don't ride in extreme heat.

TRY THE TRAINER OR CROSS-TRAINING

If riding becomes uncomfortable—physically or psychologically—don't sweat it. You can easily maintain your fitness by hopping on an indoor exercise bike or setting yours up on a stationary trainer. If that bores you, swim, hike, or dance. This is your time to take care of yourself as you like.

GET BACK IN THE SADDLE

Like pretty much everything in your pregnancy, when you get back on the bike after the baby is born is a very personal decision and depends largely on the circumstances of your delivery. Did you have a Caesarian section? Do you have stitches? Were there complications? Even if everything went swimmingly, you will be a bit uncomfortable and have some bleeding in the first days following delivery. As a general rule, your body is still in a state of great fluctuation for about 4 to 6 weeks after the baby is born. ACOG's position is that women who have no medical complications are in the clear to return to their usual activities as soon as they feel up to it, which could be within days or weeks of delivery. I've seen that to be true in my own circle of friends. I had a complication-free delivery with no tearing and was able to get on my bike for a spin around the park later that week. Other friends found that engaging in such activity too soon left them with more cramping and bleeding, so they had to lay off a little longer. Again—let common sense and your doctor's advice be your guide. They won't let you down.

CHAPTER 25

Menopause

"HEY, SELENE!"

It's my friend Clare from New York. She's a longtime cyclist, avid bike commuter, recreational racer, and not one bit shy about speaking her mind. She's in town for some races and has a bone to pick with me.

"You write about all this stuff every week, but you've never written about menopause. How come? It's a bitch, you know. It would be nice to have someone talking about it."

"Well, the cop-out answer is that I've never written about it because I haven't been through it!" I tell her honestly. But it doesn't take more than a moment's thought to realize she's right. Hot flashes, lousy sleep, and muscle loss—sound like a recipe for cycling success? Not so much. Yet, in all the years I've been writing for and reading mainstream cycling magazines, I can't recall ever seeing menopause addressed. And to point that finger right back at myself: Though I have researched and written a great deal about menopause for women's magazines like *Prevention*, I've never offered a lick of advice on it in the pages of *Bicycling*.

Time to change that. Starting now. Because when I look around the cycling community at large, from the elite racing fields to the usual shop, social, and charity riders, it's clear that there are a significant number of women who will be, if they are not already, heading into "the change."

"The Change"

That's what menopause was called for years before we got comfortable with using words like "menopause"—the change. Which is okay, but it implies just one change—the end of your menstrual periods. Of course, that alone is a pretty seismic change that is itself brought on by a series of changes, and it leads to a succeeding series of changes that go beyond simple freedom from feminine hygiene products.

Outside of the obvious—you're no longer ovulating and can no longer get pregnant—the main metabolic change many women notice is body composition. As the estrogen level drops, there's a tendency to accumulate fat in your belly and to lose lean muscle mass. That's a problem for a few reasons. If you can't maintain your muscle, you can't produce the power to push those pedals up hills or in a paceline as hard and you're bound to slow down, especially if you're also gaining body fat. Even if you aren't a racer, gaining weight and slowing down just aren't fun.

That's not all. Even if you maintain your body composition, the hormone shift with menopause brings on some permanent changes in your metabolism that can affect your training and riding and overall sense of well-being. For some advice on that front, I called up my go-to source for all things female physiology, exercise physiologist, nutrition scientist, and fellow cyclist Stacy Sims, who has devoted about 20 years to studying these issues. Here's her short list of what you can do to keep on rolling strong.

HANDLE THE HEAT

"Postmenopausal women break into a sweat later during exercise and they vasodilate longer," explains Sims. In plain language, that means your body sends more blood to the skin to get rid of heat, since it can't rely on perspiration to cool you. It's also harder for you to handle increases in your core temperature. So riding and/or racing in the heat is just plain harder.

Hydration becomes even more important during menopause and beyond. If you're going out for a long and/or hard ride in the heat, prehydrate with a sodium-rich drink before you get on the bike. Take in at least a bottle an hour while riding and grab a protein-rich recovery drink to sip on when you're done. Consider also cooling yourself before exercising in hot weather by draping a cold towel around your neck. Consume ice-cold fluid during your ride if you can. And to cool down and speed recovery, dip yourself in a cold bath or pool when you're done to help constrict those dilated blood vessels so your blood returns to your central circulation.

Speaking of heat, hot flashes are one of the hallmarks of menopause. Studies are mixed on how much exercise helps alleviate them, but most have found that active women have fewer or at least less extreme ones than those who aren't active.

CURB THE CARBOHYDRATES

You become more sensitive to carbohydrates as you enter menopause, which means you're more susceptible to blood sugar swings, and you actually need fewer carbohydrates overall, says Sims. "Eat more mixed macronutrient foods during your rides. Aiming to get about 30 grams of carbohydrate per hour"—about what's in a banana—"on long rides is probably sufficient."

GET PARTICULAR ABOUT PROTEIN

Your body uses protein less effectively as you approach menopause and in the years after, making it more difficult to maintain your muscle integrity. Recovery is harder, as is holding on to your lean muscle tissue. That means you need to be pickier about the proteins you consume.

"It's essential for menopausal and postmenopausal women to lower their postexercise stress hormones, like cortisol, as quickly as possible, since that makes you catabolic, and you can't afford to be eating into your muscle tissue at this point," says Sims. That means bathing your damaged muscle fibers in essential amino acids, which helps stop the production of cortisol and promotes muscle synthesis and repair. "You don't want soy at all," says Sims, noting that many women reach for soy proteins with the thought that they're better for women. "It may help stop cortisol, but it does nothing for muscle synthesis. You want whey and casein for the best results."

Sims recommends taking 15 grams of whey or 9 grams of BCAAs (branched-chain amino acids) about a half hour before training. You can get that in 8 ounces of Greek yogurt or two eggs. After you've racked your bike, get another 25 grams of protein (that's 3 ounces of tuna or 6 ounces of cottage cheese) within 30 minutes. If you're training hard, get another 20 to 25 grams of mixed protein 2 hours post training and 10 to 15 grams before bed.

If it sounds like you're piling on the protein, it's because you are. You need it. And it's still well within the 90 grams a day that protein researchers like the University of Illinois's emeritus professor Donald K. Layman, PhD, recommend for active women, especially those who are also watching their weight or trying to lose a few pounds. Personally, I swear by 30 grams—sometimes more—per meal, especially when I'm doing lots of riding and racing. As a bonus: Extra protein may boost your immunity to protect you from getting sick when you're training hard.

RIDE FASTER AND HARDER SOMETIMES

The speed and strength of your muscle contractions often lessen after menopause. You can counteract that by shifting your training to focus more on power—think intervals on the bike and strength training in the gym—and a bit less on those long steady, often slower, endurance rides. "Power and speed training are essential elements in a postmenopausal woman's training arsenal," says Sims.

Do the intervals starting on page 149 and the strength moves in Chapter 15. You'll be happy you did.

RECLAIM YOUR SLEEP

Insomnia is common during menopause, as are nighttime sweats, which can be extremely disruptive to sleep. And, of course, poor sleep quality is a double whammy, because you need sleep not only to fend off fatigue (which is common during menopause) but also to do the normal nighttime muscle repairs and recovery—and this is during a time when recovery is more difficult in general.

If sleep eludes you, Sims recommends topping off your evening dose of protein with 400 to 600 milligrams of valerian (an herb known for its sleep-inducing properties). "The combination helps with overnight muscle repair, keeps cortisol low (which helps keep the stimulus for developing belly fat low), and helps maintain a lower core body temperature so you're less likely to experience hot flashes."

JUST RIDE

Finally, just getting out there on your bike will help alleviate some of the nagging symptoms a woman can face during this time of hormonal havoc. While there are very few studies on menopausal athletes, there is a healthy body of research on exercise's effect on menopause. And it's overwhelmingly positive.

In one Spanish study, the scientists asked 48 women ages 55 to 72 to either exercise for 3 hours a week or go about their mostly sedentary lives as usual. At the start of the study 50 percent of the women in the exercise group and 58 percent of the non-exercisers complained of severe menopause symptoms like fatigue and insomnia. By the study's end, the percentage of women with severe symptoms dropped to 37 percent in the active group, but rose to 66 percent among the non-exercisers. The active women also reported better mood and mental well-being, while their non-exercising counterparts were having a tougher time mentally and emotionally. So even if you don't always feel like it, get out there and ride. You'll feel better for it. And that's something that even the change can't change.

Finally, skeletal health is a big concern for postmenopausal women. Your osteoporosis risk rises sharply during this stage of life. So go back to page 161 and do those resistance and plyometric moves at least twice a week to keep your structural system as strong as the rest of you.

CHAPTER 26

Lady Parts

"HEY, SELENE, GOT A MINUTE?" (**A LOT OF MY "I NEED SOME** advice" conversations begin like this, as you may have noticed.) I looked up from my yard work to see my neighbor Lani leaning over the fence, holding a saddle in her hand. *This should be good*, I thought. Lani is an avid (okay, maybe obsessive) triathlete. And as a woman who has been around the block a few times, she's got zero compunction about speaking her mind. "I have a question for you!"

I walked over to the fence and saw that she was not only holding a saddle but also, with the other hand, balancing a hot new time trial bike. "I hope I have an answer," I said. "I'll at least try."

"I finally decided to do a full Ironman. And I know you've done one or two," she said, gesturing to the bike with her saddle. "How the hell did you sit on one of these for 5 or 6 hours without everything down there going painfully numb? What saddle did you use?"

I explained that I actually was 100 percent comfortable "down there" during both of my Ironman triathlons, because I'd had a bike fitting (see Chapter 3) to make sure I wasn't smushing my lady parts for the better part of a day. I told her that her first stop should be the bike shop across town to get measured for a saddle and to dial in her position. I told her to ask for Lisa, the woman in charge, because Lisa is totally down-to-earth about all things crotch and butt related, so Lani could fire away without fear.

"Thanks! I had a fitting done years ago. And it was okay. But it was done by a guy and they don't know vaginas and I didn't feel like talking to him about mine!" she said as she saddled up and rode off.

Therein lies the problem. Or problems, I should say. First is that most bike shops are still dominated by men. And well, that bro in the bike shop probably knows less than he thinks about vaginas and vulvas and all the sensitive tissues therein. No matter how much experience he may have with the business end of female anatomy, he won't understand what it's like to sit on a saddle with any of it. And while there are certainly good male bike fitters, you as a female have to be completely comfortable talking to the fitter about those intimate parts of your anatomy.

So let's open the door on the conversation here and talk sexual health, vaginal health, and, maybe most important, how to talk about all this stuff and keep your undercarriage happy and healthy no matter how many hours you spend in the saddle.

Let's Talk about Sex

When it comes to cycling and sexual function, men have taken up the lion's share of the spotlight with their talk about numbness and erectile dysfunction. Those open discussions led to new saddle designs and general cycling advice that has helped our male counterparts keep their equipment in good working order. Well, just because we women don't have an equally obvious barometer of sexual function doesn't mean that we don't suffer our own versions of dysfunction.

In one particularly telling and very bluntly titled report, "Bicyclist's Vulva: Observational Study," published in the *BMJ*, formerly called the *British Medical Journal*, researchers found that chronic inflammation of the vulvoperineal area, which includes pretty much everything from your clitoris to your anus, was common among competitive cyclists. If left unchecked, that swelling could damage lymphatic vessels. That's bad because the lymphatic system is instrumental in removing waste from your body. Nobody wants that stuff building up anywhere, but especially down there (the article included photos—yikes).

Not surprisingly, research shows that the more stretched out and aerodynamic a woman's position is on the bike, the more pressure she is likely putting on sensitive tissues, which raises her risk for reduced blood flow and soft tissue trauma. In one scientific paper that made headlines, Yale researchers reported that competitive female cyclists have decreased genital sensation compared to runners. What's more (and likely related), 62 percent of the riders had reported feeling some saddle-related pain, numbness, and/or tingling in the previous month.

So that's the bad news. The good news is that though the cyclists had higher "vibratory thresholds" (a measurement of when sensation is felt), they had normal, healthy sexual function and there was no difference between cyclists and runners in that department. So their sex lives weren't suffering.

Still. You shouldn't be doing damage down there. These studies back up the importance of not just getting a good bike fit so your weight is on your sit bones rather than your sensitive tissues but also trying out as many different saddles as it takes to find one that fits your particular female form. It's important to note that this can also change as you age. As mentioned earlier, I have more than one friend who needed to shop for a new saddle after turning 40 because their labia had thinned, leaving them more exposed and vulnerable to pressure.

Other steps that can relieve pressure: Raising the bars a bit so they're closer to level with your saddle (don't worry, any aerodynamic benefits you lose—which are minimal—will be offset by your being able to produce more power in a more comfortable position). Stand up when riding over bumpy terrain. And get out of the saddle periodically to give your nether regions a break.

Bumps, Abrasions, and Infections, Oh My . . .

Not so funny story: A triathlete friend who spends long hours in an aerodynamic tuck developed a saddle sore, which, as it sounds, is a sore spot or inflamed bump from friction with your shorts and/or bike seat, on her labia. Her gynecologist insisted on checking her for

herpes. She declined the test, left the office, and got another gyno who not only helped her heal the sore but also gave her some pretty good advice for avoiding future bumps, boils, and abrasions.

Chafing and saddle sores can happen even if you have a perfect bike and saddle fit, especially if you put in long miles in hot weather. Your saddle, shorts, and the salt crystals from dried sweat can work together like fine sandpaper on your butt while you pedal. It's even worse if it's humid or raining, because wet skin is particularly vulnerable to chafing.

Often, you don't even realize you're rubbing yourself raw down there until you get off the bike and hit the shower (where you find out immediately). Sometimes, saddles sores can also seem to appear out of nowhere. You might notice a little skin irritation, and then bacteria take over and suddenly you have inflamed hair follicles. Left untreated, they can develop into infected boils and oozing abscesses. Not pretty, and really painful.

If the sore is significant enough that it hurts when you sit on it, take a few days off from the bike and keep the affected area clean and dry. Diaper rash and antibiotic creams can soothe the pain and speed up healing. Infected sores require a trip to the doctor and prescription antibiotics, says Gloria Cohen, MD, a former physician for the Canadian national and Olympic cycling teams.

To prevent a recurrence, take a few measures to remove all friction points with that sensitive skin. Invest in shorts with a seamless chamois, wash them between rides, and never sit around in your sweaty shorts for longer than absolutely necessary. Get out of your shorts as soon as the ride ends and at least towel off (even better, clean up with a baby wipe if you can't shower for a while). And remember: No underwear with bike shorts. I'm shocked by how many events I go to where I can spot panty lines. It's really just asking for trouble.

Also consider using chamois cream, which is a lubricant that goes between you and your chamois to reduce friction. Many contain lavender, eucalyptus, tea tree oil, aloe, witch hazel, and other natural antibacterial agents that help ward off infections before they begin. Some are creamy in texture, while others are waxy (I've found the waxy ones to be better in really humid, sweaty, wet conditions). There are even women's specific chamois creams like DZNuts Bliss, Hoo Ha Ride Glide, and Chamois Butt'r

Her' that are specially formulated to help maintain a healthy pH balance so as to not open the door to urinary tract infections. Unlike unisex (really, men's) products, which often contain heavy doses of menthol and other cooling ingredients that can cause massive amounts of unwanted tingling when they hit your vagina, women's specific creams tend to be mostly tingle free, or at most, very lightly cooling. Ultimately, the type you choose is a matter of personal preference.

Whichever type it is, apply it in liberal amounts. Start with a quarter-size dab and slather it on wherever your body meets your chamois. No need to rub it in. If I know I'm going to be out for a long ride in wet conditions, I'll smear a light coating on the chamois itself for double protection. If you shave your bikini area and are prone to red bumps and razor burn, make sure to generously coat that particular area.

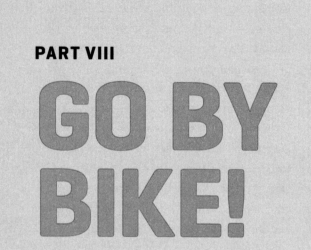

PART VIII

GO BY BIKE!

At its very essence, a bicycle is a vehicle for transportation—a wonderful machine that, when powered by a human, can take that person nearly anywhere they want to go, whether it's the summit of l'Alpe d'Huez or the coffee shop down the street. Before there were cars, bikes were how many people got around. And although cars now dominate the roadways, many people are using their bicycles not just for fun and exercise, but also as a mode of transportation. Even more special is that, unlike cars, you don't have to be a certain age to "drive" a bike. So your entire family can take adventures together.

That's what this section is all about: All the physical—and maybe spiritual— places you can go by bike, starting with work. Bike commuting is on the rise among women, and as many cities' infrastructure continues to evolve to become more bike friendly, those numbers will only grow. In the next chapter, you'll find all the tips you need, including what to wear, how to find the safest routes, and, of course, how to deal with helmet hair (admit it—it's a concern) to start and finish each day on the right pedal stroke.

Because cycling is as much a vehicle for change as it is for getting from point A to point B, there's a chapter on charity rides, which are nearly a rite of passage for cyclists. If there's a cause, you can bet there's a ride that benefits it. But all charity rides are not created equal, and just because it's a good cause doesn't mean it's a good ride. You'll learn how to evaluate rides before you register as well as how to thrive (not just survive) during them, as well as strategies for raising money for the cause, which is often far harder than the ride itself.

We'll also talk bike touring. There are more than 42,000 miles of established bike routes in North America alone. There are tens of thousands more around the globe, from the well-worn paths through rice paddies in Vietnam to the cobblestone roads of France and Belgium. No matter what level of rider you are, there are bike tours you can (and really should) do. Your packing list is in Chapter 29.

Want to bring your kids along? Chapter 30 includes clear how-to advice on getting even the youngest member of your family rolling. Hint: Ditch the training wheels; they do more harm than good. You'll also find a smart parent's guide to planning a fun family cycling outing that won't have your kids whining, "Are we there yet?"

CHAPTER 27

Commuting

"I GOT INTO CYCLING 10 YEARS AGO BECAUSE I WANTED TO GET around Philadelphia, where I live, without a car. Then I met a bunch of cyclists and saw how much fun people were having on long rides. So I got a better bike and started riding for fun and exercise as well as to get from here to there. I love the sense of accomplishment after a long hard ride. I love the freedom of just getting on my bike and going places. I love going up hills. I love being strong. I love that I can do it alone or with friends. And I love that I can go on bike rides with my dad and now my mom. It all started with just not wanting the hassle of driving around and parking in the city."

That's my friend Samantha Lockwood talking. What started as a practical commuting move ignited a huge passion for the sport of cycling. What's interesting is that so few people tend to make the shift in the other direction. There are many cyclists who love to ride for hundreds of miles all over creation, but never imagine using their bikes for transportation when they want to go somewhere.

There are many reasons for that. They think it will take too long. They worry that they'll be sweaty and messy and have bad helmet hair when they get there. Or quite frankly, it just never occurs to them to ride to all the places they usually drive to. If that's you, it's time to reconsider your transportation choices, especially for all those short trips around town we all make every day, maybe a few times a day.

A study by New York City's Transportation Alternatives shows that trips of less than 3 miles are often faster by bike, and those 5 to 7 miles in length—more than half of all Americans live less than 5 miles from where they work—take about the same time. Bike commuting is soaring in popularity now that more cities are creating bike lanes and bike share programs to deal with out-of-control traffic. Commuting can be fun and easy, and the clothes are cute, too. Here's what you need to know to get in on the trend.

> "Commuting by bike connects you to your environment. I love seeing the flowers in spring, how people decorate for Christmas, and being able to smile and say hi to people along the way. By the time I get to work, I feel wonderful."
> **—PHYLLIS LAUFER, 52, 4-H AGENT**

Ride to Work. Get Fit. Save Earth.

Let's get the first concern—time—out of the way first. Bike commuting is likely quicker than you think. As mentioned above, if you're going somewhere that's about 5 miles away, especially if it's in town where you have to wait in traffic, bike commuting is often faster. Otherwise, a good rule of thumb is that commuting by bike will take two times as long as driving.

So, okay, it might take a little longer. But do you try (and maybe not always succeed) to get to the gym every day? You won't need to carve out that extra hour if you ride your bike for 20 to 30 minutes to work and back. You'll also arrive at work with a clearer head and be able to shed the stress of the job at the end of the day as you spin home.

Even a short commute will help you stay fit. A Harvard study of more than 18,000 adult women reported that those who started biking—even for as little as 5 minutes each day—gained less weight over a 16-year period than their non-cycling peers. Women who rode more than 4 hours a week fared best and were 26 percent less likely to gain more than a few pounds over the study period. Study author Rania Mekary, PhD, sang cycling's praises in a report on the study, saying, "The more time women spent bicycling, the better. . . . This is encouraging for women with weight problems because they could substitute bicycling for slow walking or car driving," which is what commuting is all about.

So even if you opt to make just the shortest trips, like those to the library, the coffee shop, and a nearby friend's house, you're still helping your health—and that of your community as well. Another study, published last year in the *American Journal of Public Health*, concluded that "communities with more walkers and cyclists are healthier than those where people must rely on cars to get around." No surprise there.

WHAT ABOUT MY HAIR?

Unless you can wear a sweat suit and ball cap on the job, you'll want to clean up and look fresh and professional when you arrive at work. Many office buildings are equipped with showers or have a gym facility nearby that you can use for cleaning up. If yours does not, shower and take care of personal hygiene at home before you leave, then freshen up in the lavatory at work. On-the-fly styling products such as TRESemmé Fresh Start Refreshing Mist and Herbal Essences Style Refreshing Mist make it a breeze to refresh your look. Stow baby wipes and deodorant at work, too. That way, you can wipe your face, feet, underarms, and any other sticky areas and feel shower fresh in less than 5 minutes.

What you wear depends on how far and hard you plan on riding as well as the dress code in your workplace. Basically, you have two choices: Riding to work dressed for work or riding to work in your cycling clothes and changing when you get there.

If the ride is fairly short and casual, you can just wear normal clothing, like people do in countries like China and the Netherlands, where everyone rides everywhere. After all, you're not racing, you're riding. Whatever you usually wear should work just fine. Companies like My Alibi and Club Ride make minimally padded undies you can slip under even your slimmest pants for added commuting comfort. If you really get into it, you can start expanding your wardrobe with some cycling-specific gear that looks more downtown than Planet Fitness. Propelled by the advancing popularity of urban riding, along with an ever-broadening definition of how bicycles fit into our daily lives, clothing makers are throwing the boundaries of cycling's sartorial territory wide open—a tailored pencil skirt unzips to reveal a gusset for easy pedaling, a rear zipper pocket finds common ground with a shirt collar and covered button placket. Activewear from places like REI and Athleta blur the lines between fashion and function.

The new minimalist aesthetic whittles away everything but the essentials of performance and comfort. In the pursuit of design purity, fine knits, muted solids, and subtle touches such as hidden vents at the collarbones and stylish quilt stitching at the shoulder speak louder than logos—and permit a discreet and seamless transition from the road to daily modern living.

Women's riding apparel, in particular, is reclaiming the innovative spirit that fueled a fashion revolution during the first golden age of bicycling more than a century ago, when women seeking an alternative to skirts drove the popularity of bloomers. Young, often-urban entrepreneurs who are largely independent of the mainstream cycling industry are creating stylish and practical solutions to challenges they themselves encounter, from achieving flattering, day-into-night versatility to maintaining safety and visibility in traffic. For many, growing a business also means building a movement to attract more women to cycling's freedom, fitness, and fun.

Of course even the most stylish cycling attire may not work for every office environment. If you work in a starched-shirt, shiny-shoe atmosphere, you may opt to drive in once a week to deliver fresh clothes for the upcoming week and shuttle worn ones back home for laundering. Or if you have fairly wrinkle-resistant business casual clothing, you can pack things in a backpack or messenger bag and change in the restroom when you arrive.

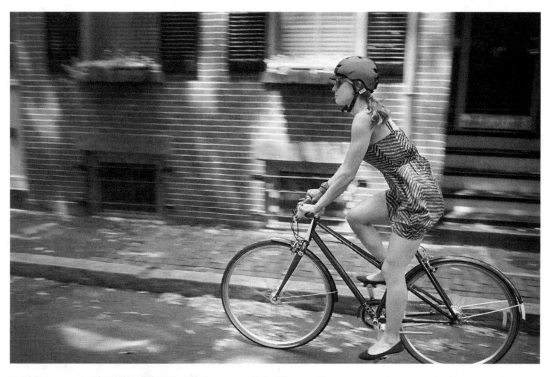

Today's commuting clothes are stylish enough to wear off the bike as well as on.

CHOOSE YOUR CARRY-ON

There are a number of ways you can carry the items you'd normally bring to work in your briefcase. One of the most popular is a simple backpack. Companies like Chrome, Dakine, and Osprey make multiuse sports-oriented backpacks that stand up to any type of weather and have smart features like integrated padded laptop sleeves and easy access pockets for your keys, cards, and cell phone.

If you have a rear rack, you can bungee-strap a bag on the back of your bike. Some commuters prefer to use panniers, bags that attach to your rack. A bike shop can show you your options.

Along with your basic necessities, such as tools, clothing, and personal hygiene items, you might consider carrying some spare cash in case of an emergency. If you have too much to carry, simply drive to work once or twice a week with a few days' worth of clothes and necessities so you carry less when you ride.

WHICH WAY DO I GO?

Depending on your current commute, you may follow the same roads on your bike that you drive, or you may need to choose a path that avoids highways or other unsafe roads. Your local bike shop can assist you in choosing the best routes to your destination. They also may have maps that show bike-friendly routes in your region, so you can try several different routes.

Another option is to visit MapQuest.com, where you can choose driving directions right from your street address to work. Once the directions come up, click on the "Avoid Highways" tab. This should give you directions for the shortest route to work using back roads. Other options include RidetheCity.com, which is a clearinghouse for safe bike routes. Get There by Bike, an iPhone app, allows you to map, record, and, share routes in 23 cities (and counting). Google Maps allows you to choose cycling options for wherever you want to go.

Can't commit to a long commute? Cut it in half. The first day, drive to work with your bike, then ride home that night. Ride to work the next morning, then drive home, and so on. Or drive halfway to work, but park at a mall or another safe place and ride the rest of the way. Many bus and rail lines allow bicyclists to bring their bikes on board (some require a permit, so check in advance), so you can ride your bike to a park-and-ride lot and catch a ride the rest of the way. Call your local transit station for ride share options in your area.

Interestingly, car drivers may even be more courteous to you as a woman cyclist on the road. A British researcher from the University of Bath recently hypothesized that cars pass an average of 5.5 inches closer to male cyclists than female cyclists. To determine this, the good scientist used an "ultrasonic distance sensor" and pedaled away as 2,500 vehicles passed. Sometimes he wore a long-haired blond wig to make drivers think he was a woman. He found that indeed, he got more riding room when the drivers thought he was a woman.

Lock It Up

At work, there are likely places where you can stash your bike out of the way for the day. If not, talk to your boss about bike parking options. Many workplaces are eager to encourage employee health and fitness because it benefits their bottom line, so he or she has some incentive to help you keep your bike safely stored while you're at work. If there's nowhere to stash the bike inside, you'll need a lock, just as you would for other rides that might involve leaving your bicycle unattended for a time.

In most areas, you only need a U-lock—a U-shaped metal ring with a removable locking crossbar that allows you to secure your bike to any sturdy post; they're available almost everywhere, from bike shops to big-box discount retailers. Double up on protection in high-theft zones by adding a cable lock: Start by parking your bike next to a rack, signpost, or other immovable object. Run the U-lock between the rack, rear wheel, and seat tube, but keep it open. Then take one end of a cable and run it through your frame and front wheel, looping it through the cable's other end to form a lasso. Finally, attach the free end of the cable to the U-lock and close the crossbar to lock the bike.

CHAPTER 28

Charity Rides

I GOT MY INTRODUCTION TO CHARITY RIDES THE WAY MANY do, as a rider in an MS 150, which for those new to the charity bike ride world is a 2-day 150-mile ride that raises money for the National Multiple Sclerosis Society. I will confess that when I signed up, I knew next to nothing about the cause or the charity. I went because my friends were doing the ride and it sounded like fun. And it *was* fun. We did 75 miles through the rolling hills of Pennsylvania Amish country, rode past a Mennonite wedding, made new friends, and drank beer and told stories in the evenings when the riding was through.

I also learned about the cause. Turned out that I had two coworkers with MS. They were extremely grateful for my fund-raising and riding efforts and were more than happy to educate me about what their lives with MS were like. Given that information, the ride became as meaningful as it was enjoyable. Being able to put human faces to a cause I now very much cared about also made it far easier to raise the $150 minimum in donations we needed to participate in the ride.

Buoyed by that positive experience, I quickly signed up for another one: the Montana AIDS Vaccine ride, 600 miles from Missoula to Billings. This time we had to raise more money—a *lot* more money. To the tune of $3,500. I was doing a lot of personal training at the time and had a number of gay clients, nearly all of whom had lost someone to AIDS and/or knew someone living with HIV/AIDS, if they weren't themselves. Through their generosity, I was able to raise the funds and do the ride, which was inspiring and amazing and simply stunning. Sadly, my elation was deflated shortly after I got home, when I read a story in the paper about how little of the funds raised actually went to the cause for those vaccine rides: 15 to 30 percent.

I felt sick to my stomach. But I'd learned a very valuable lesson. Part of my future charity ride work would go beyond putting in the miles and raising the funds to also investigating the charity putting on the ride. Happily, I'm proud to say I have never repeated that error. All the rides I've done since give the lion's share of monies raised to the cause and use only a small amount to cover overhead.

So now, instead of letting you go out and learn the hard way like I did, I'll give you the lowdown on how to choose the right ride for you, what to expect from your charity ride experience, and how to fund-raise and get fit for the big event.

Pedaling for a Purpose

The main draw of charity rides, aside from the obvious—bringing money and attention to an important cause—is the atmosphere. Charity rides draw big crowds by welcoming everyone from families out for a few miles to best friends pushing it for 7 straight days in honor of someone or something they believe in. And that's the idea: Through entry fees and fund-raising,

these events benefit cancer research, children's hospitals, humane societies, and more. Unlike a race, for which solid fitness and pack-riding skills are a must, bike rides for a cause are pleasantly noncompetitive.

For many, signing up is great motivation to enjoy time on the bike, both during the event and on conditioning rides leading up to it. Of course, that said, there will most definitely be folks on the ride who are looking to drill it to the finish and "win the ride." You can join their "race" if you choose, but you'll have plenty of pleasant company if you'd rather just ride along.

If possible, sign up to ride with at least one friend. That way you'll have a training partner and event-day camaraderie and support, and you can even combine your fund-raising efforts with things like joint raffles and yard sales. Having a buddy or two is especially useful if you're new to cycling. Stuff can go wrong at even the best-prepared event. Food trucks break down. Riders can go off course and get a little lost. People get flat tires. It's easier to conquer any challenges that come up when you're in the company of friends.

As for which event to pursue, ideally, you want to choose a charity that you feel personally connected to. But before you make a decision, consider how the beneficiary will spend your donation. Check out Charity Navigator (see "How Does Your Charity Check Out," page 276), which evaluates the financial health of more than 5,500 organizations.

Rides vary in number of days and distance. Common distances include 10 to 15, 30 to 40, and 75 to 100 miles. Obviously, if you sign up for one of the longer routes, you might need to give yourself a bit of time to train beforehand. Choose an event that allows you sufficient opportunity to get appropriately fit, as well as to raise the necessary funds. Once you make your choice, sign up before hesitation sets in. Worst case if you bail: Your registration fee will still go to the cause.

DOING THE DISTANCE

Many charity rides are long and fairly hard (or at least offer long and fairly hard options) because the point is to push outside your comfort zone and challenge yourself for a good cause. Of course, when you take chances, there are risks involved. Whether it's mechanical, a muscle mutiny, or self-doubt, things can go wrong on long charity rides. Here's how to keep your chin up and your cranks turning for even a 100-mile day in the saddle.

MILE MARKER: 20

Snag: Your lungs are paying the price for your attempt to keep up with faster riders.

Solution: Back off your speed and ride at a conversational pace. Save your energy for the remaining 80 miles. Remember, this is not a race.

MILE MARKER: 40

Snag: You're not even halfway and the finish feels impossibly out of reach.

Solution: Break the remaining ride into chunks. If you have 60 miles and two aid sta-

tions to go, focus on getting to the next stop. Nibble on the energy bars and gels you stuffed in your pockets.

MILE MARKER: 60

Snag: Your rear end is rebelling.

Solution: Rise out of the saddle often. And next time, take measures to keep it from happening in the first place: Use chamois cream to prevent chafing and find a saddle during training that you can count on for the long haul.

MILE MARKER: 80

Snag: Your back and shoulders are screaming.

Solution: Switch your hand position on the handlebars to disperse joint stress. Also, wear cycling gloves with padding to prevent numbness. If need be, stop and stretch.

RAISING THE DOUGH

Unless you're an all-star in the sales department, the hardest part of charity rides is often not the riding, but the fund-raising. It's not always easy to ask people to donate. Yet there are people who are amazingly adept at soliciting huge sums of money from friends, family, and even strangers. One such woman is Shannon Gilmartin, a fortysomething cyclist from Orchard Park, New York. She has drummed up more than $36,000 for the Dempsey Challenge (a ride founded by *Grey's Anatomy*'s Patrick Dempsey that raises funds for the Patrick Dempsey Center for Cancer Hope and Healing). Here are a few of her secrets.

SELL STUFF. People are more likely to donate if they get something in return. "I like to bake," Gilmartin says. "So I organize a Confections for Cancer Patients campaign. All proceeds from my cakes, cookies, and pies go to the Dempsey Challenge."

ORGANIZE A RAFFLE. "I had one of my most effective fund-raisers after I bought scrubs and paired them with a *Grey's Anatomy* script I won in a Twitter contest," Gilmartin says. "I took them to one of Patrick Dempsey's car races and waited in the autograph line. Then I raffled off the signed memorabilia and raised over $2,000."

BE CRAZY. The wackier you can be, the more attention you will bring to your cause. "One year I organized a Pie Me in the Face game," Gilmartin says. "People donated money for a chance to throw a whipped-cream pie at me." Share the pictures on Twitter, Instagram, and other social media sites to raise awareness and engage potential supporters.

How Does Your Charity Check Out?

Cyclists take many things into account when choosing a ride to support: personal connection to the cause, location, the size of the post-ride burrito. But also consider how the beneficiary spends your money. One of the best ways to investigate is by checking CharityNavigator.org.

Charity Navigator rates more than 7,000 US-based nonprofit organizations that receive more than $500,000 in public support each year on a scale of zero to four stars. (About 2,400 groups currently merit the highest rating.) It does not rate hospitals, private or community foundations, colleges or universities, PBS stations, land trusts or preserves, or religious organizations (such as the Salvation Army) that are exempt from filing IRS Form 990, which Charity Navigator uses to determine ratings.

Even if your cause of choice isn't listed, you can ask questions to determine a nonprofit's worthiness. (Federal law requires that charities make 3 years of financial data publicly available.) Here are some factors Charity Navigator takes into account.

ORGANIZATIONAL EFFICIENCY: What percentage of expenses relate to programs, as opposed to administration and fund-raising? Ideally, it's 75 percent or more.

FUND-RAISING EFFICIENCY: How many cents does the organization spend to raise each dollar? Fewer than 10 is commendable.

GROWTH: Are revenues—and services—increasing over time?

WORKING CAPITAL: How long could the charity sustain its programs without raising more money? The answer should be at least a year.

CHAPTER 29

Bike Touring

THE REAL BEAUTY OF BICYCLING IS THAT IT CAN TAKE YOU TO all kinds of spectacular places, and there is absolutely no better way to see a place than from the saddle of a bike. It's faster than walking, so you can cover dozens of miles, yet you're still immersed in the elements, so you can feel, hear, see, and smell your surroundings, be they crashing ocean waves, fields of wildflowers, tall pines, or red rock canyons.

That's why I encourage everyone I know to take a bike tour if they can. It's an experience of a lifetime that I think can be particularly transformative for women. My friend Kate Veronneau, who works for Thomson Bike Tours, says she has witnessed many transformations firsthand.

"It's exhilarating and empowering to crest giant mountains and cover all this terrain on your own two wheels," says Kate. "Women come for all reasons. Maybe they just got divorced. Or they're rewarding themselves for hitting a big weight-loss goal. Or they've always wanted to see a particular country, but they don't want the typical vacation. They want to be challenged and grow. And they do. They meet new people and they feel strong and independent and worldly . . . just on top of the world physically and mentally. There's an awful lot for women to gain from the experience. And hey, it's a vacation where you can eat and drink what you want and still come back leaner and stronger for it. How often can you say that?"

Pick Your Type

Convinced? Of course you are. The first thing to consider when deciding to take a bike tour is what type you want to take. Bike touring covers a huge spectrum, from the pick-a-route, grab-a-friend-or-two, pack-and-carry-all-your-stuff-and-go variety to the kind where you plunk down your credit card to have everything but the actual pedaling handled for you. There are obvious pros and cons to each. You just have to ask yourself a few key questions.

HOW MUCH CAN YOU OR ARE YOU WILLING TO SPEND?

Fully guided, supported tours range in price from about $900 all the way up to $9,000. As you'd imagine, the tours at the two price extremes put you up in radically different accommodations. On lower-budget tours you'll likely camp (which can be quite awesome, depending on where you are) and be responsible for much of your own gear. On the high end, you'll get laundry service and a chocolate on your pillow at a luxury inn.

If you go fully DIY, you'll still have some expenses, even if you pitch a tent every night. Factoring in campsite fees and/or motel rooms, meals, and gear, figure on at least a few hundred dollars.

WHERE DO YOU WANT TO GO?

Want to go somewhere exotic you've never been where nobody speaks your language? Might be better to find a guided, supported tour. Want to explore some popular destinations in the United States? It's pretty easy to do it yourself or with a small group. The Adventure Cycling Association (adventurecycling.org) has established a cycling route network with more than 42,000 miles of routes throughout North America. They sell maps for these routes, which are traveled by thousands of cyclists each year.

HOW MUCH GEAR ARE YOU WILLING TO CARRY?

This is a biggie. If you and your friends are doing this on your own, that means you'll have to carry everything you need—rain gear, bike repair gear, maybe camping gear. It's a lot of stuff that all requires packs and panniers. It's also the type of trip that demands that you perform an extra level of preparation, as you need to practice packing and riding with that much stuff. You can lessen the load by "credit card touring," which means carrying only what you really need and paying for the rest (i.e., food, lodging, etc.). If you prefer to carry nothing but your phone and maybe a vest, a supported tour is the way to go.

HOW LONG AND FAR DO YOU WANT TO RIDE?

The longer you want to go, the more you'll need to take, and the greater the likelihood that you'll encounter some adversity like bad weather or bike mechanical issues. In those situations, it's always nice to have a support van that's not too far away. You'll also cover more ground in any given amount of time when you're carrying less.

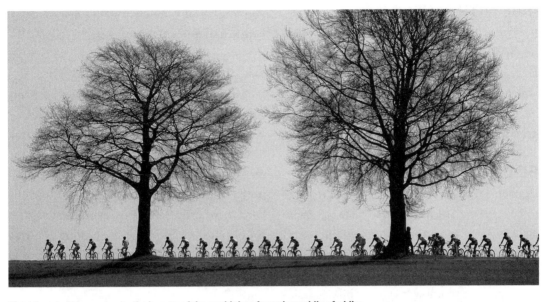

There is no better way to see the beauty of the world than from the saddle of a bike.

WHAT'S YOUR PRIORITY?

If you decide on a guided tour, know what your priority is before you pick one. Some focus on low mileage on the bike to give you a chance to do other sightseeing for the bulk of the day. Others are very ride focused, so you'll be on the bike the majority of the day. There are culinary tours where eating plays as large a role as riding. All types can be amazing. It's just a matter of picking the one that's right for your priorities.

Tour Preparation

Whenever I tell people about the multiday tours and races I've done, the first question they ask is, "How do you train for that?" Not surprisingly, that's the number one worry on the minds of many of Kate's clients as well. "Women will look at the mileage and elevation profiles [graphs that show how much you're going to be climbing] and get apprehensive," she says. "They're worried that they won't be able to get fit enough."

Fact is, you don't have to go out and do hill repeats or lots of crazy interval training to tour. You need to get comfortable on your bike, says Kate. "I tell people to just get as much saddle time as possible. Get really comfortable spending a lot of time on your bike. You don't need to go really fast. You just need to be able to keep pedaling along. It's touring."

There are some special things you should practice, however, that you might not think of. Here's what she recommends for maximum tour enjoyment.

RIDE WITH OTHERS

Ride with groups that include people of various levels of ability so you'll be comfortable with faster people, slower people, and people who have a different riding style than you do. Nearly any charity ride can serve as good practice.

GO OUT IN THE RAIN

Of course you don't want to. But if you're going to be covering any measurable distance, especially if you're going through mountainous terrain where the weather is capricious at best, you might get caught in some wet weather, so it's important to know how your bike handles and how to dress. Likewise, go out in the cold and the heat. Figure out how to layer for wide temperature variations and you'll be more comfortable on nearly any tour.

STOP AND GO

Sounds funny, but the hardest part of touring can be all the stopping. When you stop, blood sort of pools in your legs and you stiffen up a little. Getting going again, especially if you've just sat down to eat for an hour or so, can be harder than you'd think. Prepare for it with a little practice. Go out with a friend and ride to lunch and back. Get used to eating and drinking and riding pretty much all day long.

All the Places You Can Go

Anywhere you can tour by car (and many places you can't), you can tour by bike. But just to give you a taste of popular touring destinations, here are some cycling favorites.

CALIFORNIA WINE COUNTRY

I did a women's tour through Napa and Sonoma Valleys about 8 years ago, and it still stands as one of the most scenic rides I've ever been on. California wine country is a classic destination for cyclists of all stripes for a reason: It's stunning. You see it all—panoramic views of the Pacific, towering redwoods, quaint towns, lush rolling hills. And, of course, along the way there are copious amounts of amazing food and wine.

ITALY

Italy is a bike rider's dream destination. There's food. There's wine. The breathtaking scenery serves up rides that satisfy every type of rider. Hard-core cyclists can tackle the soaring massif walls of the Dolomites, while beginner riders can have an easy day skirting the country's famously hard hills by hugging the coastline and pedaling along the Mediterranean and Adriatic Seas.

HOLLAND AND BELGIUM

Spinning through the Dutch countryside is like pedaling through a picture book. Holland and Belgium are renowned cycling territory, and the whole region is cycling mad. Everyone has a bike, and they ride everywhere because the pastoral landscape is so sweet and easy for riders of all abilities. You can fill up on fresh mussels, fine beer, and, of course, chocolate, and then

Pack It All

The secret to bike touring success is packing the right stuff. "Pack it all!" is Kate Veronneau's advice. She's actually not kidding. Unless you're heading somewhere where the weather never changes, you'll likely need clothes to keep you comfortable in a wide range of temperatures and conditions. "Weather, especially in the mountains, can be very unpredictable," she warns. "It can be hot and sunny and cold and wet all in the same day!" Here's the packing list she dishes out to her clients at Thomson Bike Tours.

- Cycling shoes
- Cycling socks
- Shorts
- Shortsleeve jerseys
- Longsleeve jerseys
- Wind jacket
- Fleece jacket
- Rain jacket
- Undershirts
- Summer gloves
- Winter gloves
- Leg warmers
- Winter tights
- Arm warmers
- Shoe covers
- Helmet
- Helmet cap
- Cleat covers
- Sunglasses
- Chamois cream
- Small backpack to store spare clothes in the sag van (for a supported tour)

soak up windmills, canals, and endless fields of flowers.

FRANCE

Home to the big Tour, France is a cycling mecca. There are the Alps and the Pyrenees and all the storied climbs along the way. Riding through France is like taking a trip through history, as the countryside is riddled with castles and architectural wonders. Like other famous European destinations, each day's riding is also rewarded with lots of great food, in this case cheese, bread, and wine.

VERMONT

No need to jet to the far-flung corners of the world for unprecedented beauty. New England has plenty to offer, and bucolic Vermont is top on the list for cyclists. The landscape is marked by quiet farms, beautiful rivers, and of course, if you go in the fall, eye-popping foliage. You'll also get to enjoy the world's best maple syrup every morning.

UTAH

Mountain bikers can tour too, and there are companies that specialize in off-road adventures. There might be no better destination than Utah. Moab is synonymous with mountain biking. There's no place like it on Earth. Canyonlands National Park offers jaw-dropping views around every bend. The whole state offers hundreds of miles of trails that are as mellow or as death-defying as you'd like.

CHAPTER 30

Cycling as a Family Affair

I LIVE IN A VERY ENTHUSIASTIC CYCLING COMMUNITY. WE ALL met and were riding together long before many of us were in serious relationships, let alone had families. But then time passed, people got pregnant; bike seats, bike trailers, trikes, tandems, and scoot bikes were bought. Races became even more fun, as we got to cheer for moms and dads and kids alike.

Sure, not all the kids ended up being cyclists. Mine sure hasn't. And that's okay. But we have a tandem, and it's a fun day out for all of us when my husband and daughter truck out the tandem and I pedal along with them on one of our local charity rides or out to grab brunch on a Sunday morning.

And that's the cool thing about riding. It really is something you can share with your family and do with your kids, if you have kids. Some of my friends even ended up taking very cool cycling vacations where the kids get a kids' ride and other fun stuff to do during the day while the parents go out for some all-day epic.

Getting Them Started

Of course, before you can ride with your kids, you need to teach them how to ride. Helping your son or daughter learn to ride a bike is a milestone, and trust me, there's nothing quite like seeing them pedal off unassisted for the first time. But it doesn't happen overnight and, like everything, some kids pick it up more (or less) easily than others.

That's why, with the help of some experts, *Bicycling* developed its own method, which differs from the traditional run-beside-the-bike way most of us were taught. They found that it results in fewer crashes and a shorter learning time—many kids begin spinning on their own within 15 or 20 minutes. Here's what they recommend.

1. Remove the training wheels from your kid's bicycle. Lower the seat so she can put her feet flat on the ground while seated.

2. Find a grassy slope with a gentle downhill of 30 yards or so. If possible, use a hill that ends with a flat stretch or a slight uphill, to help your rider slow down at the bottom.

3. Strap on your child's helmet and tuck in her shoelaces.

4. Walk halfway up the hill and hold the bike while your child gets on. Have her sit on the saddle with her feet on the ground.

5. Make sure your rider is as relaxed as possible, with loose elbows and a light grip on the handlebars. Explain that it will be easier to balance if she's looking ahead, not down.

6. Tell your child to lift her feet and coast down the hill without pedaling. Remind her that she can put her feet down to slow the bike if she gets scared. (If the pedals get in the way, remove them for this step.)

7. Repeat steps 4 through 6 until your child can reach the bottom of the hill without putting her feet down.

8. Next, have her coast down the hill with her feet on the pedals, but not pedaling.

9. After several runs, have your child begin pedaling as she rolls. Once she's comfortable, move farther up the hill for a few more runs.

10. Raise the saddle and go to a flat area to ride loops and practice turning, braking, and starting from a standstill.

Helpful Hints

The learning process is a parent–child bonding moment like no other, so don't rush—enjoy it!

GIVE HER SPACE

Run behind, not beside, your child so you don't distract her. Don't hold on to the bike. Let her feel balance on her own.

CRASHES HAPPEN

Be ready to comfort, coerce, cheerlead, and bandage—and possibly wait for another day.

TAKE YOUR TIME— AND KEEP IT FUN

Depending on the child, learning to ride a bike can take as little as a few minutes or as long as several days. If she seems scared or frustrated, pack it in for the day and try again later.

Once she's gotten the hang of pedaling and balancing without toppling over, you can advance her to a few of the finer skills of riding a bike.

How to start pedaling from a standstill

TELL 'EM: Start with one pedal pointing to the handlebar.

WHAT YOU SHOULD KNOW: This puts the pedal at roughly 2 o'clock, which lets her give a solid pedal stroke to power the bike and keep it steady until her other foot finds its pedal.

How to ride straight

TELL 'EM: Look straight ahead.

WHAT YOU SHOULD KNOW: When a novice rider turns her head, her arms and shoulders follow, causing the bike to swerve. Next lessons: Keep the elbows and knees loose, and pedal smooth circles.

How to corner

TELL 'EM: Slow down before you turn.

WHAT YOU SHOULD KNOW: Slowing before entering a corner leaves room for error in cornering—as confidence grows, your child will learn to position the inside pedal upward and look through the turn to the exit.

How to ride in traffic

TELL 'EM: Ride like a car.

WHAT YOU SHOULD KNOW: This keeps your kid from swooping and swerving on roads, running stop signs, and riding on the wrong side of the road. It also reminds her to hold a line in groups.

How to stop

TELL 'EM: Squeeze both brake levers at the same time.

WHAT YOU SHOULD KNOW: This provides maximum braking and control. Jamming on the front brake alone can launch Junior over the handlebars, while using only the back brake limits the rider to just 20 to 40 percent of braking power and makes the bike more likely to skid.

Let's Go Ride!

The kid is pedaling like a champ. You're stoked. It's summer vacation time. And wouldn't it be awesome to plan a few kid-friendly bike getaways? With the rise of bike lanes, greenways, and bike paths, it's easier than ever. You just need to take a few simple steps first.

DO YOUR HOMEWORK

Before your trip, call a bike shop or cycling club near your destination. Specify the age and riding ability of your kids and ask about flat, scenic, low-traffic rides with plenty of places to eat, play, and sightsee along the way. If you'll be doing a short ride on a long trip, consider renting bikes and trailers or tag-alongs to avoid the hassle of wrangling and hauling your own. (If you plan to rent a trailer, make sure it has a five-point harness, a roll bar, ventilation, and a sunshade.)

ALWAYS HAVE A PLAN— AND A PLAN B

Schedule riding time after meals and naps. Low blood sugar coupled with fatigue can turn a family joyride into the Tour de Meltdown. Kids (and some spouses) bonk faster than experienced cyclists, so carry extra food and water. Communicate your plan to the whole family so no one has to ask, "Are we there yet?" But have a secret backup plan: If you're riding dirt, find a trail with loops of manageable distances or multiple bailout points close to a road. Touring a new town? Be ready to pull over if you spot something that looks fun. If all else fails, leave your spouse with the kids while you get the car.

PICK BIKE ROUTES THAT HAVE REWARDS

While the ride itself might be a treat for you, your family may need goals and a more tangible payoff. It might be breathtaking views that unfold around every bend or an ice cream shop or a playground. If it's safe, let the kids lead: They'll set the pace that works best for them, and you'll be able to keep an eye on their fatigue level. Provide fun checkpoints to break the ride into segments, or turn it into a scavenger hunt. Keep a few special treats in your jersey pocket to share when the group reaches its goal.

Four Fam-tastic Cycling Routes

There are undoubtedly great places to ride close to your back door. But if you want to get really adventurous, here are a few of the ones that *Bicycling* likes best of all.

GOLDEN GATE PARK

The San Francisco park is home to attractions including a playground, the California Academy of Sciences, and a Dutch windmill. Bonus: Sections of JFK Drive are closed to traffic on Sundays.

GREAT SMOKY MOUNTAINS NATIONAL PARK

Cars aren't allowed on the 11-mile Cades Cove loop in Tennessee until 10:00 a.m. on Saturdays and Wednesdays from May through October.

KATY TRAIL

Rail trails (former railways converted into bike paths) are usually flat and car free. This one in Missouri connects charming small towns filled with shops, parks, wineries, and B&Bs.

ZION NATIONAL PARK

Traffic is limited to bikes and eco-friendly buses on some park roads from April to October, ensuring empty ribbons of scenic byway winding through Utah's psychedelic canyon lands.

PART IX

MAINTAINING YOUR MACHINE

knew a woman who was an accomplished athlete and owned a high-end road bike suitable for long rides and racing, yet the vast majority of her time riding it was when it was hooked up to her indoor trainer. Not because she lived in some far-flung corner of Siberia—she kept her beautiful bike inside because she had a nearly pathological fear of flat tires. They brought her literally to tears.

She even wrote a story about it for *Bicycling*, in which she talked about her maiden voyage on her sweet new ride.

I felt invincible pedaling across the George Washington Bridge [over the Hudson River] on my brand-new, triple-chainringed red Cannondale, the first bike I'd owned since my three-speed Schwinn 15 years prior. The day before, I had taken a few laps of Central Park, clicking my first pair of cleats into and out of the pedals, the only mechanical skill I thought I needed for my new wheels. I was reveling in seeing the pavement fly beneath me, until I heard a "psssst" coming from my front wheel. The thought crossed my mind that it wasn't a good noise, so I turned around but kept pedaling, confident I could cover the 5 or so miles back home to New York City. Wrong. Within a few more pedal strokes I stopped dead on the rim. I clacked 400 yards to a gas station, tears streaming down my cheeks, feeling as if I was stranded with nobody around for hundreds of miles, and not in suburban New Jersey on Route 9W, cars flying past.

I stood at the station for a while, wondering if the air pump could somehow reinflate my tire. [I had no idea there was a tube in there, or that it had something called a "Presta valve," which wasn't compatible with the pump's chuck.] Too embarrassed to ask for mechanical help from the attendant—a good decision, in hindsight—I asked him for a phone book. Twenty minutes later I stuffed my bike, wheels not released [I had no idea they did that], into the back seat of a taxi, jumped into the front seat and bit my cheeks so I wouldn't cry in front of the cab driver.

When I told my boyfriend, Grant, about my adventure over the phone, he didn't judge me for being so—what's the word?—stupid. Instead, that night, he brought over a seatbag, a minipump, tire levers and spare tubes for my new red ride. He knew enough about me, still clearly stinging from my ignorance, not to offer instruction; instead, he quietly fixed my flat. I can't remember if I had told him at that point in our relationship that I loved him, but I definitely knew for sure then. He eventually became my husband and, not surprisingly, my bike mechanic.

The story went on, spanning a solid decade in which she lived in cloistered fear of flats, had her husband pump her tires for her, and finally, after growing weary of not being able to reach her full potential as a cyclist because she couldn't venture too far from home, she went to her local shop to learn how to change a tube in her tires.

It wasn't easy. It took tons of practice. But she did it, and though she still "sucks" at fixing flats (her word, not mine), she feels less fearful wandering out on her own out of cell phone range because she knows that when push comes to shove, she can take care of herself.

That's important for all of us—men and women—but I suspect it's even more so for women. I know that for many years whenever I got a flat, some guy on the ride would chivalrously step in and fix it. And I let him. I knew how, but I didn't want to. Ditto with more complicated fixes like bent derailleurs, broken chains, and the like.

It was all good until I started racing. Because guess what? When you get a flat tire in a race, some nice man doesn't pull over and sacrifice his race to put a fresh tube in for you. And if you haven't practiced, you lose a *lot* of time—and definitely the race—because you're fumbling around for 20 minutes doing a job that you could do in less than 3 with practice.

I also started leading some women's rides on the mountain. Suddenly I was the expert and when one of the women broke her chain, I had to step in and fix it. To this day, I'm not sure how I knew what to do—osmosis from watching others over the years, I imagine—but I did. Then I went to a Park Tool class to learn basic bike maintenance and repair so I could race, ride, and enjoy my bike everywhere and anywhere with the peace of mind of knowing that I could take care of myself if something went awry.

That's the goal of this section. I'm not looking to turn you into a professional wrench. And I'm not going to go super in depth on bleeding brakes, pulling apart suspension forks, or high-level mechanical fixes and maintenance that, frankly, are best left to professionals. But when you're done, you should feel like you know what to do if something minor goes wrong.

CHAPTER 31

Basic Maintenance and Repair

BIKES ARE MACHINES, AND MACHINES REQUIRE SOME BASIC maintenance to work best. I'll be the first to admit, I'm pretty awful about maintaining mine. But after putting a few unnecessary dents in my bank account replacing pricey parts that went bad prematurely because of neglect, I've learned to become somewhat better about taking care of the essentials. And truly, it's really not that hard. Here's what you need to know.

Create Your Tool Kit

Unless you live next to a bike shop (and even if you do), you'll need a few tools and supplies to keep your bike tuned and ready to roll. Here are the basics *Bicycling* recommends.

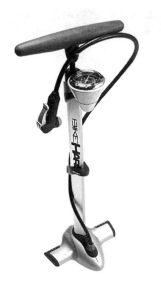

A floor pump lets you inflate your tires to the proper pressure with just a few easy strokes.

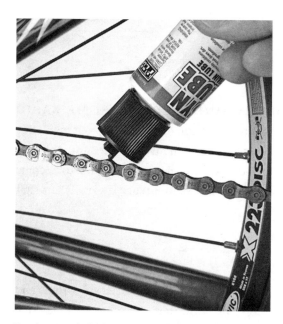

Keeping your chain clean and well lubed makes your bike run better and extends the life of your drivetrain.

FLOOR PUMP

Even if you never actually get a flat by puncturing your tube, your tires will eventually go flat if you don't pump them up. That's because the rubber is slightly porous and naturally loses air, even in as little time as overnight. You'll want to have a standard floor pump (not just a mini-pump) to inflate your tires with on a regular basis. I make it a habit to pump up my tires before just about every ride, or at least every other ride. A good pump will have a gauge that tells you your tire pressure, and many also have convenient markings right on the gauge indicating the appropriate pressure for road, mountain, and hybrid bikes.

LUBE

Chain lube reduces the friction of metal on metal that can grind down and wear out your bike's drivetrain prematurely. It also helps keep your bike pedaling quietly and shifting smoothly. There are many types of lubes for all sorts of riding conditions. I like "self-cleaning" varieties, which means the lube acts like a solvent that cleans the chain of debris and old lube while it lubricates. (See "Love Your Drivetrain," page 294 for more on how to lube that chain properly.)

TIRE LEVERS

You can't fix a flat if you can't get the tire off the rim. And though it's sometimes possible to do it with your bare hands, it's *far* easier with a set of tire levers. The mechanics I know like Mavic levers because they have a broad, flat blade and rigid plastic build that make them kind to tires, tubes, and rims, yet still effective for peeling off stubbornly tight tires.

HEX KEYS

Also known as Allen wrenches, these are a must-have for any avid cyclist.

Bicycle-specific toolmakers make sets, but good-quality metric keys from a hardware store work fine. Bondhus ($20) is a popular brand, known for its often-copied ball-shaped tip, which allows you to easily spin bolts from an angle when access is limited. Get the following wrench sizes: 1.5, 2, 2.5, 3, 4, 5, 6, 8, and 10 millimeters. These will work with tiny setscrews on suspension-fork adjuster knobs, crank arm fixing bolts, and everything else.

TORX KEYS

You definitely still need your hex keys, but there's another type of hardware taking over the cycling world called Torx bolts that are shaped more like stars than hexagons. Disc brake rotor hardware is nearly all Torx already, and Campagnolo uses Torx on many of its newest components, as do SRAM for its XX group and FSA for its chainring bolts. Three sizes—T-10, T-25, and T-30—are all you need for now. Park Tool makes a folding set (the TWS-2, $19) that has these sizes and more.

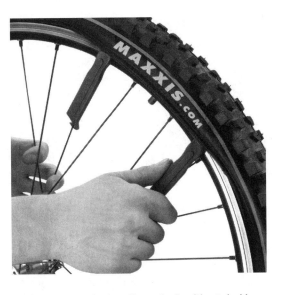

Tire levers let you change a flat on the fly without pinching your fingers and destroying your nails.

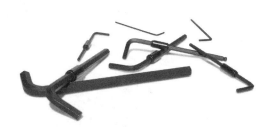

A good set of Allen wrenches are a must for keeping the bolts on your bike nice and tight.

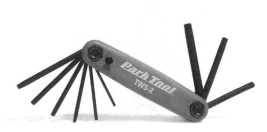

A good tool can keep all your wrenches in one place.

MULTI-TOOL

Mentioned earlier, but it bears repeating: A good multi-tool can mean the difference between making a swift, easy midride adjustment or repair and suffering with poorly working equipment or, worse, whipping out your cell phone and waiting for a ride home. Always carry a palm-sized workshop like the Lezyne RAP 13 ($25), which boasts eight sizes of hex and Torx keys, a Phillips screwdriver, a chain tool, and even spoke wrenches.

SHOCK PUMP

If mountain biking is your thing, you'll need a shock pump, which, as it sounds, is a pump that allows you to put air in your suspension fork and rear shock. You won't need to use it as much as your floor pump for your tires, but it's still useful to have one of your own to keep your suspension set to the proper psi (more on this later). One that's popular with mechanics is the Fox Digital High Pressure Shock Pump, which can hit pressures between zero and 300 psi. At less than 100 psi, it measures in increments of half a pound; at more than 100, it measures in 1-psi increments. The pressure is shown on an easy-to-read display, the body is made from durable aluminum, and it features a hose that swivels 360 degrees. If you overinflate, a pressure release button lets you back off. The digital readout displays in psi, bars, kilopascals, and kilograms per square centimeter, and it shuts off automatically after 1 minute of inactivity.

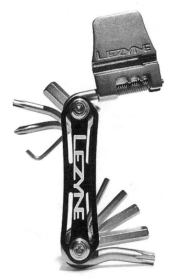

One good multitool can be all you need for most basic maintenance.

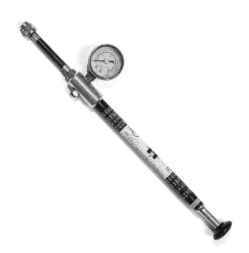

If you ride a mountain bike with suspension, you'll want a shock pump to keep your fork and rear shock inflated to the proper pressure.

Fast Flat Fixes

It's a fact: You will get a flat tire in your lifetime. So be prepared. All you need to get yourself out of a jam and back on the roll is a mini-pump (or another type of inflation device, such as a CO_2 cartridge), a spare tube or patch kit, tire levers, and a little patience. When your ride goes flat, here's what to do.

REMOVE THE TIRE

Hook the rounded end of one tire lever under the bead (the outer edge) of the tire to unseat it. Hook the other end onto a spoke to hold the lever in place and to keep the unseated tire from popping back into the rim. Hook the rounded end of the second lever under the bead next to the first and walk it around the tire and rim clockwise until one side of the tire is off the rim. For particularly tight tires, a third lever might be necessary to fully pry the tire from the rim.

FIND THE CULPRIT

Remove the tube and pump air into it to find the leak. Two holes side by side is a pinch flat—the tube got pinched between the tire and rim. A single hole was most likely caused by a sharp object such as a thorn or a piece of glass. Carefully run your fingers along the inside of the tire to make sure the foreign object is no longer there. If you don't, it could cause another flat.

IF YOU PATCH

Clean the punctured area of the tube with an alcohol prep pad and roughen the surface with an emery cloth or fine-grit sandpaper. For a glueless patch, simply stick it over the hole and press firmly. For a patch that requires glue, apply a thin layer of glue to the tube and the patch. Wait for the glue to get tacky, then apply the patch and press firmly until it adheres. If you don't patch, stuff the tube in your bag and fix it when you get home. It could be good for another season or more of use.

INSTALL THE TUBE

Inflate either your patched or new tube just a little, until it holds its shape, and then insert it into the tire. With the valve stem installed straight, work the tire back into the rim with your hands by rolling the bead away from yourself. (Do not use levers to reseat the tire, as you could puncture the tube.) When you get to the valve stem, tuck both sides of the tire bead low into the rim, then push upward on the stem to get the tube up inside the tire. Inflate completely, checking that the bead is seated correctly.

CUT TIRE OR RIPPED SIDEWALL

When the tire tears, the inner tube usually pops through the gash and then explodes. To fix this, besides installing a new tube, you need to boot—reinforce—the tire. Anything that will withstand the pressure of the tube in the tire will work as a boot. Mylar wrappers from gels and nutrition bars, as well as duct tape, even folded paper money can do the trick. Locate the cut in the tire (and mark it somehow if you can, for easy reference), then remove one side of the tire from the rim and replace the punctured tube with a fresh one. Put enough air in the tube to give it shape, then tuck the boot inside the tire so it covers the hole. The semi-inflated tube should hold it in place. Press the rest of the tire back on the rim, then inflate the tube enough to hold your weight and allow you to ride. Don't forget to replace the tire when you get home.

TLC to Maintain the Machine

Bikes require very little maintenance to keep them rolling along smoothly. Much of it you can do yourself with a little know-how. Here is what you need to know.

LOVE YOUR DRIVETRAIN

A friend of mine once wisely described the drivetrain (the chain and gears) as the bike's kitchen—even if the rest of the house is a mess, you want that area clean. Same is true for your bike. It might not look nice to have dust and dirt on the frame, but it really won't hurt anything. A dirty chain, however, can lead to rough shifting and shorten the life span of your drivetrain. So if you do nothing else, keep your chain clean.

Complicated methods abound: Remove the chain and soak it overnight; disassemble and clean each roller with a cotton swab; do something else involving pipe cleaners and a toxic solvent. I believe in making things simple. So try this lazy chain cleaner's process. Buy a chain cleaner such as Park Tool's Cyclone Chain Scrubber and fill it with Pedro's Oranj Peelz Citrus Degreaser. Attach the device to your chain, turn the crank 15 revolutions, and let the brushes scrub away grime (shown). Remove the chain cleaner and wipe the chain dry with a clean rag. No chain cleaner? Spray Finish Line Speed Degreaser onto the chain, focusing on small sections at a time (it evaporates quickly), and wipe clean with a dry rag. Apply lube when you're done.

How much and what kind? Depends on the conditions you ride in. If you ride on wet roads or muddy trails, you should opt for a wet lube, which has a thicker consistency so it won't wash away in a downpour. For more arid conditions, try a thinner, dry lube. Buy one of each so you're ready for any weather, but thoroughly clean your chain before switching.

Many lubes come in squirt bottles, which allow you to deliver a precise dose to each link of your chain. Less common (and sometimes less effective) are aerosol spray-ons, which disperse the lube into every nook and cranny. Be careful not to accidentally coat your rims or rotors, which could impair braking.

Lube your chain about every 100 miles or whenever your bike gets wet. For every minute you spend greasing it, spend 2 holding a rag lightly against both sideplates of the links as you spin the chain backward. Excess oil attracts dirt, and over time that dirt will work its way to the moving parts inside, leaving you with a

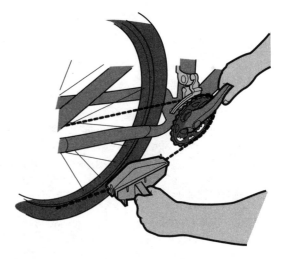

Built-up grit and grime increases the wear and tear on your gears. Clean your drivetrain regularly, especially after riding in the rain.

gritty mess that creates almost as much damage as no lube at all. With proper care, your chain should last 1,500 to 2,000 miles.

KEEP YOUR TIRES INFLATED

Proper tire pressure lets your bike roll quickly, ride smoothly, and fend off flats. Narrow tires need more air pressure than wide ones: Road tires typically require 80 to 130 psi, mountain tires 30 to 50 psi, and hybrid tires 50 to 70 psi. To find your ideal pressure, start in the middle of these ranges, then factor in your body weight. The more you weigh, the higher your pressure needs to be. For example, if a 165-pound rider uses 100 psi on his road bike, a 200-pound rider should run closer to 120 psi, and a 130-pound rider could get away with 80 psi. Never go above or below the manufacturer's recommended pressures.

Sounds easy right? It is. But I have more than one friend who has confessed to me that she has never inflated her own tires and makes her husband do it, which is all well and good, but if he's not around, she doesn't ride. And frankly, that's not all well and good. So in case you've never done it, here's how it's done.

There are two kinds of valves on tubes: Presta (found on most bikes) and Schrader (the kind found on your car tires). They're different sizes, and most pumps will have a setting for each. For the Presta valve, you need to unscrew the top nut and give it a little tap with your finger to open it up and ready it for inflating. Then install the pump head onto the valve and lock it in place (there is generally a lever or switch) and pump to the desired pressure. After you're done, unlock the pump head and pull it off straight, so you don't bend the valve. Then screw the top nut tight. A Schrader valve is inflated the same way, but you don't need to open and close it; it does it automatically.

KEEP YOUR SHIFTING SMOOTH

Over time—especially if your bike is new—your cables can stretch, causing sloppy shifting. And what good is a clean chain if it jumps around and skips gears? With your bike in a repair stand, shift to the smallest cog. Turn the barrel adjuster on the rear derailleur one-half turn clockwise (shown on page 295). Then, as you rotate your pedals, shift once. If the chain doesn't jump to

Tubeless Technology

If you're a mountain biker, running tubeless tires (tires that are sealed to the rims sans tubes and that use a liquid sealant to self patch small punctures) is a game changer. They allow you to drop your pressure for greater traction without pinch flatting. But they're not maintenance free. Routinely inspect your sidewalls for wear and tear (too worn tires tear easily) and make sure the sealant inside them is fresh (it dries over time). Simply put your ear by the wheel and shake it (off the bike, of course). If you hear sloshing, you're good to go. Silence, take it to the shop for a sealant recharge. They can also help you buy what you need to do it yourself at home.

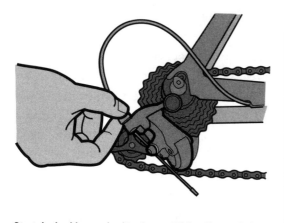

Stretched cables can lead to sloppy shifting. If your chain is skipping around on the cassette, you can tune it back in line with a twist of the barrel adjuster.

the next cog, make another half-turn. If the chain starts to jump two cogs for every one shift, you went too far. Back it down a half-turn. Don't turn the barrel adjuster more than halfway at a time. You may end up with too much tension, which will make your shifting just as bad or worse than when you started.

CLEAN CAREFULLY

I did a race in West Virginia once where they offered a bike cleaning service. I handed my bike to a nice young man wearing waders and he handed it back to me 30 seconds later after blasting it with a pressure hose. When I got home and pulled the bike out a few days later, I couldn't budge the cranks—the whole drivetrain was seized. That's because he'd blasted through the seals in the bottom bracket, driving in the grit and pushing out the grease, leaving the bearings inside to rust. The take-home lesson: Spray down your bike gently. Use

Tools to Carry on a Ride

I asked my friend and *Bicycling* mechanic Mike Yozell what tools of the trade he carries on every ride in case of emergency. The list may seem long, but he showed me how neatly it fits into a wallet-sized bag that he tucks into the center pocket of his jersey. I confess I don't always carry a patch kit or zip ties, but I do generally have the rest on hand, especially when I'm riding alone, because you just never know.

➤ **A laminated card with emergency contact numbers and personal identification**

➤ **18-piece multi-tool that includes a chain breaker and 8- and 10-millimeter hex wrenches**

➤ **4 zip ties**

➤ **2 tire irons (I use King Cage titanium tire levers)**

➤ **A patch kit (I like Rema Tip Top) into which I also put a 40-millimeter valve extender so I can inflate deep rims, and SRAM quick links for 9-, 10-, and 11-speed chains**

➤ **$20, in denominations of $10, $5, and five ones; if you only bring one bill and have to use it to boot your tire, forget about a midride lunch or post-ride espresso**

a hose running not much harder than your granny's watering can. Or use a bucket with soapy water, a sponge, and an assortment of brushes—even old dishwashing scrubbers and toothbrushes.

CHAPTER 32

Shop Talk

BICYCLING RECENTLY DID AN ONLINE SURVEY THAT REVEALED that 86 percent of their women readers enjoyed shopping in bike shops. I confess to being extremely pleasantly surprised. For a long time, way too many (but not all) bike shops were the equivalent of "no girls allowed" clubhouses, where women walked in and got condescending glances and cold shoulders.

About 10 years ago, I witnessed firsthand how my friend Joyce, who was clearly very inexperienced but had about five grand burning a hole in her pocket, was treated at a shop run by snobby racer dudes. They barely acknowledged her and seemed almost annoyed by her questions. We walked out and kept pounding the pavement until we found a shop where they greeted her with a smile and spent time fielding her questions and helping her find the right bike—which she promptly bought, shelling out all five grand for the bike as well as shorts, jersey, saddlebag, tools, and pump.

So I was happy to see so many women were clearly having positive experiences. But then I read through the survey comments and saw that those who did not enjoy shopping at bike shops were unhappy because they'd received treatment similar to what Joyce got at the snobby shop.

Among positive comments like "Endless possibilities," "Learn a lot talking to the employees," and "You can try everything," were more than a few like this: "They make me feel dumb and insecure. Also the (usually male) employees are always eager to talk down to me and assume I don't know anything just because I don't have their same priorities (expensive racing bikes)" and "I found a local family-owned and -run bike shop where I feel comfortable. I don't get 'the looks' [from] the employees because I'm female and big."

Shop Around

The take-home message is that though bike shops have definitely gotten better at welcoming women, there are still some bad apples in the bunch. And frankly, it's not necessarily just women those shops treat poorly. It tends to be anyone who doesn't seem "core" (read: not a racer, a hipster, fit, or cool) enough. I've heard complaints from many men who have gotten their unfair share of attitude and nonexistent service.

Making matters worse is that a shop that caters mostly to a male clientele simply may not carry bikes in your size if you're a small woman. "I decided I wanted a road bike with at least Shimano 105 components. With $1,500 in my pocket (not a lot when it comes to bikes, but it was a lot to me), I went to every bike shop in Lincoln, Nebraska, where I live, and was ignored at each AND there was not a single bike I could try in my size—I'm 5 feet, 4 inches tall," said Valerie Hynes Wolf. Though it was hardly convenient, she made the trip to Omaha, where she found two shops that stocked a fleet of bikes including her size, treated her well, and were helpful.

The right bike shop is like a community center for cyclists. You go there and feel at home, meet other riders, hang out and shoot the breeze, maybe even sit down and do a little work if they have Wi-Fi. You should feel comfortable and confident there. Here's how to find that home away from home and how to make the most of your bike shop relationship.

TEST THE WATERS

Just as you would test-drive a car, "try a shop before you commit," advises Liza LeClaire, chief operating officer of Wheel and Sprocket, a retail chain in Wisconsin and Illinois. Walk in and browse around. Make small talk with the employees. Join a shop ride, take a maintenance class, or just stop by and browse. Buy from the store where you have the best connection and experience, she says.

If you plan on making a major purchase—like a bike—at this shop, ask lots of questions before you even get to the bike part. It will help determine what level of service you can expect. Here are a few to jot down and take with you.

1. WILL YOU BUILD ME A TEST RIDE?

Always ride before you buy. If a shop doesn't have your size on display, ask to have a sample built (that's what putting all the components on a bare frame is called). Or, test a similar model by that brand; product lines often share geometries, or even whole frame designs.

2. WHAT ABOUT PARTS SWAPS?

Not all saddles and stems work for everyone. A shop should be willing to swap a part here and there to ensure proper fit, and it may offer upgrades at a discount.

3. DO YOU USE A FIT SERVICE?

A good shop uses a recognized fit service, like Fit Kit, TruFit, Retül, BG Fit (Body Geometry Fit by Specialized), or another reputable fit system. A fit session will cost between $40 and $200, depending on the complexity of service you want, but it can be a worthwhile investment. At the very least the shop should be knowledgeable about bike fit and help set you up so you are 100 percent comfortable out of the gate.

4. IS THERE A FIT GUARANTEE?

Some elements of bike fit, such as the reach to the bars, bar height, and cleat position, manifest themselves only over time. Is the shop prepared to help you dial in those issues as part of your bike-buying investment? Look for a written guarantee that lasts at least 30 days.

WARNING SIGNS

Most bike shops are great, but beware if you encounter any of these things.

THEY SAY NO TEST RIDES. A few shops have stopped offering test rides for liability reasons. We recommend steering clear of them because not trying out a bike could lead to potential future headaches on fit issues.

YOUR OBJECTIONS ARE OVERRULED. If a salesperson insists a frame is the right size and you think it's not, seek a second opinion at another shop. The first shop may be trying to get rid of old inventory. A key tip-off here is having just a few bikes out as floor stock, especially if you're considering a discounted model from last year.

YOU GET ATTITUDE, OR IGNORED. If the salesperson seems uninterested in you, go elsewhere.

How to Buy a Bike

So you know where you want to buy and, hopefully based on what you learned from taking the quiz "What Bike Should I Buy?" on page 32, what (or at least pretty close to what) you want to buy. Now the question is how to go about buying it. Don't worry, it's nowhere near as stressful as the experience you have at haggle-happy car dealerships. But there are still a few tips to know.

KNOW THE BASICS

A bike shop can help you narrow down your selection to the perfect bike if you can answer basic bike-buying questions. They will ask questions much like the ones in the quiz on page 32, so be prepared to answer the following. Commit the answers to memory before you go.

—What will you (or do you) use your bike for?

—When, where, and how often will you ride?

—How much can you spend?

This exercise should help you—and the shop staff—focus on your needs, whether you're buying your first bike, or new pedals or bar tape for your existing ride.

RIDE BIKES

If you're buying a bicycle, you should test-ride a few. (If the shop doesn't allow this, go to one that does.) Touch and feel accessories so you know exactly what you're getting. "Turn on lights, try on shoes, turn shorts inside out," says LeClaire.

BE ASSERTIVE

It's easy to feel put off by shop employees who rattle off jargon. Even helpful, friendly staff can unwittingly talk over your head, making you feel dumb when that's not their intention. "Don't be afraid to ask them to slow down and speak in language you understand," says bicycle retail consultant Ray Keener. Most will be happy to help. "Remember that you are in control of the situation," Keener says. After all, you have the money.

PLAY FAIR

Your local bike shop is not the place to haggle. With so many online outlets competing with their business, brick-and-mortar retailers must keep their prices competitive. Profit margins on bike sales are razor thin. It's not uncommon for a shop to net more money on the extras—helmet, pedals, computer, and so on—than on the bike sale itself. For this reason, dealers are often more willing to throw in a free seat bag or bottle cage than to give you a deal on the bike. Service is an area where you can seek out value: It's common for shops to provide a year of free basic adjustments on your new bike, so it's worth asking for this if your shop offers less.

Another way to potentially save some cash is by joining your local advocacy group. Many shops discount their prices for members. If you really don't like the deal offered by a shop, then quietly go elsewhere. You may find a better price in a nearby town, but remember, it's not always worth driving an hour to save a few bucks. In the end, having a good local bike shop will save you time and money on service and any warranty issues. Shops tend to go the extra mile for you if they know you bought the bike there (and it doesn't hurt to tip your mechanic!).

Finally, eBay is good for many purchases, but bikes aren't one of them. Yes, it's possible to buy a bike online (though *Bicycling* doesn't recommend it). And many reputable sellers offer new and used bikes online, if that's the way you really want to go. But steer clear of ads that are vague or downright shady, like one we saw on eBay that read, "not recommended for the Pittsburgh area," presumably because that's where the bike had been stolen. When you venture online, you're on your own. If you know your preferred frame angles, top tube length, and stem and handlebar sizes, you might find a barely used dream ride and save hundreds. It's happened. But if those measurement terms mean nothing to you, visit a bike shop for help. Otherwise, you'll get a bargain online but spend twice the savings trying to make the bike fit, and it may never feel right. We see that happen all the time. Also, please don't test a bike at your local shop and turn around and buy it online. That's just bad juju.

SHOP SMART

Just because you shouldn't haggle with your shop doesn't mean you can't get a good bargain on a new bike. Like shoes, cars, and clothing, bikes are seasonal. New models arrive on the bike shop sales floor each year, typically in the fall, as the riding season winds down. This is the best time to look for deals, because shops don't want soon-to-be-year-old inventory lingering through the slower winter months. While hot models in popular sizes will sell out over the summer, you may get lucky and find last year's model at a discount, but do your homework before buying: Models often get dramatic redesigns only every few years, so if the new model just has different paint and minor parts tweaks, you'll save on last year's bike. But if the new model has big frame changes or parts upgrades, then it can be worth paying for the new model. Beware of bikes that are more than a few seasons old. Advances in frame materials and component technology happen quickly, so a seemingly great deal may be only an average one.

Acknowledgments

I APPRECIATE THE SUPPORT AND ASSISTANCE OF THE FOLLOWING PEOPLE in compiling this book:

Matt Allyn	Emily Furia
Andy Applegate	Cristina Goyanes
Kelly Bastone	James Herrera
Neil Bezdek	Joe Lindsey
Chris Cassidy	Lou Mazzante
Ben Christopher	Jen Sherry
Alan Cote	Jenny Skorcz
Kim Cross	Anne Stein
Brian Fiske	Alex Stieda
Leah Flickinger	Susi Wunsch
Paige Fowler	Allison Young

Also, thanks to you, the reader, for perusing these pages. Keep pedaling and always enjoy the ride.

Index

Boldface page references indicate photographs. <u>Underscored</u> references indicate boxed text or tables.

A ctive Hydration drink, 220
Active rest, 152
Acute Recovery drink, 223
Adrenaline, 6
Adventure Cycling Association, 4, 278
Aerobic enzymes, 143
Air brake, 96
Alcohol, avoiding while cycling, 104
"All-arounder" bikes, 21, **21**
Allen, Hunter, 146, 224–25, 229
Allen wrenches, 291, **291**
Aluminum bike material, <u>36</u>
Anaerobic system, 142
Ankle pain, preventing, <u>42</u>
"Ankling," 79–80, 91–92
Anthony, Susan B., <u>xi</u>, xii
Applegate, Andy, 84–85, 89, 96
Arm warmers/knee warmers, 56–57, **56**
Avocado, 209

B ackpacks, 271
Back pain, preventing, <u>43, 160</u>
Base layer clothing, 57–58, **57**
BCAAs, 207, 210, 219–20
"Being doored," 102
Belgium bike tour, 280–81
Bell peppers, <u>222</u>
Belly breathing, 86
Berries, <u>222</u>
Beta-alanine, 243
Bibs, 50
Get There by Bike (iPhone app), 272

Bike fit
aero, 38–39
basic, 39–40
bike shop and services for, 299
detailed, 39
fitter for, finding, 40
frame size and, 41
guarantee, 299
handlebar reach and, 29, 41, 44
importance of, 38–39
pain and, avoiding, <u>42–43</u>
pedals and, 44
performance of bike and, 39
recommendation for, 40
saddles and, 28–29, 41, 44–46
seat height and, 41
stem and, 30
Bikes. *See also* Bike fit; *specific type or parts of*
brakes, 29–30, <u>79</u>
buying, 26–27, <u>32–35</u>, 36–37, <u>37</u>, 298–301
carry-on for, 271
checking before century ride, 196
cleaning, 296
cranks, 29
current, 16
cycling needs and, 16
cyclocross, 22–24, **23**, 123, 126
gravel, 22, 24–25, **25**
for gravel grinding, 128
grips, 29
handlebars, 29
hybrid, 25–26, **25**
locks for, 62, **62**, <u>272</u>

maintenance and repair of, 289–92, <u>293</u>, 294–96, **294**, **295**, <u>296</u>
materials for constructing, 17, <u>36</u>
mountain, 20–22, **20**, **21**, **22**
performance of, fit and, 39
racks for, 271
retrofitting, 38
road, 17–19, **17**, **18**, 25, **25**
shifters, 29
stem, 30
suspension, 30
track, 134
variety of, 15
weight of, 28, 87
women-specific design, 26–31, 113
Bike shops, navigating, 297–303
Blood pressure, 212
Blood sugar levels, 10, 285
Blumenthal, James, 7
Body fat, 143, 225. *See also* Weight loss
Body image and cycling, 6–7
Body temperature and sleep, 155
Body weight and cycling technique, 83–84
Bomber bikes, 21–22, **22**
Bonci, Leslie, 153, 204, 240, 242
Bone density, 159, 261
Booties, 58, **58**
Bottle cage, 60, **60**
Brain diseases, preventing, 9
Brain growth and cycling, 9
Brakes, 29–30, <u>79</u>
Braking, 78–79, <u>79</u>, 90–91, 96, 114

Branched-chain amino acids
(BCAAs), 207, 210, 219–20
Breast cancer, preventing, 10
Breathing, 86, 89, 94
Brick roads, 106
Brinton, David, 105–6
Brown, John, 30–31, 37–39, 44

Cadence, 77, 86
Caffeine, 155, 219–20, 244–45, 245
Calories, 204–5, 230–31
California wine country bike tour, 280
Cannabinoids, 7
Cantrell, Carl, 92
Carbohydrates, 152, 205–6, 206, 211, 260
Carbon fiber bike material, 36
Carry-on, bike, 271
Carver, Todd, 79–81
Casa, Douglas, 218–19
Cassette gear, 76
Catabolic reaction, 207
Catcalls while road riding, 105
Celery, 222
Celiac disease, 215
Century rides, 195–99, 197, 198
Chafing, 264
Chainline, 77
Chain mark, avoiding, 74
Chainrings, 76
Chains, avoiding dropped, 77–78
Challa, Shekhar, 239
Chamois, 50
Chamois creams, 265
"Change, the," 258–61
Charity Navigator, 274, 276
Charity rides, 185, 273–76, 276
Children, cycling with, 65–66, 282–85,
285
Chip-sealed roads, 105
Chocolate, dark, 209
Chocolate milk, 152, 211
Christie, Brian, 9
Chromoly bike material, 36
Cleaning bike, 296
Cleat tension, 60, 82
Climbing hills, 84–88, 84, 96–97
Clipless pedals and cleats, 44, 59–60,
59, 81
Clothing, x, 48. See also specific type
Club Ride undies, 270
CO₂ cartridge pump, 61–62, 293
Cobbled roads, 106
Cold bath, 154
Colds, 239
Commuting by bike, 4, 19, 19, 67, 68,
269–72, 271, 272
Compression clothing, 154
Computer, cycling, 62–63, 63
Cornering bike, 78–79, 91–92, 91, 105

Cortisol, 6, 153, 244, 260
CPSC, 48
Cracks, danger of parallel, 106
Cranks, 29
Crashing bike, 118, 192, 283
Cravings, food, xii
Credit card touring, 278
Criterium ("crits"), 186–87
Cross-country (XC) bikes, 21, 21
Cross-country (XC) races, 188–89
Cross-training, 257
Cruiser bikes, 26, 26
Cucumber, 222
Cup, the, 253
Curves, flattening road, 92
Cycling. See also Commuting by bike;
Racing; Touring by bike
body image and, 6–7
brain growth and, 9
with children, 65–66, 282–85, 285
empowerment and, 5–6
energy levels and, 7–8
with family, 65–66, 282–85, 285
fatalities from, 100
freedom and, xi, 1–2, 4–5
groups, 69
growth of sport, 11
happiness and, 7
health and, general, 9–10
in heat, 212, 259
historical perspective of, xi
Internet and, 69, 272
lifestyle, 64–69
mental acuity and, 8–9
mood and, 7
motivation for, 68–69
planning ride and, 65
reasons for, 1
safety of, 100–101
self-awareness and, 10–11
sexual function and, 263–65
sleep and, 8
social media and, 69
socialness of, 93, 140
stress management and, 6
support for, 65–66
3-foot laws and, 101
time for, selecting, 66–68
for transportation, 267
weight loss and, 224–25
"Cycling kit." See Clothing
Cyclists' characteristics, ix. See also
Women cyclists
Cyclocross races
bikes for, 22–25, 23, 123, 126
describing, 190
dismounting bike in, 124, 124
experience of, 123–24
fun of, 123
historical perspective of, 122–23

hydration during, 126
pit crew and, 126
portage in, 124–25, 124
practice laps before, 125
remounting bike in, 125, 125
shouldering bike in, 125, 125
tires of bike and, 126
warmup before, 126
women cyclists in, increase of, 4
Cyclosportif races, 184–85

Davison, Lea, 112–13, 118
Dehydration, 212
Dempsey Challenge, 275
Derailleur, front, 76–77
Descending hills, 88–91, 91
Dietary fats, 10, 208–9
Diet. See Nutrition; specific food
Digestive problems, 239
Disc brakes, 30
Dismounting bike in cyclocross, 124, 124
DivaCup, 253
Dogs, danger of, 107
Donovan, Leigh, 113, 115, 117
Dopamine, 214
Double riding, 97–98, 97
Double-sided pedals, 60
Downhill bikes, 21–22, 22
Downhill races, 190
Downhills, 88–91, 91
Drafting, 186
Drills, cycling, 92, 129
Drivetrain maintenance and repair,
294–95, 294
Drop-offs and mountain biking, 119–21
Dropped chains, avoiding, 77–78
Duct tape, 62

Easy interval training, 147–48
Eating. See Nutrition
Eating disorders, 231
Einstein, Albert, 8–9
Electrical muscle stimulation (EMS),
155
Electrolytes, 198, 217–18
Emergency stops, 79
Emery, Brent, 74
Empowerment and cycling, 5–6
EMS, 155
Endorphins, 7
Endurance races, 189–90
Endurance training, 147
Enduro races, 21, 190
Energy levels, 7–8, 97, 142
Enthusiast/endurance bikes, 18, 18
Equipment, x, 13–14, 47–49, 54, 59.
See also specific type
Estrogen, 209–10

Evening bike rides, 67
Exercise. *See also* Cycling; Flexibility
    training; Strength training
    aerobic, 9–10
    brain and, 8–9
    breast cancer prevention and, 10
    foam roller, 172, **180–82**, <u>180–82</u>
    menstrual cycle and, 252
    plyometrics, 170–71, **170–71**
    triglyceride levels and, 10

Family, cycling with, 65–66, 282–85,
    <u>285</u>
Fast-twitch muscle fibers, 142–43, 158
Fat bikes, 22, **22**
Fatigue and sedentary lifestyle, 7–8
Fatty acids, 10
Feathering brakes, 90–91, 96
Female anatomy, 14, 262–65
Fermented foods, 215
Fitness, 137–39. *See also* Flexibility
    training; Strength training;
    Training
"Fixies" (single-gear track-style
    bikes), <u>31</u>
Fix-it kit, 61–62, **61**, 289–92, <u>296</u>
Flat bar road bikes, 25, **25**
Flat pedals, 59
Flat tires, 61–62, 287–88, <u>293</u>
Fleshner, Monika, 6
Flexibility training
    exercises, 174–79, **174–79**, **180–82**,
    <u>180–82</u>
    with foam roller, 172, **180–82**,
    <u>180–82</u>
    importance of, 173
    muscles and, 173
    power position and, 173
    range of motion and, 172–73
    science of stretching and, <u>180</u>
"Float," cleat, 60
Floor pump, 290, **290**
Flu, 239
Foam rollers, <u>154</u>, 172, **180–82**,
    <u>180–82</u>
Follicular hormone phase, 209
Foodborne illness, 214
Food labels, reading, 212
Foot, dominant, 74–75
Foot pain, preventing, <u>42</u>
Fox Digital High Pressure Shock
    Pump, 292
Frames, bike, 27–29, 41
France bike tour, 281
Freedom and cycling, <u>ix</u>, 1–2, 4–5
Freeride mountain bikes, 21–22, **22**
Friel, Joe, 87–88, 205–6, 208–9, 228
Fruits, 204–5, <u>206</u>. *See also specific type*
Fundraising for charity rides, 275

Garmin GPS, 63
Gear, x, 13–14, 47–49, 54, 59. *See also*
    specific type
Gears, 75–76, **75**. *See also* Shifters;
    Shifting
Gender differences, cycling, ix–xii, 13–14,
    183. *See also* Women cyclists
Getzin, Andrew, 212
Gibbons, Michael, 127
Gidus, Tara, <u>222</u>
Glasses, 53–54, **54**, 54
Glass, J. David, 7
Gloves, 53, **53**
"Glueless" tire patches, 61
Gluten-free diet, 212, 215
Golden Gate Park cycling route, <u>285</u>
Google Maps, 272
GPS units, 63, **63**
Grains, 207, <u>222</u>
Gran fondo races, 184–85
Gravel bikes, 22, 24–25, **25**, 128, 130–31,
    190
Gravel grinders, 24, 127–31
Gravelly roads and corners, 105
Gravel World Championships, 129
Great Smoky Mountains National
    Park cycling route, <u>285</u>
Grips, handlebar, 29
Group riding, 93–95, 97–99, **98–99**,
    199. *See also* Pacelining
Guzman, Anne, 21, 214–15, 231

Hair issues and cycling, 269–70
Half wheeling, avoiding, 98
Handlebars, 29, 41, 44, 102–3, 264
Hand pain, preventing, <u>43</u>
Hand signals, directional, 103, **103**
Happiness and cycling, 7
Health, cycling and general, 9–10
Heart rate, 85, 141–42, 144
Heart rate monitor, 85, 144–46
Heat, cycling in, 212, 259
Helmet, 48–49, **49**
Herbal Essences Style Refreshing
    Mist, 270
Hex keys, 291, **291**
HGH, 155
High-intensity interval training
    (HIIT), 143
Hilly Bill Roubaix (West Virginia)
    race, 130
Hinton, Pamela, 218
Hip pain, preventing, <u>43</u>
Hogg, Steve, 38–39
Holding a straight line while road
    biking, 102
"Hole shot," 189
Holland bike tour, 280–81
Holz, Scott, 173

Hormones, x, xii, 6, 209–11, 214
Hot flashes, 259
Hot spots in foot, <u>42</u>, 44
Hughes, Dan, 130–31
Human growth hormone (HGH),
    155
Hybrid bikes, 25–26, **25**
Hydration
    caffeine and, 155, 219–20
    during century ride, 198
    during cyclocross, 126
    drinks, 152, 208, 219–21, 223
    electrolytes and, 198, 217–18
    foods for, <u>222</u>
    heat and, 259
    hyponatrema and, avoiding, 218
    importance of, 202, 216–17
    while pacelining, 97
    perspiration and, 217–19, <u>221</u>
    pregnant cyclists and, 256–57
    protein and, 219
    during recovery, 152
    sports drinks, 219–21, 223
    thirst and, 217
    for women cyclists, 220–21, 223
Hydration pack, 58–59, **58**
Hyponatremia, 218

Ibuprofen, <u>243</u>
Ignosh, Ray, 95–96
Imagery, 11
Individual pursuit races, 135
Inflammation, 154, 263
Injuries, gender differences, xi
Inner tube, 61, **61**
Insomnia, health risks of, 8
Internet and cycling, 69, 272
Intersections, navigating, 98–99,
    <u>104</u>
Interval training, xi, 147–51, <u>149</u>
Ironman triathlons, 262
Iron supplement, 211
Ischial tuberosities, 30, 45, 264

Jackets, 55–56, **55**
Jerseys, 49–50, **49**
Johnson, Evan, 218
Jumping drills, 170–71, **170–71**

Katy Trail cycling route, <u>285</u>
Keirin races, 134
KIND bars, 215
Kings Gap downhill, 88–89
"Kitchen sink" supplements, 242
Knee pain, preventing, <u>42</u>, 80
Kovarik, Chris, 118
Kramer, Arthur, 9

Lactate, 142
Lactate threshold (LT), 144, 146–47
Lactic acid, 147, 154
Layman, Donald K., 207, 260
League of American Bicyclists
    statistics, 3, 11
LeMond, Greg, 81
Lentz, Douglas, 159
L'étape race, 184–85
Lettuce, 222
Leucine, 207, 210
Licenses, racing, 186
Lifestyle, cycling, 64–69. *See also*
    Commuting by bike
Locking retention system on helmet,
    49
Locks, bike, 62, **62**, 272
Long ride, 196, 197
Looking behind, 103
LT, 144, 146–47
Lubes, 290, **290**, 294
Lunch break bike rides, 66–67
Luteal phase, 209, 220

Macrobiotic diet, 215
Macronutrient foods, 260
Maintenance and repair of bikes,
    289–92, 293, 294–96, **294**,
    295, 296
MapMyRide (mobile phone app), 63
Marathon races, 189
Massage, 153, 154
Match sprint races, 134
Mavic levers, 291
Maximum heart rate (MHR), 141–42,
    145
Max training, 146
Max VO$_2$, 146
Meditation, 85
Melatonin, 155–56
Melons, 222
Menopause, xii, 258–61
Menstrual cycle, 211, 249–53
Mental acuity and cycling, 8–9
Metabolism, 142, 259
MHR, 141–42, 145
Microadjusting while pacelining, 96
Milk, 152, 207, 211
Minkin, Mary Jane, 254–55
Miss and out races, 134
Mitochondria, 143, 153
Mobile phone apps, 63, 272
Monounsaturated fatty acids
    (MUFAs), 209
Montana AIDS Vaccine ride, 273–74
Mood and cycling, 7
Morning bike rides, 66
Motivation for cycling, 68–69
Mountain bike races, 188–90, **188**

Mountain bikes, 20–22, **20**, **21**, 24, 31,
    115–18
Mountain bike shoes, **51**, 52, 60
Mountain biking
    better riders and, riding with, 117
    bike selection for, 115–18
    braking while, 114
    cornering while, 91, 118
    crashing while, 118
    drop-offs and, 119–21
    obstacles and, overcoming, 118, 119
    overthinking while, avoiding, 115
    pedaling while, 118
    position for, proper, 113–14
    relaxing while, 112, **113**, 118
    scanning ahead while, 113
    standing up while, 113–14
    strength training for, 117
    trails for, finding, 120
    weight shifts while, 114, 118, 120
    women cyclists and, 111–12
Mounting bike, 74
MS 150 ride, 273
MUFAs, 209
Multi-tool, 62, 292, **292**
Muscles, 142–43, 153, 154, 158, 173,
    207, 213
My Alibi undies, 270
Myerson, Adam, 124–25
MyNetDiary (mobile phone app), 225

Neck pain, preventing, 43
Neurons, growth of, 9
Neurotransmitters, 9
Nutrition. *See also specific food*
    balanced, 212–13
    calories and, 204–5
    carbohydrates, 152, 205–6, 206,
        211, 260
    for century ride, 196, 198
    cravings and, xii
    dietary fats, 10, 208–9
    for endurance rides, 210, 237
    evolving information on, 203
    food labels and, reading, 212
    during gravel grinders, 128, 131
    medical research on, 201–2
    during pacelining, 97
    pregnant cyclists and, 256–57
    preride, 210, 237
    protein, 152, 207–8, **208**, 211, 213, 260
    during recovery, **151**, 152–53
    during ride, 210, 237
    salt and, 210–12, 213, 218
    special diets, 212–15
    trial-and-error with, 203–4
    women cyclists and, 209–11
Nuts, 209
NuvaRing, 251

Obstacles, overcoming mountain
    biking, 118, 119
Oils, 209
Olives, 209
1X (one-by) shifters, 31
Open road races, 187
OptygenHP, 243–44
Osmo Nutrition, 223
Osteoporosis, 242, 261
Overlapping wheels, avoiding, 96
Overthinking while mountain biking,
    avoiding, 115

Pacelining, 94–99, **95**, **97**
Pacing while climbing hills, 85
Packing lists, 191, 281
Pack riding. *See* Group riding;
    Pacelining
Pads, menstrual, 253
Pain, bike fit and avoiding, 42–43
Paleo diet, 214
"Paperboy" move, 87
Park Tool's Cyclone Chain Scrubber,
    294
Partner, cycling, 129
Pasricha, Sant-Rayn, 211
Passing during race, 194
Patch kit, 61, **61**
Peat, Steve., 119–21
Pedaling, 74–77, 79–81, 80, **80**, 85–87,
    96, 98, 118
Pedals, 29, 44, 60, 75
Pedal systems, 59–60, **59**, 81–82
Pedro's Oranj Peelz Citrus
    Degreaser, 294
Pelvis, female, 14, 262–65
Perceived exertion, rate of, 85, 144,
    229, 230
Performance, 39, 154
Performance enhancers. *See* Special
    diets; Supplements
Period, menstrual, 211, 249–53
Perspiration, 217–19, 221
Phillips, Shane A., 153
Physique, female, x, 13–14
Pill, the, 250–51
Pink, Victoria, 74
Planning bike rides, 65
"Plush" bikes, 18, **18**
Plyometrics, 170–71, **170–71**
PMS, 251
Points races, 134–35
Portage in cyclocross, 124–25, **124**
Potholes, danger of, 106
PowerBar, 240
Power meter, 145–46
Power position, 85–86, 173
Power-to-weight ratio, 87–88
Pregnancy, 254–57

PreLoad Hydration product, 220–21, 223
Premenopause, 211
Presta valves, 295–96
"Primes" (prizes), 187
Probiotics, 239–40
Progesterone, 210
Progressive relaxation, 85
Protein, **151**, 152, 207–8, <u>208</u>, 211, 213, 219, 260
Pruitt, Andy, 30, 46
"Pull your parachute" position, 90

"Qigong climbing," 85
Quinoa, 207

"Race against the clock," 135, 185–86
"Race of truth, the," 135, 185–86
Racing. *See also specific race*
　advantages of, 183–84, **185**, 194
　bikes, 18, **18**
　clubs, <u>186</u>
　crashing during, <u>192</u>
　drafting and, 186
　fun of, 184
　gender differences in, 183
　learning from, 194
　licenses, <u>186</u>
　mountain bike, 188–90, **188**
　packing list, 191
　passing during, 194
　readiness on day of, 191–94
　road races, 184–87, **185**
　rules, <u>186</u>
　settling in, 192–94
　signing in before, 191–92
　teams, <u>186</u>
　warming up before, 191–92
Racks, bike, 271
Range of motion, 172–73
Ratcheting pedals, 118
Rate of perceived exertion (RPE), 85, 144, 229, <u>230</u>
Raw food diet, 214–15
Recessed cleat shoes, **51**, 52
Recovery drinks, 152, 208
Recovery from training, 151–57, **151**, <u>154</u>, <u>155</u>
Recreation bikes, 18, **18**
Relaxing while cycling, 85, 89, 91, 94, 112, 118
Remounting bike in cyclocross, 125, **125**
REM sleep, 156
Rest, 152. *See also* Recovery
Resting heart rate, 142
Retrofitting bikes, 38
Rhodiola, 244
"Right rear" mnemonic, 76–77

Riptide Cycling team, 6
Road bikes, 17–19, **17**, **18**, **19**, 25, **25**
Road biking
　"being doored" while, 102
　car lane and, riding in, 102
　courtesy and, showing, 103–4
　danger zones and, <u>104</u>
　dog issues while, <u>107</u>
　drinking alcohol and, avoiding, 104
　eye contact with car drivers and, 103
　front wheels of cars and, watching, 102
　handlebars and, holding, 102–3
　line and, holding, 102
　looking behind, 103
　low-traffic routes for, 104, 271–72
　mirrors and rear window of cars, scanning, 102
　on no-shoulder roads, 102
　pacelining and, 94–99, **95**, **97**
　paying attention and, 104
　riding single file, 103
　safety statistics on, 100–101
　sharing road and, 101–4, **103**
　signaling direction and, 103, **103**
　stoplights and, 102
Road hazards, 92, 97–99, <u>104</u>, 105–6, <u>105</u>, <u>107</u>
Roadkills, danger of, 106
Road races, 184–87, **185**
Rocks, navigating danger of, 106, 118
Rodale, Bob, 132
Rodale Corporate Challenge race, 132
Rolling out on bike, 74–75
Rotational weight, 30
RPE, 85, 144, 229, <u>230</u>
Ryan, Monique, 217, <u>222</u>

Saddlebag, 61
Saddles, 14, 28–30, 41, 44–46, 80
Saddle sores, 264
Salt, 210–12, <u>213</u>, 218
Sass, Cynthia, 204–6
Scanning ahead, <u>75</u>, 89–90, 92, 113, 131
Schrader valves, 296
Schwinn, Anna, 13–14, 26–27
Scratch races, 134
Seats. *See* Saddles
Seat tube angle, 28–29
Sedentary lifestyle, 7–8, 261
Seeds, 209
Self-awareness and cycling, 10–11
Self-massage, <u>154</u>
Serotonin, 214
Sexual function and cycling, 263–65
Sharing road with car drivers, 101–4, **103**
Shifters, 29, <u>31</u>, 296

Shifting, 76–78, 86–87, 89, 131
Shirts, 49–50, **49**
Shock pump, 292, **292**
Shoes, 51–53, **51**, <u>52</u>, 60
Shorts, 50–51, **50**, 264–65
Short track races, 189
Shouldering bike in cyclocross, 125, **125**
Sims, Stacy, 201, 210–11, 220, 223, 243–44, 259–61
Single-file road biking, 103
Single-sided pedals, 60
Single-speed bikes, <u>31</u>
Sit bones, 30, 45, 264
Skout Organic Trailbars, 215
Sleep, 8, 154–57, 261
Slippery conditions, 92, 105–6
Slowing down bike, 78–79, 90
Slow-twitch fibers, 143
Smith, Caroline, <u>221</u>
Social media and cycling, 69
Socks, 54–55, **55**
Sodium, 210–12, <u>213</u>, 218
Softcup, 253
Soft pedal, 96, 98
Soup, <u>222</u>
Special diets, 212–15
Specialized Venge bike, 15
Speed ride, 196, <u>197</u>
SportLegs, 244
Sports drinks, 219–21, 223
Sports-specific supplements, 242–45
Spray Finish Line Speed Degreaser, 294
Stage races, 187, 189
Standard shifters, <u>31</u>
Staring at wheel in front of you, avoiding, 95–96
Stationary trainers, 126, 257
Steady ride, 196, <u>197</u>
Steel bike material, <u>36</u>
Stem, bike, 30
Stevens, Evie, xii
Stieda, Alex, 78, 84, 89, 90–91, 128
Stopping bike, 78–79. *See also* Braking
Strava (mobile phone app), 63
Strength training
　bone density and, 159
　controversy surrounding, 158–59
　core exercises, 160–65, **161–65**
　joint health and, 159
　leg exercises, 166–71, **166–71**
　for mountain biking, 117
Stress management and cycling, 6
Stretching. *See* Flexibility training
Suicide shift, 77–78
Sunglasses, 53–54, **54**, <u>54</u>
Supplements, 238–45, **240**, <u>241</u>, <u>243</u>, <u>245</u>
Suspension, 30, 115–16
Sweating, 217–19, <u>221</u>

"Tacking" move, 87
Tampons, 253
Technique, cycling, 71–74, 83–84. *See also specific type*
Tempo training, 147
Tension, cleat, 60, 82
Terry, Georgena, 45
Testosterone, xii
"Third eye" (navel), 92
Thirst, 217
3-foot laws, 101
Threshold heart rate, 85
Threshold training, 146
Time for cycling, selecting, 66–68
Time trial (TT), 146
Time Trial races, 135, 185–86
Time trial/triathlon bikes, 18–91, **19**
Tire levers, 61, **61**, 290–91, **291**
Tire pumps, 61–62
Tires
    cyclocross bike, 126
    flat, 61–62, 287–88, 293
    gravel bike, 130
    inflating, 295–96, 295
    mountain bike, 116–17
    patch kit, 61, **61**
    pressure of, 116–17
    selecting, 117
    tubeless, 61, **61**
Titanium bike material, 36
Toe clips, 59
Tool kit, 61–62, **61**, 289–92, 296
Torx keys and bolts, 291
Touring by bike, 267, 277–81, **279**, 281
Touring/commuting bikes, 19, **19**
Toxic shock syndrome (TSS), 253
Track bikes, 134
Track races, 187
Track riding, 132–35
Trail/all mountain bikes, 21, **21**
Trail riding. *See* Mountain biking
Trails, finding, 120
Training
    advantages of, 142–43
    for century rides, 195–96, 197, 198
    easy interval, 147–48
    endurance, 147
    fun of, 140–41
    gender differences, xi–xii
    hard interval, 147, 149–50
    high-intensity interval, 143
    interval, 147–51, 149
    long ride, 196
    max, 146
    mix-and-match, 146, 148, 148

monitoring efforts, 143–46
need for, 140
power, 260–61
purpose of, 141–42
recovery from, 151–57, 154, 155
speed, 260–61
speed ride, 196
steady ride, 196
stopping, reasons for, 156
tempo, 147
threshold, 146
zones, 147, 148, 149–51, 149
Trash, danger of, 106
TRESemmé Fresh Start Refreshing Mist, 270
Triathlons, 140, 255, 262
Triglycerides, 10
Triple shifters, 31
TSS, 253
TT, 146
Tubeless tires, 61, **61**, 295
Turkey sandwich, 212, **212**
24-hour races, 189–90
Twenty-Four Hours of Canaan race, 84
2X (two-by) shifters, 31
Two-abreast riding, 97–98, **97**

U-locks, 272
Ultracross/gravel races, 190–91
Underwear, 265, 270
Uphills, 84–88, **84**, 96–97
USA Triathlon, 4
US Consumer Product Safety Commission (CPSC), 48

Vagina, 262–65
Valley Preferred Cycling Center (T-Town), 132
Vegan diets, 213
Vegetables, 204–5, 206. *See also specific type*
Veloci-SRAM Pro Cycling team (formerly known as Specialized-lululemon), xiii
Velodrome riding, 132–35
Vests, 56, **56**
Visualization, 11
Vitamins, 213, 239–40, 241, 242

"Wall" (hill of 10 percent or higher), 87
Water bottles, 60

Weekend bike riding, 67–68
Weight distribution, gender differences in, x
Weight loss
    calories and, 230–31
    cycling and, 224–25
    digestive health and, 239
    gender differences, xii
    Go Faster Eating Plan for, 231, 232
    options for targeting, 226–29
    recipes for, 233–37
    sweet spot of cycling, 225–26
    2-week plan, 229–30
    unhealthy, 231
Weight shifts while cycling, 78–79, 114, 118, 120
Wet roads, 92, 105–6
Wheels, 24, 30–31
Women cyclists
    bikes designed for, 26–31, 113
    clothing for, 49–59
    connotative meaning of term, x
    cycling and, relationship to, x
    in cyclocross, increase in, 4
    historical perspective of, xi
    hydration for, 220–21, 223
    increase in number of, xiii, 3–4, 11, 69
    injuries, xi
    issues facing, overview of, x–xi
    menopause and, xii, 258–61
    menstrual cycle and, 211, 249–53
    motivations for, 3
    mountain biking and, 111–12
    nutrition and, 209–11
    physique of, 14
    pregnancy and, 254–57
    premenopause and, 211
    proportions of, 13
    respect and, desire for, xii–xiii
    saddles and, 14
    statistics on, xiii
Women's Cycling Association, xiii

XC bikes, 21, **21**
XC races, 188–89

Yozell, Mike, 296

Zabriskie, David, 212
Ziesing, Hunter, 185
Zigzagging across uphill road, 87
Zion National Park cycling route, 285